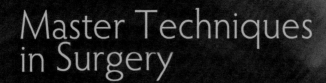

Master Techniques
in Surgery

GASTRIC SURGERY

Master Techniques in Surgery

Series Editor: Josef E. Fischer

Also available in this series:

Breast Surgery

Kirby I. Bland
V. Suzanne Klimberg

Colon and Rectal Surgery:
Abdominal Operations

Steven D. Wexner
James W. Fleshman

Colon and Rectal Surgery:
Anorectal Operations

Steven D. Wexner
James W. Fleshman

Esophageal Surgery

James D. Luketich

Hepatobiliary and Pancreatic Surgery

Keith D. Lillemoe
William R. Jarnagin

Hernia

Daniel B. Jones

Master Techniques in Surgery

GASTRIC SURGERY

Edited by	*Series Editor*
Michael S. Nussbaum, MD, FACS	**Josef E. Fischer, MD**
Professor and Chair, Department of Surgery	William V. McDermott Professor of Surgery
University of Florida College of Medicine—	Harvard Medical School
Jacksonville	Chair, Department of Surgery
Jacksonville, Florida	Beth Israel Deaconess Medical Center, Emeritus
	Boston, Massachusetts

Illustrations by: BodyScientific International, LLC.
Anne Rains, Arains Illustration, Inc.
Sara Krause, MFA, CMI

 Wolters Kluwer | Lippincott Williams & Wilkins
Health

Philadelphia • Baltimore • New York • London
Buenos Aires • Hong Kong • Sydney • Tokyo

Acquisitions Editor: Brian Brown
Product Manager: Brendan Huffman
Production Manager: Bridgett Dougherty
Senior Manufacturing Manager: Benjamin Rivera
Marketing Manager: Lisa Lawrence
Design Coordinator: Doug Smock
Production Service: Aptara, Inc.

Printed in China

Library of Congress Cataloging-in-Publication Data

Gastric surgery / edited by Michael S. Nussbaum.
        p. ; cm. – (Master techniques in surgery)
    Includes bibliographical references and index.
    ISBN 978-1-4511-1297-9 (hardback)
    I. Nussbaum, Michael S.   II. Series: Master techniques in surgery.
    [DNLM: 1. Stomach–surgery.   2. Gastrectomy–methods.
3. Gastroplasty–methods.   4. Laparoscopy–methods.   5. Peptic
Ulcer–surgery.   6. Vagotomy, Truncal–methods. WI 380]

    617.5′53–dc23

                              2012020564

Care has been taken to confirm the accuracy of the information presented and to describe generally accepted practices. However, the authors, editors, and publisher are not responsible for errors or omissions or for any consequences from application of the information in this book and make no warranty, expressed or implied, with respect to the currency, completeness, or accuracy of the contents of the publication. Application of the information in a particular situation remains the professional responsibility of the practitioner.

The authors, editors, and publisher have exerted every effort to ensure that drug selection and dosage set forth in this text are in accordance with current recommendations and practice at the time of publication. However, in view of ongoing research, changes in government regulations, and the constant flow of information relating to drug therapy and drug reactions, the reader is urged to check the package insert for each drug for any change in indications and dosage and for added warnings and precautions. This is particularly important when the recommended agent is a new or infrequently employed drug.

Some drugs and medical devices presented in the publication have Food and Drug Administration (FDA) clearance for limited use in restricted research settings. It is the responsibility of the health care provider to ascertain the FDA status of each drug or device planned for use in their clinical practice.

To purchase additional copies of this book, call our customer service department at (800) 638-3030 or fax orders to (301) 223-2320. International customers should call (301) 223-2300.

Visit Lippincott Williams & Wilkins on the Internet: at LWW.com. Lippincott Williams & Wilkins customer service representatives are available from 8:30 am to 6 pm, EST.

10 9 8 7 6 5 4 3 2 1

Dedication

He who combines the knowledge of physiology and surgery, in addition to the artistic side of his subject, reaches the highest ideal in medicine.
—Christian Albert Theodor Billroth

This book is dedicated to the three most important women in my life. My wife, Dr. Sue Nussbaum, inspires me daily with her wisdom and passion for always doing what is right. My wonderful and gifted daughters Jaclyn and Rachel thoroughly amaze me with their talents and creativity.

Wasef Abu-Jaish, MD, FACS
Assistant Professor of Surgery
Department of Surgery
Minimally Invasive and Bariatric Surgery
Fletcher Allen Health Care
University of Vermont College of Medicine
Burlington, Vermont

Bestoun H. Ahmed, MD, FRCS
Assistant Professor
Department of Surgery
University of Florida College of Medicine—Jacksonville
Jacksonville, Florida

J. Wesley Alexander, MD, ScD, FACS
Professor Emeritus
Department of Surgery
Director Emeritus, Transplantation Division
Director Emeritus, Center for Surgical Weight Loss
University of Cincinnati Medical Center
Cincinnati, Ohio

Stanley W. Ashley, MD
Frank Sawyer Professor of Surgery
Chief Medical Officer
Division of General and Gastrointestinal Surgery
Department of Surgery
Brigham and Women's Hospital
Harvard Medical School
Boston, Massachusetts

Kevin E. Behrns, MD
Edward R. Woodward Professor and Chairman
Department of Surgery
University of Florida
Gainesville, Florida

Kfir Ben-David, MD, FACS
Assistant Professor of Surgery
Chief, Minimally Invasive, Gastroesophageal, and
  Bariatric Surgery Service
Department of Surgery
College of Medicine
University of Florida
Gainesville, Florida

Edward C. Borrazzo, MD
Attending Surgeon
Department of Surgery
Fletcher Allen Health Care
Associate Professor of Surgery
University of Vermont College of Medicine
Burlington, Vermont

Markus W. Büchler, MD
Professor and Chair
Department of General, Visceral and
  Transplantation Surgery
University of Heidelberg
Heidelberg, Germany

Angel M. Caban, MD
Assistant Professor
Department of Surgery
University of Florida
Gainesville, Florida

Keyur Chavda, MD
Fellow, Minimally Invasive Surgery
Department of Surgery
University of Florida College of Medicine—Jacksonville
Jacksonville, Florida

Thomas E. Clancy, MD
Assistant Professor of Surgery
Division of Surgical Oncology
Department of Surgery
Brigham and Women's Hospital
Harvard Medical School
Boston, Massachusetts

Daniel T. Dempsey, MD, MBA
Chief of Gastrointestinal Surgery
Assistant Director of Perioperative Services
Hospital of the University of Pennsylvania
Professor of Surgery, University of Pennsylvania
Philadelphia, Pennsylvania

Mark Alan Dobbertien, DO, FACS
Fellow, Minimally Invasive Surgery
Department of Surgery
University of Florida College of Medicine—Jacksonville
Jacksonville, Florida

E. Christopher Ellison, MD, FACS
Associate Vice-President Health Sciences and
  Vice-Dean for Clinical Affairs
Chair, Ohio State University Physicians Board
Robert M. Zollinger Professor and Chair
Department of Surgery
Ohio State University Medical Center
Columbus, Ohio

Jameson Forster, MD, FACS, FRCSC
Professor
Department of Surgery
University of Kansas Medical Center
Kansas City, Kansas

Matthew R. Goede, MD
Assistant Professor of Surgery
Division of Gastrointestinal and Minimally Invasive Surgery
Department of Surgery
University of Nebraska Medical Center
Omaha, Nebraska

Eric S. Hungness, MD, FACS
Assistant Professor of Surgery
Division of Gastrointestinal and Oncologic Surgery
Department of Surgery
Feinberg School of Medicine
Northwestern University
Chicago, Illinois

Mustafa Hussain, MD
Assistant Professor of Surgery
Minimally Invasive GI and Bariatric Surgery
University of Chicago Medical Center
Chicago, Illinois

Woo Jin Hyung, MD, PhD
Associate Professor of Department of Surgery
Director of Robot and Minimally Invasive Surgery Center
Yonsei University College of Medicine
Seoul, South Korea

Namir Katkhouda, MD, FACS
Professor of Surgery
Vice Chairman, Clinical Affairs
Director, Bariatric Surgery Program
Keck School of Medicine
University of Southern California
Los Angeles, California

John C. Lipham, MD
Chief, Division of Upper GI and General Surgery
Associate Professor of Surgery
Department of Surgery
Keck Medical Center of USC
University of Southern California
Los Angeles, California

Andrew M. Lowy, MD
Professor of Surgery
Chief, Division of Surgical Oncology
Moores Cancer Center
University of California San Diego
San Diego, California

David W. McFadden, MD, MBA
Professor and Chairman
Department of Surgery
University of Vermont
Surgeon-in-Chief
Fletcher Allen Health Care
Burlington, Vermont

David W. Mercer, MD
Chairman and Professor
Department of Surgery
University of Nebraska Medical Center
Omaha, Nebraska

Thomas A. Miller, MD
Ammons Distinguished Professor of Surgery
Department of Surgery
Virginia Commonwealth University
    School of Medicine
Chief of General Surgery
Hunter Holmes McGuire Veterans Affairs Medical Center
Richmond, Virginia

Michael W. Mulholland, MD, PhD
Professor of Surgery and Chair
Department of Surgery
University of Michigan Medical School
Ann Arbor, Michigan

Vladimir Neychev, MD, PhD
Chief Surgery Resident
Department of Surgery
Danbury Hospital
Danbury, Connecticut

Ninh T. Nguyen, MD, FACS
Professor of Surgery and Chief
Division of Gastrointestinal Surgery
University of California Irvine Medical Center
Orange, California

Michael S. Nussbaum, MD, FACS
Professor and Chair
Department of Surgery
University of Florida College of Medicine—Jacksonville
Jacksonville, Florida

Kazutaka Obama, MD, PhD
Assistant Professor
Department of Gastrointerological Surgery
Kyoto University Hospital
Kyoto, Japan

Brant K. Oelschlager, MD
Byers Endowed Professor of Esophageal Research
Chief of Gastrointestinal Surgery
Department of Surgery
University of Washington
Seattle, Washington

Rebecca P. Petersen, MD, MSc
Assistant Professor
Division of General Surgery
Department of Surgery
University of Washington
Seattle, Washington

Melissa S. Phillips, MD
Assistant Professor
Division of General Surgery
Department of Surgery
University of Tennessee Health Science Center
Knoxville, Tennessee

Alfons Pomp, MD, FACS, FRCSC
Leon C. Hirsch Professor
Vice Chairman, Department of Surgery
Chief, Section of Laparoscopic and Bariatric Surgery
NewYork-Presbyterian Hospital
Weill Medical College of Cornell University
New York, New York

Jeffrey L. Ponsky, MD
Oliver H. Payne Professor and Chairman, Department of Surgery
University Hospitals Case Medical Center
Case Western Reserve University
Cleveland, Ohio

Mitchell C. Posner, MD, FACS
Thomas D. Jones Professor and Vice-Chairman
Chief, Section of General Surgery and Surgical Oncology
University of Chicago Medicine
Knoxville, Tennessee

Aurora D. Pryor, MD, FACS
Division Chief
General Surgery, Durham Regional Hospital
Associate Professor of Surgery
Division of General Surgery
Department of Surgery
Duke University Medical Center
Durham, North Carolina

K. Roggin, MD
Associate Professor of Surgery and Cancer Research
Program Director, General Surgery Residency Program
Department of Surgery, Surgical Oncology
University of Chicago Medical Center
Chicago, Illinois

Raul J. Rosenthal, MD, FACS, FASMBS
Professor of Surgery and Chairman
Department of General Surgery
Section of Minimally Invasive Surgery
Bariatric and Metabolic Institute
Program Director
Fellowship in Minimally Invasive Surgery
Cleveland Clinic Florida
Weston, Florida

Alan A. Saber, MD, FACS
Associate Professor of Surgery
Case Western Reserve University School of Medicine
Director of Bariatric and Metabolic Surgery
University Hospitals Case Medical Center
Surgical Director, Bariatric Surgery, Metabolic and Nutrition Center
University Hospitals Digestive Health Institute
Cleveland, Ohio

George A. Sarosi Jr, MD
Associate Professor of Surgery
Surgery Residency Program Director
Robert H. Hux, MD, Professor of Surgery
University of Florida College of Medicine
NF/SG VA Medical Center
Gainesville, Florida

Michael G. Sarr, MD
Consultant
Gastroenterology Research Unit, Division of Gastroenterologic and General Surgery, Department of Surgery
James C. Masson Professor of Surgery
Mayo Clinic
Rochester, Minnesota

Jeannie F. Savas, MD
Associate Professor of Surgery
Department of Surgery
Virginia Commonwealth University School of Medicine
Chief of Surgery
Hunter Holmes McGuire Veterans Affairs Medical Center
Richmond, Virginia

Bruce Schirmer, MD
Stephen H. Watts Professor of Surgery
University of Virginia Health System
Charlottesville, Virginia

Carol E.H. Scott-Conner, MD, PhD, MBA
Professor of Surgery
University of Iowa Carver College of Medicine
Iowa City, Iowa

Sunil Sharma, MD
Assistant Professor
Department of Surgery
University of Florida College of Medicine—Jacksonville
Jacksonville, Florida

Brian R. Smith, MD, FACS, FASMBS
Assistant Professor of Surgery
Associate Residency Program Director
Division of Gastrointestinal Surgery
University of California Irvine Medical Center
Long Beach, California

Helen J. Sohn, MD
Department of Surgery
Sharp Grossmont Hospital
La Mesa, California

Vivian E. Strong, MD, FACS
Associate Attending Surgeon
Memorial Sloan-Kettering Cancer Center
Associate Professor of Surgery
Weill Medical College of Cornell University
New York, New York

Ranjan Sudan, MD
Vice Chair Surgical Education
Associate Professor of Surgery and Psychiatry
Department of Surgery
Duke University Medical Center
Durham, North Carolina

Hop S. Tran Cao, MD
Research Fellow
Department of Surgery
University of California San Diego
San Diego, California

Richard H. Turnage, MD
Professor and Chairman
Department of Surgery
University of Arkansas for Medical Sciences
Little Rock, Arkansas

Carmine Volpe, MD, FACS
Associate Professor of Surgery
Chief, Division of Surgical Oncology
Department of Surgery
University of Florida College of
    Medicine—Jacksonville
Jacksonville, Florida

R. Matthew Walsh, MD
Professor of Surgery and Chairman
Department of General Surgery
Case Western University Lerner College of Medicine
Rich Family Distinguished Chair of Digestive Diseases
Cleveland Clinic Foundation
Cleveland, Ohio

Thilo Welsch, MD
Assistant Professor
Department of General, Visceral and Transplantation
    Surgery
University of Heidelberg
Heidelberg, Germany

Yanghee Woo, MD
Instructor of Clinical Surgery
Division of GI/Endocrine Surgery
Department of Surgery
Columbia University College of Physicians and Surgeons
New York, New York

Joerg Zehetner, MD, MMM
Assistant Professor of Surgery
Division of Upper GI and General Surgery
Department of Surgery
Keck School of Medicine of USC
University of Southern California
Los Angeles, California

This series of mini-atlases, of which this is the fourth, is an outgrowth of *Mastery of Surgery*. As the series editor, I have been involved with *Mastery of Surgery* since the third edition, when I joined two greats of American surgery Lloyd Nyhus and Robert Baker who were the editors at that time. At that time, in addition to *Mastery of Surgery*, which really was, almost in its entirety, an excellent atlas of how to do operations, atlases were common and some quality atlases which existed at that time by Dr. John Madden of New York, Dr. Robert Zollinger of Ohio State, and two other atlases, with which the reader may be less familiar with is a superb atlas by Professor Pietro Valdoni, Professor of Surgery at the University of Rome, who ran ten operating rooms simultaneously, and as the Italians like to point out to me, a physician to three popes. One famous surgeon said to me, what can you say about Professor Valdoni: "Professor Valdoni said to three popes, 'take a deep breath,' and they each took a deep breath." This superb atlas, which is not well known, was translated by my partner, when I was on the staff at Mass General Hospital, Dr. George Nardi from Italian. Another superb atlas was that by Dr. Robert Ritchie Linton, an early vascular surgeon whose atlas was of very high quality.

However, atlases fell out of style, and in the fourth and fifth edition of *Mastery of Surgery*, we added more chapters that were "textbooky" types of chapters to increase access to the increasing knowledge base of surgery. However, atlases seem to have gone out of favor somewhat. In discussing with Brian Brown and others of Lippincott, as well as some of the editors who have taken on the responsibility of each of these mini-atlases, it seemed that we could build on our experience with *Mastery of Surgery* by having individual books which were atlases of 400 to 450 pages of high quality, each featuring a particular anatomical part of what was surgery and put together an atlas of operations of a sharply circumscribed area. This we have accomplished and all of us are highly indebted to a group of high-quality editors who will have created superb mini-atlases in these sharply circumscribed areas.

Why the return of the atlas? Is it possible that the knowledge base is somewhat more extensive with more variations on the various types of procedures, that as we learn more about the biochemistry, physiology, genetics, and pathophysiology in these different areas, there have gotten to be a variation on the types of procedures that we do on patients in these areas. This increase in knowledge base has occurred simultaneously when the amount of time available for training physicians—and especially surgeons—has been diminished and continues to do so. While I understand the hypothesis that brought the 80-hour work week upon us, and that limits the time that we have for instruction, and I believe that it is well intentioned, but I still ask the question: Is the patient better served by a somewhat fatigued resident who has been at the operation, and knows what the surgeon and what he or she is worried about, or a comparatively fresh resident who has never seen the patient before?

I do not know, but I tend to come down on the side that familiarity with the patient is perhaps more important. And what about the errors of hand off, which seem to be more of an intrinsic issue with the hand off which we are not able to really remedy entirely rather than poor intentions.

This series of mini-atlases is an attempt to help fill the voids of inadequate time for training. We are indebted to the individual editors who have taken on this responsibility and to the authors who have volunteered to share their knowledge and experience in putting together what we hope will be a superb series. Inspired by their experience of teaching residents and medical students, a high calling, matched only by their devotion and superb care they have given to thousands of patients.

It is an honor to serve as the series editor for this outstanding group of mini-atlases, which we hope will convey the experiences of an excellent group of editors and authors to the benefit of students, residents, and their future patients in an era in which time for education seems to be increasingly limited.

Putting a book together, especially a series of books, is not easy, and I wish to acknowledge the production staff at Lippincott, Wolters Kluwer's including Brian Brown, Julia Seto, Brendan Huffman, and many others, and my personal staff in the office who include Edie Burbank-Schmitt, Ingrid Johnson, Abigail Smith, and Jere Cooper. None of this would have been possible without them.

Josef E. Fischer, MD, FACS
Boston, Massachusetts

It is a most gratifying sign of the rapid progress of our time that our best text-books become antiquated so quickly.

—*Christian Albert Theodor Billroth*

When I was an intern at the University of Cincinnati, **Master Techniques in Surgery** series editor Dr. Josef Fischer was the chairman of the department. Every Monday afternoon we had Professor's Hour with Dr. Fischer where we would present cases to him and he would use the opportunity to teach us the nuances of surgical care that is exemplified in this series. One day, early in that year, one of the chief residents presented a case of giant duodenal ulcer; an entity that was new to me. Near the end of the session, Dr. Fischer asked for a resident volunteer to review the Cincinnati experience with giant duodenal ulcer. Fellow resident Mark Schusterman and I volunteered and thus began my academic career as a gastrointestinal surgeon.[1] Flash forward 30 years and I am now a department chair, holding my own Professor's Hour on Monday afternoons. Once again I find myself completing a project for Dr. Fischer related to gastric surgery as both editor and author in *Master Techniques in Surgery: Gastric Surgery* (see Chapter 14. *Operation for Giant Duodenal Ulcer*).

I trained during the era when gastric operations were common. Peptic ulcer and the inherent complications were frequent problems that we faced on a daily basis. The training opportunities for residents in gastric surgery have diminished over the ensuing years due to the advent of antisecretory therapy, the discovery of helicobacter pylori, and advances in therapeutic endoscopy. However, as this volume exemplifies, benign and malignant gastroduodenal disease continues to provide challenges to the practicing surgeon. A thorough knowledge of the various approaches and techniques are essential components in anyone's armamentarium. Further confounding these issues are the growing opportunities to apply minimally invasive approaches in certain circumstances. To be a complete gastric surgeon, one must be comfortable with both minimally invasive and open approaches, depending upon the underlying situation. In this text, where appropriate, we detail both the open and minimally invasive approaches, including laparoscopic as well as robotic applications.

The objective of the **Master Techniques in Surgery** series is to provide authoritative descriptions and illustrations of the management of each theme. This volume serves to supplement and augment the other resources available to surgeons-in-training as well as practicing surgeons faced with gastroduodenal pathology. The authors represent a truly global expertise in this field and they address the many operations and approaches in the management of benign, functional, and malignant gastric pathology. *Master Techniques in Surgery: Gastric Surgery* is intended to provide detail and clarity in the approaches to very specific diagnoses and procedures. Each chapter makes liberal use of color illustrations and photographs to elucidate important anatomical relationships and key operative steps. Further, the book comes with an associated Web site with fully searchable text and procedural videos. This volume should be useful for comprehensive review as well as a ready preoperative resource in preparation for specific gastric operations.

---

[1]Nussbaum, M.S., Schusterman, M.A.: Management of giant duodenal ulcer. *Am. J. Surg.* 1985;199:357–361.

Once again, I am indebted to my mentor and colleague, Josef Fischer, for asking me to take on this task and allowing me to contribute as the editor of this important volume in the **Master Techniques in Surgery** series. Under Dr. Fischer's stewardship, **Mastery of Surgery** continues to withstand the test of time as an essential resource for any serious student of surgery. The **Master Techniques in Surgery** series will certainly add to that predominance as both an enhancement as well as an amplification of the body of knowledge on the subject matter.

Finally I want to thank Brian Brown and Editorial Product Manager Brendan Huffman at Lippincott, Williams & Wilkins as well as Associate Project Manager Ruchira Gupta at Aptara, Inc. for all of their insight, diligence, and support of this project. Their help and advice was invaluable to all of the authors and me. This has been a true labor of love and I hope that you find the book to be enlightening, informative, and enjoyable.

Michael S. Nussbaum, MD, FACS
Professor and Chair Department of Surgery
University of Florida College of Medicine—Jacksonville
May 2012

▰▰▰ ▰▰▰ ▰▰▰

PART I: PROCEDURES FOR ULCER DISEASE

PART IV: BARIATRIC

PART V: OTHER GASTRIC OPERATIONS

1 Truncal Vagotomy with Gastrojejunostomy

Richard H. Turnage

INDICATIONS/CONTRAINDICATIONS

Indications

Gastrojejunostomy is most commonly used to treat patients with gastric outlet obstruction (GOO) of whom nearly two-thirds will have malignancies of the distal stomach, pancreas, or duodenum. The most common benign causes of GOO are peptic ulcer disease (PUD), caustic strictures, and Crohn's disease. Less common benign etiologies include tuberculosis, chronic pancreatitis, benign gastric polyps, and Bouveret's syndrome (i.e., obstruction of the pylorus by a gallstone). Although not amenable to gastrojejunostomy, systemic medical diseases, most notably diabetes mellitus, are important causes of impaired gastric emptying.

Complete resection is the treatment of choice for patients with upper gastrointestinal (UGI) malignancies. Unfortunately, locally advanced or metastatic disease precludes this approach in a significant percentage of these patients. Although noncurative gastric resection is an important option for managing symptomatic patients with advanced gastric cancer, this approach is less often feasible for patients with advanced pancreatic cancer. Endoscopic stenting of malignant obstructions of the distal stomach and duodenum is an important option in managing patients with GOO who have relatively short life expectancies, such as those with metastatic disease or poor performance scores. Advances in imaging with multidetector computed tomography have significantly improved preoperative identification of patients with advanced disease such that gastrojejunostomy is now used most often for symptomatic patients with unresectable cancer for whom endoscopic stenting has been unsuccessful or patients who are unexpectedly found to have advanced disease during exploratory laparotomy for cure.

PUD is the most common benign cause of mechanical GOO. Medical management combined with endoscopic balloon dilation results in durable relief of obstructive symptoms in about 70% of cases. This approach is particularly effective for patients with GOO due to *Helicobacter pylori*-associated ulcers. In contrast, NSAID-induced ulcers seldom resolve with nonoperative approaches. Young age, long duration of symptoms, the need for repeated endoscopic balloon dilatations, and the continuous use of NSAIDs predict the need for surgical management. Surgical approaches to patients with GOO from PUD include truncal vagotomy and antrectomy or truncal vagotomy and a drainage procedure (either pyloroplasty or gastrojejunostomy). Truncal vagotomy and antrectomy has the lowest rate of recurrent ulcer disease. The magnitude of the operation and the consequent operative risk necessitates other strategies in patients with significant medical comorbidities as well as those patients who are found intraoperatively to have significant inflammation and scarring of the distal stomach and duodenum. Truncal vagotomy and pyloroplasty is suitable for patients with minimal inflammation or deformity of the pylorus or proximal duodenum, thereby permitting a tension-free transverse closure of the pylorus. Unfortunately, this is often not the case, making truncal vagotomy and gastrojejunostomy (TV & GJ) the best option.

Lastly, the ingestion of strong acidic solutions causes strictures in the prepyloric region of the stomach leading to GOO. Kochhar et al. have described excellent short- and intermediate-term outcomes with endoscopic balloon dilation of caustic-induced gastric strictures. Others have managed these patients with distal gastrectomy. Thus, gastrojejunostomy is reserved for those patients with prepyloric strictures who have failed endoscopic balloon dilation and are poor operative candidates for distal gastrectomy.

Contraindications

The principal contraindications to the performance of a TV & GJ are technical. If a truncal vagotomy is required in a patient who has had a previous operation in the esophageal hiatus (e.g., fundoplication or prior vagotomy), a thoracoscopic approach to vagotomy may be preferable to allow dissection in tissue planes free from scarring and inflammation. In patients with ulcer disease or other benign causes of GOO, the enlarged stomach makes the performance of a tension-free gastrojejunostomy relatively straightforward. However, peritoneal metastases in patients with gastric or periampullary cancers may cause foreshortening of the small bowel mesentery, rendering it difficult to achieve a tension-free anastomosis between the stomach and the jejunum.

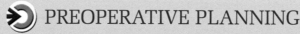

PREOPERATIVE PLANNING

The initial management of a patient with GOO consists of intravascular volume and electrolyte resuscitation, nutritional repletion, and identification of the underlying cause of the obstruction. Significant intravascular volume depletion and electrolyte abnormalities, especially hyponatremia, hypokalemia, and hypochloremia, are common and are readily corrected by the intravenous infusion of a normal saline solution with potassium chloride. The loss of gastric secretions from persistent vomiting may also cause a significant metabolic alkalosis which will correct with the administration of normal saline and potassium chloride. Gastric aspiration via a nasogastric (NG) tube will decompress the dilated atonic stomach and improve the patient's abdominal discomfort, nausea, and vomiting. The intravenous administration of a proton pump inhibitor will reduce gastric acid secretion, and the administration of total parenteral nutrition via a central venous catheter will begin to correct the patient's calorie and protein deficits.

After resuscitating the patient, esophagogastroduodenostomy should be performed to determine the etiology of the obstruction. An ulcer or mass in the stomach or a suspicious lesion in the duodenum necessitates endoscopic biopsy. Biopsy of the gastric mucosa will document the presence of *Helicobacter pylori*—eradication of which will facilitate healing of benign ulcers and in many cases relieve the patient's obstruction. If a malignancy is identified or if endoscopy is indeterminate, computed tomography will characterize the lesion by determining its size, relationship to surrounding structures, and the presence or absence of visceral metastases.

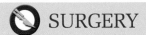 SURGERY

Patients should receive a prophylactic dose of antibiotics intravenously 30 to 60 minutes prior to the incision. It is the author's preference to use cefoxitin in those patients who are not beta lactam allergic. Subcutaneous injection of 5,000 units of heparin sulfate administered preoperatively will reduce the risk of postoperative pulmonary embolism. The risk of aspiration during the induction of anesthesia and intubation may be diminished by the evacuation of gastric contents via the NG tube and posterior pressure on the cricoid cartilage.

Positioning

TV & GJ may be performed by either a laparoscopic or an open approach. Depending on the surgical approach, the patient can be placed in the supine or lithotomy position. For minimally invasive gastric approaches, if the patient is in a supine position, the operating surgeon stands on the right side of the patient while the assistant is on the contralateral side. If the lithotomy position is used, the surgeon stands between the legs. The patient is secured to the table with two safety straps, a foot board, and all of their bony prominences are well padded. For an open approach the patient is placed in the supine position with the head of the operating table elevated to facilitate exposure of the organs within the upper abdomen. The lower chest and entire abdomen is prepped with a chlorhexidine-alcohol solution and then draped with sterile towels and sheets.

Technique

The open approach will be presented in detail, but, ultimately, the same operative steps are generally true for a laparoscopic approach (for details on placement of laparoscopic trocars and specific techniques see Chapters 4, 6, and 7). When the laparoscopic approach to this procedure is used, a low threshold for conversion to an open procedure should exist when visualization of important structures are impaired. Standing on the patient's right side, the surgeon makes an upper midline incision from the xiphoid to the umbilicus. The incision is extended through the subcutaneous tissue and linea alba until the peritoneal cavity is entered. The ligamentum teres is ligated with 2-0 silk and divided and the falciform ligament is released from the anterior abdominal wall. The abdominal cavity is carefully explored and then attention is directed to the upper abdomen. In patients with GOO from ulcer disease, the location of the ulcer, extent of inflammation, and the patient's general medical condition will influence the choice of gastric resection versus a drainage procedure. For patients with malignancies, the first steps of the operation are to determine the resectability of the tumor and document the presence or absence of peritoneal or visceral metastases. The ability to mobilize an adequate length of jejunum for the performance of a tension-free gastrojejunostomy is ascertained at this time.

Truncal Vagotomy

A self-retaining abdominal wall retractor is placed to allow lateral retraction of the rectus abdominis muscles and anterior and superior retraction of the costal margins. The left lobe of the liver is mobilized by incising the avascular left triangular ligament with an electrocautery. This is facilitated by downward traction on the left lobe of the liver with the right hand while the index finger is placed behind the triangular ligament to protect the underlying structures. The triangular ligament is incised from lateral to medial until the left lobe of the liver can be folded upon itself thereby exposing the underlying gastroesophageal junction. The liver is covered with a moist laparotomy sponge and a Harrington-type blade for the self-retaining abdominal wall retractor is used to hold the left lobe of the liver to the patient's right side. In a laparoscopic approach the triangular ligament is left intact and the lateral segment of the left lobe of the liver is elevated with a self-retaining retractor such as a Nathanson retractor.

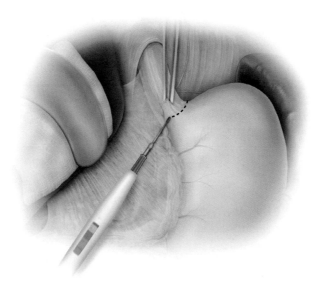

Figure 1.1 Transverse incision of the peritoneum and phrenoesophageal ligament to expose the underlying intra-abdominal esophagus and esophageal hiatus.

The peritoneum overlying the distal esophagus is grasped with DeBakey forceps and incised perpendicular to the long axis of the esophagus with Metzenbaum scissors or the electrocautery. The peritoneum and the underlying phrenoesophageal ligament are incised sufficiently to allow identification and mobilization of the esophagus (Fig. 1.1). This will usually include opening the medial most aspect of the gastrohepatic ligament on the right. The left gastric artery and its esophageal branch are left undisturbed. It is not necessary to divide the short gastric vessels on the left. By opening the incised peritoneum and phrenoesophageal ligament, the surgeon is able to free the distal 5 or 6 cm of the esophagus from the surrounding tissues by blunt dissection with his/her index finger. Once completed, the esophagus may be encircled with the index finger passed from the patient's left side to the right (Fig. 1.2). The esophagus with the NG tube is felt anterior to the surgeon's finger and the abdominal aorta is appreciated posterior. A 1-inch Penrose drain is then passed behind the esophagus to encircle it. Downward and slight anterior traction on the esophagus using the Penrose drain will facilitate blunt dissection of the distal 8 to 10 cm of esophagus from surrounding soft tissue, thus exposing the right crus of the diaphragm and the tissue lateral and posterior to the esophagus.

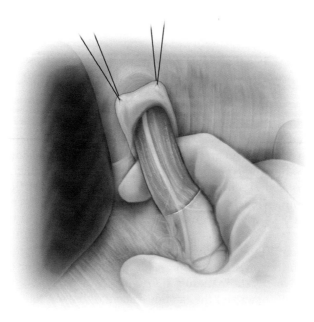

Figure 1.2 Mobilization of the distal 5 to 6 cm of esophagus from the soft tissue of the esophageal hiatus by passing the surgeon's index finger from the left to the right side of the esophagus.

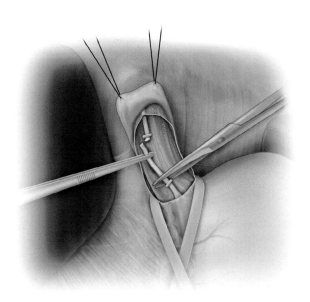

Figure 1.3 Identification of the left vagus nerve on the anterior surface of the esophagus, just to the right of the midline. The nerve is clipped with a medium stainless steel clip and then divided.

Identification of the vagus nerves is accomplished by passing the tip of the index finger over the anterior surface of the esophagus while placing downward traction on the Penrose drain. The vagus nerve fibers will present as tense, wire-like structures passing parallel to the long axis of the esophagus; the nerve fibers have been likened to "banjo strings." In addition to the larger left and right vagus nerves, there are often multiple smaller nerve fibers traversing the surface of the esophagus and the esophageal hiatus. In an anatomic study of the vagus nerve at the esophageal hiatus, Skandalakis et al. found four or more vagal trunks in 12% of their dissections.

The left vagus nerve is usually found on the anterior surface of the esophagus just to the right of the midline. A left truncal vagotomy is performed by lifting the nerve off the surface of the esophagus with a nerve hook or a long right angle clamp. It is freed of surrounding soft tissue for a distance of 5 to 6 cm with long Metzenbaum scissors. The proximal most portion of the nerve is then clipped with a medium stainless steel surgical clip and divided at the upper margin of the dissection just distal to the clip. The distal portion of the nerve is grasped and then clipped and divided 2 to 3 cm from the cut proximal margin (Fig. 1.3).

The right vagus nerve can be found by lifting the esophagus anteriorly while maintaining downward traction on the encircling Penrose drain. Although the nerve may be found on the posterior surface of the esophagus, it is more commonly displaced posteriorly during the process of mobilizing the distal esophagus. In this case, the nerve is found to the right of the midline resting against the posterior wall of the esophageal hiatus, anterior to the aorta. The right vagus nerve is resected as described for the left vagus by elevating the nerve trunk, applying a surgical clip to the proximal-most portion of the nerve, and then excising a 2 to 3 cm section of the nerve (Fig. 1.4). The right and left vagal trunks are sent for histologic confirmation.

With the right and left vagal nerve trunks divided, a careful search for additional nerve fibers is undertaken. This is best accomplished by downward traction on the Penrose drain and careful palpation of the anterior and posterior surfaces of the esophagus. The distal 5 to 6 cm of the esophagus and the surrounding tissue must be carefully inspected to identify and divide any small nerve fibers that may have branched from the vagal trunks in the chest, such as "the criminal nerve of Grassi" which arises from the right vagal trunk to innervate a portion of the posterior gastric fundus. The Penrose drain is then removed and the esophagus allowed to fall back toward the esophageal hiatus. The operative field is then carefully inspected for bleeding which is readily controlled with the electrocautery. The incised peritoneum and phrenoesophageal ligament are not reapproximated.

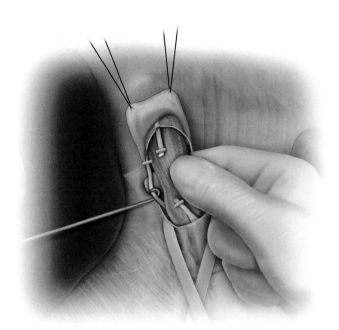

Figure 1.4 Identification of the right vagus nerve posterior to the esophagus on the right side of the esophageal hiatus.

Gastrojejunostomy

The gastrojejunostomy may be constructed on either the anterior or the posterior surface of the distal stomach. The optimal site will be influenced by the amount of scarring and deformity in the distal stomach or duodenum in patients with benign strictures and by the location of the tumor in patients with malignancies. There is no evidence that anterior, antecolic gastrojejunostomy is superior to posterior, retrocolic gastrojejunostomy or vice versa. The easier anterior gastrojejunostomy is most commonly performed and hence it is this anastomosis that is described.

Hand-sewn, Anterior or Antecolic Gastrojejunostomy

With the self-retaining abdominal wall retractor in place, the greater omentum and transverse colon are elevated to reveal the ligament of Treitz just to the left of the midline at the base of the transverse mesocolon. The proximal jejunum is brought onto the anterior surface of the stomach and oriented such that the afferent limb is adjacent to the body of the stomach and the efferent limb is juxtaposed to the distal stomach. The length of the afferent limb should be as short as possible to reduce the risk of afferent limb obstruction. The surgeon must be careful to avoid twisting of the bowel or placing tension on the anastomosis.

Stay sutures of 3-0 silk are placed through the seromuscular layers of the stomach and the jejunum at the proximal and distal ends of the anastomosis, about 8 cm apart from one another. The ends of these sutures are secured with a hemostat and brought out the left and right side of the operative field. This maneuver orients the anastomosis horizontally allowing the surgeon to sew toward himself or herself.

The back row of the anastomosis is constructed by placing interrupted 3-0 silk Lembert sutures through the serosa and muscularis of the juxtaposed stomach and the jejunum about 8 mm behind the planned gastrotomy and enterotomy. The sutures extend from the right stay suture to the left and are placed about 8 mm apart from one another. The sutures are tied after the entire row has been placed. The middle suture is not cut at this time but left long to aid in the placement of the inner posterior row of sutures. The full thickness of the stomach is then incised with the electrocautery parallel to and 8 mm from the back row of silk sutures. Fluid within the stomach is aspirated and a matching incision is made through the adjacent jejunal wall. The gastrotomy and jejunotomy should be approximately 1 centimeter shorter than the site of the silk stay sutures (Fig. 1.5).

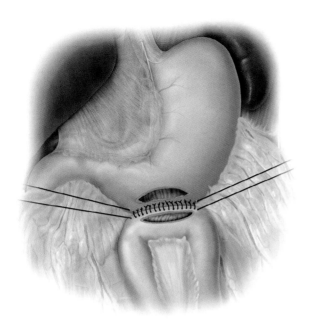

Figure 1.5 Construction of the outer layer of the back wall of an anterior or antecolic gastrojejunostomy using interrupted 3-0 silk Lembert sutures.

The inner layer of the anastomosis is constructed by sewing the juxtaposed gastric and jejunal walls together with two running, spiral sutures of 3-0 polyglycolic acid. The sutures are started at the midpoint of the back wall of the anastomosis and continued around the corners until the front wall is closed. The stitch is placed about 4 to 5 mm from the cut-edge of the bowel and incorporates the full-thickness of the gastric and jejunal walls. Elevating the serosal edge of the jejunum (or stomach) with DeBakey forceps 1 cm from the site of the planned stitch will help to incorporate all the layers of the bowel in the stitch. At the corner of the anastomosis, slightly more serosa than mucosa is included in the stitch to facilitate the invagination of the mucosa within the lumen of the anastomosis. As each stitch is placed, the edges of the anastomosis are gently drawn together. Ultimately, the inner layer of the anastomosis is completed and only the seromuscular edges of the stomach and the jejunum are visible (Fig. 1.6).

The front wall of the anastomosis is now completed by placing interrupted seromuscular Lembert sutures of 3-0 silk between the gastric and the jejunal walls. These stitches are placed several millimeters from the inner layer of the anastomosis

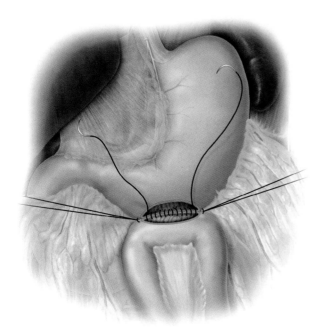

Figure 1.6 Construction of the inner layer of the back wall of anterior gastrojejunostomy using a continuous 3-0 polyglycolic acid suture placed through all layers of the juxtaposed stomach and jejunum.

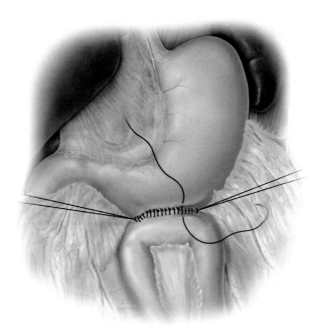

Figure 1.7 Construction of the outer layer of the front wall of the anterior gastrojejunostomy using interrupted 3-0 silk Lembert sutures placed 7 to 8 mm from one another. This row of sutures should completely bury the completed inner layer of the anastomosis.

and about 7 to 8 mm apart. This layer should bury the inner layer from view (Fig. 1.7). The corners of the anastomosis can be completed by either tying the stay sutures or by placing a new Lembert stitch in each corner to completely cover the inner layer of the anastomosis. The lumen of the anastomosis should be readily palpable either through the gastric or the jejunal wall. The operative field is inspected for evidence of bleeding or injury and the self-retaining retractor is removed. The linea alba is closed using a running suture of no. 1 polydioxanone, and the skin is closed with a skin stapler.

Stapled, Anterior Gastrojejunostomy

The orientation of the stomach and jejunum and the placement of the 3-0 silk stay sutures at the corner of the proposed anastomosis is as described earlier. A small gastrotomy and jejunotomy are made about 1 cm from the stay suture at the proximal corner of the anastomosis. One limb of a 60-mm linear stapling device (endoscopic linear stapler in laparoscopic) is inserted into the jejunum and the other limb

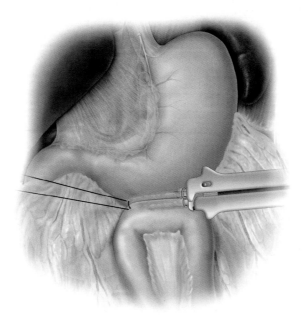

Figure 1.8 Construction of anterior gastrojejunostomy using a GIA 60 stapler inserted through a small gastrotomy and matching enterotomy. Stay stitches of 3-0 silk are placed at the proximal and distal margins of the proposed anastomosis.

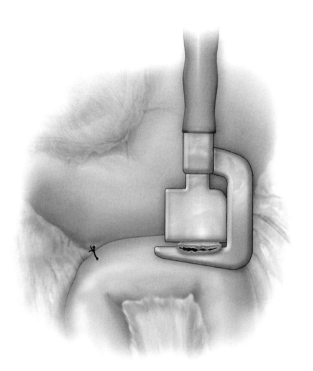

Figure 1.9 Completion of the stapled anterior gastrojejunostomy by closing the insertion site of the GIA stapler using a TA 30 stapler.

is inserted into the stomach. The device is locked and the site inspected to ensure that no tissue other than the stomach and jejunum is included within the stapler (Fig. 1.8). The stapler is then fired and removed from the operative field. The staple line is then carefully inspected for bleeding. Exposure of the staple line can be facilitated by gentle retraction with the long arm of an Army–Navy retractor. Bleeding from the staple line can be controlled with either the electrocautery or the placement of a 4-0 polyglycolic acid suture. The remaining defect in the anastomosis is grasped with several Allis clamps and a TA-30 or TA-50 stapler is aligned behind the clamps (endoscopic linear stapler or intracorporeal interrupted sutures in laparoscopic approaches). The TA stapler is then fired and the redundant tissue is excised with the scalpel before removing the stapler. The staple line is inspected for bleeding which is controlled with the electrocautery or a 4-0 polyglycolic acid suture (Fig. 1.9).

 POSTOPERATIVE MANAGEMENT

Most patients undergoing a TV & GJ may be safely managed in the general surgical ward. Intravenous fluid administration with an isotonic solution for the first 24 hours will maintain a normal intravascular volume. Generally patients will mobilize their third-spaced fluids on postoperative day 3 and the infusion of 5% dextrose/0.45% sodium chloride solution will allow the maintenance of normal intravascular volume until the patient is able to resume oral intake. Antibiotics are not administered postoperatively unless there is clinical evidence of infection. Urine output may be a useful guide to the patient's volume status in the first day or two postoperatively; thereafter, the catheter is removed. The NG tube is removed when the output is less than 300 mL per 8-hour period. If the patient is nauseated or has a distended abdomen the tube is left in place for a longer period of time. As described subsequently, poor gastric emptying is a relatively common early complication necessitating longer periods of NG aspiration. A clear liquid diet is started when the NG tube has been removed and the patient is passing flatus. If liquids are tolerated for 24 hours, the patient is allowed a regular diet and the parenteral nutrition is stopped.

Adequate pain management is an important part of the postoperative care of these patients. The upper abdominal location of the incision is painful especially when the patient takes deep breaths. Poor pain relief will diminish inspiratory volume and promote the development of atelectasis and pneumonia. Patient-controlled analgesia (PCA) with morphine, hydromorphone, or meperidine provides excellent pain relief. The epigastric location of the incision makes the use of postoperative epidural analgesia less useful.

The patient is instructed in the use of an incentive spirometer preoperatively, and it is used throughout the patient's postoperative course to reduce atelectasis and minimize the risk of pneumonia. Subcutaneous heparin injections, also started preoperatively, are continued in the postoperative period to minimize the risk of pulmonary emboli. The patient is ambulated on the first postoperative day and daily thereafter. If a truncal vagotomy has not been performed, the patient should receive a proton pump inhibitor intravenously in the early postoperative period and then orally as he or she tolerates a diet.

COMPLICATIONS

The incidence of intraoperative complications during TV & GJ is low with the most common being hemorrhage from a retraction injury to the liver or spleen during the performance of the vagotomy or injury to the middle colic vein during the gastrojejunostomy. Bleeding from the liver may be avoided by careful mobilization of the left lobe and gentle retraction. Bleeding from the spleen necessitating splenectomy can be minimized by avoiding traction on the short gastric vessels or spleen.

The early postoperative complications of gastrojejunostomy for treating patients with benign or malignant GOO are shown in Table 1.1. With the exception of the study by Kim et al., most of the patients in these studies underwent gastrojejunostomy alone, without truncal vagotomy. Overall, the rate of complications following gastrojejunostomy is relatively high, ranging from 22.7 to 62.5% (median = 32%). Most complications were relatively minor, although wound infections, delayed gastric emptying, and

TABLE 1.1	Complications of Gastrojejunostomy for Gastric Outlet Obstruction in Patients with Benign or Malignant Diseases			
Study Design	**Sample Size**	**Mortality Rate (%)**	**Morbidity Rate**	**Complications**
Retrospective comparison of Lap TV + GJ vs. Open TV + GJ in patients with PUD with GOO, patients accrued between 1999 and 2005	8	0	62.5	Delayed gastric emptying (50%); atelectasis (12.5%)
Retrospective review of patients with Crohn's disease and duodenal obstruction, patients accrued between 1995 and 2006	11	0	36	GJ leak (9%) GJ bleeding (9%) Early SBO (9%)
Retrospective review of GJ in patients with pancreatic cancer with GOO (66 patients) and without GOO (447 patients), patients accrued between 1996 and 2010	513	1.6	36.7	Wound infections (4.3%) Pleural effusion (2.5%) Cholangitis (2%)
Prospective comparison HJ alone in patients with pancreatic cancer with GOO (HJ + GJ) and without GOO (HJ alone), patients accrued between 1992 and 1995	44	9	22.7	Delayed gastric emptying (11%) Wound infection (9%) Intra-abdominal abscess (4.5%)
Single-center randomized trial, GJ vs. no GJ in patients with unresectable pancreatic cancer without GOO, patients accrued between 1994 and 1998	44	0	32	Cholangitis (9%) Wound infection (5%) Delayed gastric emptying (2%)
Multicenter, randomized trial of GJ vs. stent for patients with GOO from UGI cancers, patients accrued between 2006 and 2008	18	0	33	Delayed gastric emptying (11%) Wound infection (5%) UTI (5%)
Prospective, randomized trial of HP + GJ vs. HJ alone for patients with advanced periampullary cancers without evidence of GOO at presentation, patients accrued between 1998 and 2002	36	3	31	Delayed gastric emptying (17%) Cardiac complications (11%) Wound infection (8%)

Lap TV + GJ, laparoscopic truncal vagotomy and gastrojejunostomy; Open TV + GJ, truncal vagotomy and gastrojejunostomy performed through a laparotomy; GOO, gastric outlet obstruction; PUD, peptic ulcer disease; GJ, gastrojejunostomy; HJ, hepatojejunostomy.

anastomotic leak or intra-abdominal abscess occur with significant frequencies. The 30-day mortality rate associated with this operation ranged from 0 to 9% (median = 0).

Long-term complications specific to TV & GJ may be categorized as physiologic or mechanical. The physiologic complications include delayed gastric emptying, early satiety and weight loss, cholelithiasis, chronic diarrhea, dumping syndrome, and iron and calcium malabsorption resulting in anemia and osteoporosis, respectively. Patients in whom vagotomy was not performed or those in whom the vagotomy was incomplete are at risk for peptic ulceration of the jejunal side of the anastomosis. This condition is termed marginal ulceration and may cause life-threatening GI hemorrhage or obstruction of the anastomosis. In patients undergoing gastrojejunostomy without vagotomy this complication is prevented by the administration of proton pump inhibitors or histamine-2 receptor antagonists. The mechanical complications of this procedure include obstruction of the afferent or efferent limb, stenosis or kinking of the anastomosis, and small bowel obstruction.

RESULTS

The results of performing a gastrojejunostomy for patients with benign or malignant GOO are shown in Table 1.2. As alluded to in the previous paragraph, delayed gastric emptying in the early postoperative period is a significant problem associated with this procedure. The median time to tolerating a diet is 8.15 days (range = 4.4 to 8.5 days). The median length of hospitalization is 12.2 days (range = 8 to 21 days). The advantage of gastrojejunostomy over the placement of endoscopic stents or endoscopic dilation is a very low rate of persistent or recurrent GOO requiring remedial therapy. The median rate of patients requiring reoperation for either persistent or recurrent GOO is 0% (range = 0 to 5% and 0 to 16.7%, respectively). Of those patients undergoing gastrojejunostomy for malignant GOO the median survival was 3.8 months (range = 2.1 to 7.2 months).

TABLE 1.2	Results of Gastrojejunostomy in Patients with Benign and Malignant Gastric Outlet Obstruction					
Study Design	Sample Size	Length of Hospitalization (days)	Time to Diet (days)	Persistent GOO/ Reoperation (%)	Recurrent GOO (%)	Survival
Retrospective comparison of Lap TV + GJ vs. Open TV + GJ in patients with PUD with GOO, patients accrued between 1999 and 2005	8	21	8.5	0	0	n/a
Retrospective review of patients with Crohn's disease and duodenal obstruction, patients accrued between 1995 and 2006	11	12.2	4.4	9	0	n/a
Retrospective review of GJ in patients with pancreatic cancer with GOO (66 patients) and without GOO (447 patients), patients accrued between 1996 and 2010	513	8	n/a	0	3.1	6 mo
Prospective comparison, HJ alone in patients with pancreatic cancer with GOO (HJ + GJ) and without GOO (HJ alone), patients accrued between 1992 and 1995	44	21.5	8.3	0	0	4.8 mo
Single-center randomized trial, GJ vs. no GJ in patients with unresectable pancreatic cancer without GOO, patients accrued between 1994 and 1998	44	8.5	n/a	0	0	8.3 mo
Multicenter, randomized trial of GJ vs. stent for patients with GOO from UGI cancers, patients accrued between 2006 and 2008	18	15	8	16.7	5	2.6 mo
Prospective, randomized trial of HP + GJ vs. HJ alone for patients with advanced periampullary cancers without evidence of GOO at presentation, patients accrued between 1998 and 2002	36	11	n/a	0	5.5	7.2 mo

Lap TV + GJ, laparoscopic truncal vagotomy and gastrojejunostomy; Open TV + GJ, truncal vagotomy and gastrojejunostomy performed through a laparotomy; GOO, gastric outlet obstruction; PUD, peptic ulcer disease; GJ, gastrojejunostomy; HJ, hepatojejunostomy.

✦ CONCLUSIONS

TV & GJ is used to manage patients with GOO from PUD who have not responded to medical management and endoscopic dilation. Gastrojejunostomy (without vagotomy) is used to treat patients with UGI malignancies and impending or actual GOO who are discovered during exploratory laparotomy to have advanced or unresectable disease. Technically the operation is relatively straightforward requiring access to the esophageal hiatus and the ability to create a tension-free anastomosis between the stomach and the proximal jejunum. Early postoperative morbidity rates are relatively high when compared to the significance of these patients' underlying illness and other medical comorbidities. Delayed gastric emptying is a common complication prolonging hospital stay. Patients who undergo gastrojejunostomy without vagotomy require acid suppression to prevent marginal ulcers.

Recommended References and Readings

Ananthrakrishnan N, Parthasarathy G, Kate V. Chronic corrosive injuries of the stomach – a single unit experience of 109 patients over thirty years. *World J Surg.* 2010;34:758–764.

Boylan JJ, Gradzka JI. Long-term results of endoscopic balloon dilatation for gastric outlet obstruction. *Dig Dis Sci.* 1999;44:1883–1886.

Cherian PT, Cherian S, Singh P. Long-term follow-up of patients with gastric outlet obstruction related to peptic ulcer disease treated with endoscopic balloon dilation and drug therapy. *Gastrointest Endosc.* 2007;66:491–497.

Gibson JB, Behrman SW, Fabian TC, et al. Gastric outlet obstruction resulting from peptic ulcer disease requiring surgical intervention is infrequently associated with *Helicobacter pylori* infection. *J Am Coll Surg.* 2000;191:32–37.

Jeurnink SM, Steyerberg EW, van Hooft JE, et al. Surgical gastrojejunostomy or endoscopic stent placement for the palliation of malignant gastric outlet obstruction (SUSTENT study): a multicenter randomized trial. *Gastrointest Endosc.* 2010;71:490–499.

Jeurnink SM, Steyerberg EW, Vieggaar FP, et al. Predictors of survival in patients with malignant gastric outlet obstruction: a patient oriented decision approach for palliative treatment. *Dig Liver Dis.* 2011;43:548–552.

Jeurnink SM, van Eijck CHJ, Steyerberg EW, et al. Stent versus gastrojejunostomy for the palliation of gastric outlet obstruction: a systematic review. *BMC Gastroenterology.* 2007;7:18–28.

Kim S-M, Song J, Oh SJ, et al. Comparison of laparoscopic truncal vagotomy with gastrojejunostomy and open surgery in peptic pyloric stenosis. *Surg Endosc.* 2009;23:1326–1330.

Kneuertz PJ, Cunningham SC, Cameron JL, et al. Palliative surgical management of patients with unresectable pancreatic adenocarcinoma: trends and lessons learned from a large, single institution experience. *J Gastrointest Surg.* 2011;15:1917–1927.

Kochhar R, Kochhar S. Endoscopic balloon dilation for benign gastric outlet obstruction in adults. *World J Gastrointest Endosc.* 2010;16:29–35.

Kochhar R, Poornachandra KS, Dutta U, et al. Early endoscopic balloon dilation in caustic-induced gastric injury. *Gastrointest Endosc.* 2010;71:737–744.

Lillemoe KD, Cameron JL, Hardacre JM, et al. Is prophylactic gastrojejunostomy indicated for unresectable periampullary cancer? a prospective randomized trial. *Ann Surg.* 1999;230:322–330.

Shapiro M, Greenstein AJ, Byrn J, et al. Surgical management and outcomes of patients with duodenal Crohn's disease. *J Am Coll Surg.* 2008;207:36–42.

Shone DN, Nikoomanesh P, Smith-Meek MM, et al. Malignancy is the most common cause of gastric outlet obstruction in the era of H2 blockers. *Am J Gastroenterol.* 1995;90:1769–1770.

Shyr Y-M, Su C-H, Wu C-W, et al. Prospective study of gastric outlet obstruction in unresectable periampullary adenocarcinoma. *World J Surg.* 2000;24:60–65.

Skandalakis JE, Rowe JS, Gray SW, et al. Identification of vagal structures at the esophageal hiatus. *Surgery.* 1974;75:233–240.

Soreide K, Sarr MG, Soreide JA. Pyloroplasty for benign gastric outlet obstruction – indications and techniques. *Scand J Surg.* 2006;95:11–16.

Van Heek NT, De Castro SMM, van Eijck CH, et al. The need for a prophylactic gastrojejunostomy for unresectable periampullary cancer: a prospective randomized multicenter trial with special focus on assessment of quality of life. *Ann Surg.* 2003;238:894–905.

2 Truncal Vagotomy and Pyloroplasty

David W. McFadden, Edward C. Borrazzo, and Vladimir Neychev

Introduction

The word *vagotomy* technically means vagal nerve transection, thus interrupting sensory and motor impulses to the stomach and gastrointestinal tract. However, a 1- to 2-cm section of each nerve is usually resected. Although the proper term for resection should be "vagectomy," *vagotomy* is the much more commonly used term (Fig. 2.1). Its purpose is the elimination of direct cholinergic stimulation of gastric acid secretion. Vagal fibers innervate the stomach and play a major role in the cephalic phase of gastric acid secretion by their release of acetylcholine, which stimulates acid secretion from the parietal cell. The distal portion of the anterior and posterior vagal trunks also sends motor branches to the antrum and pylorus. The celiac branch of the posterior vagus stimulates small intestine motility as well. Gastric motility is affected by the antral and pyloric branches of the vagus that stimulate peristaltic activity of the antrum and pyloric relaxation. The vagus also stimulates receptive relaxation of the fundus, resulting in accommodating intake with no corresponding pressure increase.

Vagotomy results in a 75% decrease in basal acid secretion and a 50% decrease in maximum acid output. Additionally, due to the loss of reflex relaxation of the gastric fundus, increased gastric capacity after eating is attended by a rise in pressure, resulting in rapid emptying of liquids. Vagotomy also disturbs distal stomach motility, resulting in difficulty in emptying solids. Because of these changes, approximately 20% to 30% of vagotomy patients develop gastric atony, which may lead to stasis and chronic abdominal pain and distention. Hence, it is surgical dogma that after truncal vagotomy patients require a "drainage" procedure to offset the nonrelaxing, obstructing pylorus. Although four kinds of vagotomy have been described in the surgical literature—*truncal, selective, highly selective,* and *supradiaphragmatic*—truncal and highly selective vagotomy are generally used to treat peptic ulcer disease. Selective and supradiaphragmatic vagotomies are rarely used.

In Dragstedt's initial and seminal series of truncal vagotomy for the treatment of duodenal ulcer disease in 1943, nearly one-third of his patients experienced postoperative nausea, vomiting, and distention. His subsequent investigations revealed that truncal vagotomy denervated the antrum and pylorus resulting in a functional gastric

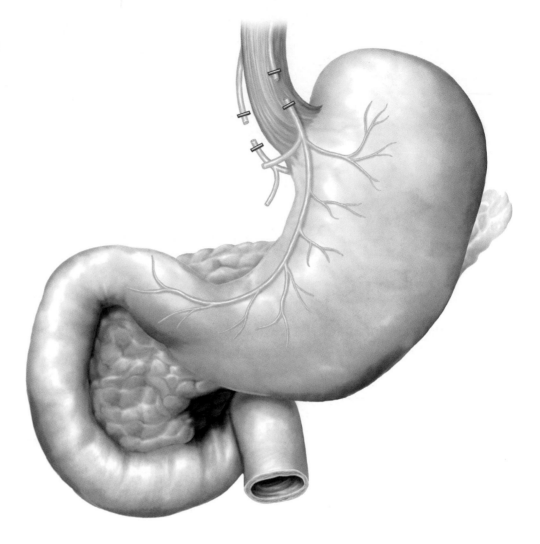

outlet obstruction. It became apparent that a "drainage" procedure was necessary to avoid the symptoms of gastric stasis. Therefore, any patient who undergoes truncal, selective, or supradiaphragmatic vagotomy should undergo a drainage procedure to facilitate gastric emptying. Drainage procedures can be divided into two categories: pyloroplasties and gastrojejunostomy. Pyloroplasty is the favored approach as it maintains the original anatomy, is simple, and is accompanied by less bile reflux than gastrojejunostomy. Currently over 90% of all drainage procedures are variations of pyloroplasty. Pyloroplasty was originally described independently by two surgeons, Heineke and Mikulicz, in 1888, decades before its routine application for drainage after vagotomy. The Heineke–Mikulicz (HM) pyloroplasty is popular because it is technically uncomplicated, widely applicable, and associated with few complications. In children with pyloric stenosis, pyloromyotomy is usually performed, leaving the mucosa intact. This approach in adults is often unsuccessful as the duodenal mucosa is more adherent to the muscle layer and the intestinal lumen is often entered during the myotomy.

Management

Three different types of pyloroplasty have been described. Truncal vagotomy and pyloroplasty is a relatively simple procedure, but there are some nuances that will prevent recurrences and complications. It can be performed laparoscopically or with open surgical technique. Indications most often include persistent ulcer disease refractory to medical therapy.

Vagotomy

Exposure is through an upper midline incision for the open technique or with five trocars positioned in a similar way as for any laparoscopic foregut operation (see Figs. 2.1 and 2.2). First, attention is turned toward the gastroesophageal junction. We use a Thompson retractor to elevate the left lateral segment of the liver when performing surgery laparoscopically, or a Bookwalter or Omni retractor for open surgery. For open surgery, the left triangular ligament is incised using cautery to allow medial retraction of the left lateral segment of the liver. This step is not necessary in the laparoscopic approach since the liver is elevated in a cephalad direction to attain access to the diaphragm hiatus. The gastrohepatic ligament is divided. Also, division of the superior attachments of the gastrosplenic ligament makes encircling the esophagus easier. The esophagus is then encircled with a Penrose drain for retraction. The crura are separated from the esophagus, and the esophagophrenic ligament is incised to expose the anterior esophagus. This step is especially important in patients with hiatal hernia. Occasionally, the gastroesophageal fat pad must be dissected if prominent, exposing the GE junction anteriorly. Again, if the lower esophagus is exposed in the mediastinum, the vagotomy may be performed superior to the GE junction fat pad.

Attention is then turned toward the anterior branch of the vagus nerve (Fig. 2.2). It is easily found traversing from left to right at the distal esophagus. Dissection of the adventitia off the anterior esophagus allows exposure of the anterior vagus nerve, which can be lifted with the help of a right-angled dissector. A short length is dissected, clips are placed proximally and distally, and a segment of the nerve is resected with scissors if clips are used. Otherwise use of ultrasonic energy facilitates ligation. If any concern exists that the resected tissue is not the vagus nerve, this small segment of tissue can be sent to pathology for frozen section to confirm nerve.

Next, the esophagus is retracted, usually anteriorly and toward the left, exposing the posterior esophagus. Since it is larger than the anterior branch, the posterior vagus nerve is usually easier to find and dissect off the esophagus (Fig. 2.3). Similar to the anterior vagus, the posterior branch is hooked with a right-angled dissector, clipped,

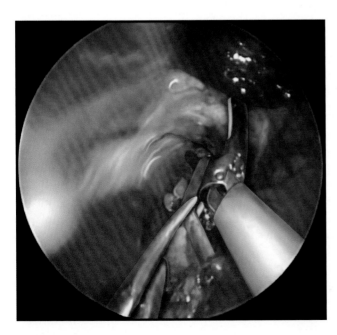

Figure 2.2 Anterior vagotomy. The esophagus is encircled with a Penrose drain for retraction. The esophageal fat pad is retracted inferiorly and the adventitia of the esophagus is cleared. The vagus nerve is dissected off the esophagus and a segment is ligated between clips or, as in this case, using ultrasonic shears.

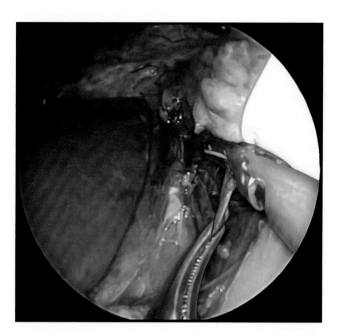

Figure 2.3 Posterior vagotomy. The esophagus is retracted anteriorly, and the vagus nerve is dissected. This image depicts the ligation of the posterior vagus nerve using ultrasonic energy.

and ligated and a portion of the nerve is resected. The Penrose drain and liver retraction are then released, and attention is turned toward the pylorus. Remember, additional vagal trunks are present in nearly 20% of patients and must be identified and transected.

Pyloroplasty

There are several methods for performing pyloroplasty. The most common is the HM pyloroplasty (Fig. 2.4). First, a Kocher maneuver is performed, mobilizing the duodenum from its retroperitoneal attachments. This ultimately helps take tension off the suture line. The pyloric muscle is easily palpated between the surgeon's thumb and index finger. Stay sutures of 3-0 silk are placed with a seromuscular bite through the pylorus just superior and inferior to the anterior aspect of the pylorus. A longitudinal incision is made in between the two stay sutures using a needle-tip electrocautery pencil or ultrasonic energy source. Care is taken to avoid making the incision longer than necessary to prevent tension on the suture line. We recommend extending it between 1 and 2 centimeters past the pyloric muscle proximally and distally (Fig. 2.5). The stay sutures are distracted, and the suture line is closed transversely (Fig. 2.6).

Many different methods exist for closing the pyloroplasty, including single-layer suture closure (with or without imbricating stitch), double-layer closure, or even stapled closure. We prefer a single-layer closure with interrupted 3-0 silk sutures using a Gambee stitch to imbricate the suture line, opposing serosa to serosa (Fig. 2.7). This allows secure closure without narrowing the lumen. Care is taken to avoid missing the mucosa, especially at the corners of the suture line as the pylorus is pushed away from the serosa by the large, thick sphincter muscle layer. If the pyloroplasty is performed laparoscopically, we prefer to use a free needle as opposed to automated suture systems for accurate needle placement. We start from the corners and work toward the middle of the suture line. If possible, the last three sutures should be tied only after all sutures are placed to facilitate assurance of mucosal bites in each stitch. The suture line can be tested by occluding the duodenum and instilling 500 to 1,000 mL of methylene blue down the orogastric tube. Omentum can be placed overlying the suture line and sutured in place if there is any concern regarding suture line integrity.

Another very quick and easy way of performing the HM pyloroplasty is with a stapling device. This is much easier to perform using open rather than laparoscopic

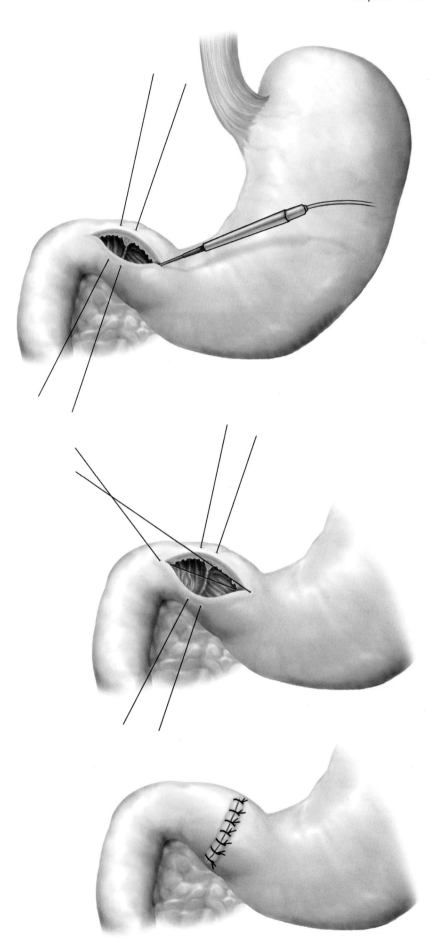

Figure 2.4 Schematic of Heineke–Mikulicz pyloroplasty. The pylorus is incised longitudinally and closed transversely.

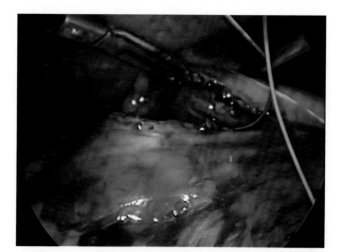

Figure 2.5 Pylorus incised and opened. Stay sutures are placed at each corner to hold the pylorus open.

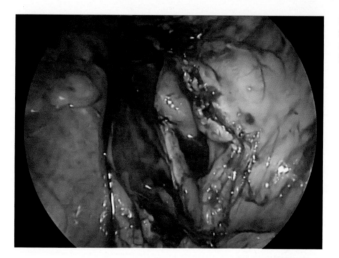

Figure 2.6 Pylorus pulled open prior to closure. The pylorus is incised completely from the prepyloric region into the duodenum.

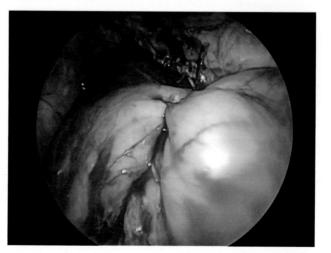

Figure 2.7 Pylorus closed transversely and defunctionalized.

technique. This technique works well if the pylorus is short and soft without scarring. The enterotomy through the pylorus can be closed transversely with a linear stapler. The thickness and the ends of the staple line may need oversewing since the pylorus is of much thicker tissue than the other parts of the stomach and the duodenum. Integrity of the staple line may also be checked with blue dye.

Alternatively, a circular stapler can be used, where a portion of the pylorus is resected. This is usually a very quick procedure useful for patients with other medical comorbidities. An enterotomy is made in the body of the stomach anteriorly, large enough to fit a 25-mm circular stapler. The stapler is opened and positioned traversing the pylorus muscle with the distal end just in the first portion of the duodenum. The stapler is lifted anteriorly while simultaneously dunking the pylorus muscle posteriorly. Care is taken to avoid catching the pylorus posteriorly. The stapler is closed and fired, creating a partial resection of the pylorus muscle with opposition of the serosa. The staples through the pylorus are then reinforced with one suture on each end of the staple line. The stapler is then removed, and the patency of the pylorus is checked by directing the orogastric tube already in place or passing a flexible dilator through the gastric enterotomy distally into the duodenum. The enterotomy in the body of the stomach is closed using a linear stapler. Although one drawback in this technique is the creation of two separate staple lines, the staple line on the body of the stomach rarely causes a leak or stricture and is usually safe to perform. The integrity of both staple lines can be checked using blue dye as described above.

Although rarely necessary, Jaboulay pyloroplasty, a gastroduodenostomy in actuality, can be performed if significant scarring exists making HM pyloroplasty difficult with a high chance of leakage. Again, the first step is always a Kocher maneuver to mobilize the duodenum. The duodenum is apposed to the antrum along the greater curvature of the stomach with seromuscular bites of 3-0 silk suture, usually in an interrupted fashion. Matching enterotomies approximately 5 cm long are made in the stomach and duodenum just anterior to the apposed serosa. The end sutures are left long to hold as stays. The anastomosis is then created by suturing the duodenum to the stomach with full thickness bites of tissue to include mucosa. This is done in a running fashion along this posterior wall. A new stitch is run from the corner anteriorly half the length of the enterotomies, while another stitch is taken from the opposite corner. This anterior stitch can be an inverting stitch to oppose the serosa. If not, we suggest interrupted Lembert stitches anteriorly using 3-0 silk suture. Again a leak test is performed with blue dye in the stomach down the orogastric tube.

Finney pyloroplasty is rarely performed today but allows excellent drainage for chronically obstructed stomach. A Kocher maneuver is performed, followed by traction sutures of 3-0 silk as with HM pyloroplasty. A 10 to 12 cm inverted U-shaped incision is made from the lumen of the stomach, across the pylorus, and into the second portion of the duodenum (Fig. 2.8). A two-layer closure is performed. First, the posterior septum between the posterior walls of the stomach and duodenum are sutured, using a 3-0 continuous absorbable hemostatic suture (Fig. 2.9). This suture begins at the pyloric aspect of the posterior wall and continues anteriorly to secure the anterior walls of the stomach and duodenum (Fig. 2.10). An outer layer of 3-0 silk Lembert sutures completes the procedure (Fig. 2.11).

Alternatively, a stapled technique can be performed here as well. After mobilization of the duodenum, enterotomies are made in the duodenum and stomach approximately 5 cm distal and proximal to the pylorus, respectively. Limbs of the linear cutting stapler are inserted into the openings positioned toward pylorus, and the stapler is fired. The common enterotomy is then closed with linear stapler and excess tissue is trimmed and the staple line is checked for hemostasis and integrity. Again, a leak test can be performed.

Postoperative nasogastric decompression is used occasionally, especially if there is a gastric outlet obstruction from long-standing disease and scarring. Closed suction drainage is rarely used.

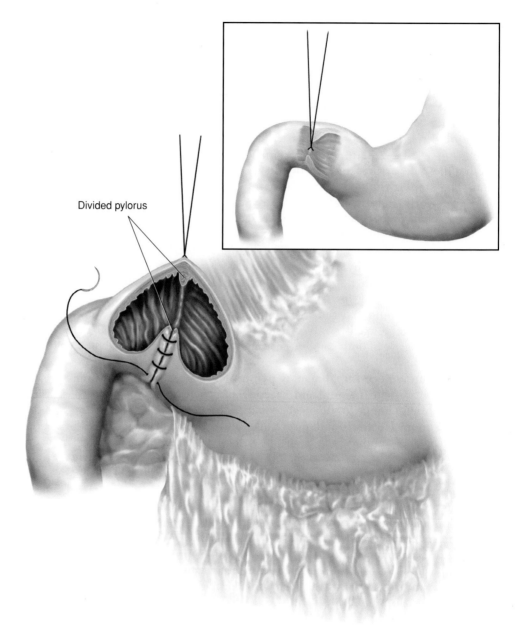

Divided pylorus

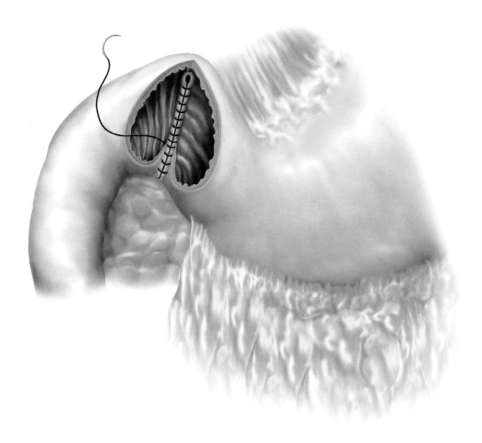

Figure 2.9 The inner row of running suture is usually of a 3-0 absorbable variety in the Finney pyloroplasty.

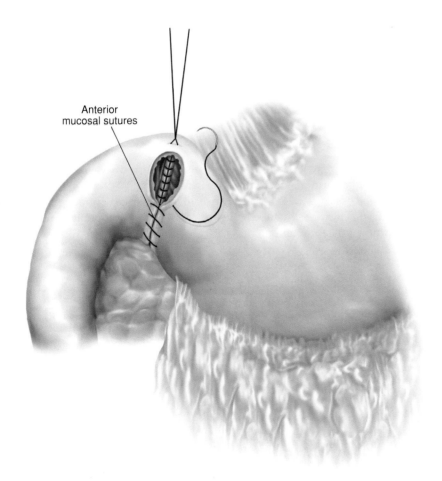

Anterior
mucosal sutures

Figure 2.10 The running inner suture line continues from superiorly and inferiorly to end anteriorly.

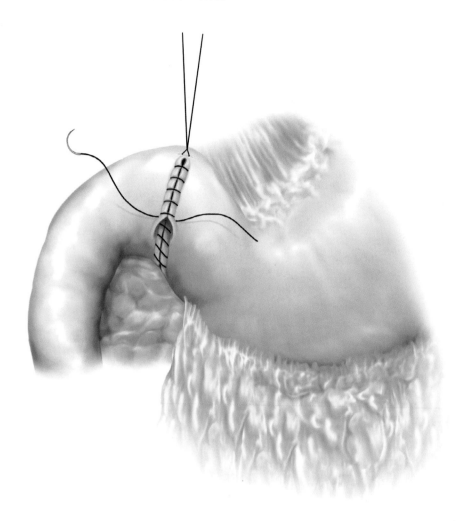

Figure 2.11 Interrupted 3-0 silk Lembert sutures completes the Finney pyloroplasty.

❖ CONCLUSION

Although an uncommon procedure today, surgeons should have vagotomy and pyloroplasty in their operative armamentarium for treatment of peptic ulcer disease. Often, this procedure is necessary emergently, as in a bleeding ulcer refractory to medical management, and familiarity with this procedure will decrease operative time, which may be important for unstable patients.

Recommended References and Readings

Broderick TJ, Matthews JB. Vagotomy and drainage. In: Yeo CJ, ed. *Shackleford's Surgery of the Alimentary Tract.* 6th ed. Philadelphia, PA: Saunders/Elsevier; 2007:811–830.

Kauffman GL. Duodenal ulcer disease: treatment by surgery, antibiotics, or both. *Adv Surg.* 2000;34:121–135.

Mulholland MW. Atlas of gastric surgery. In: Bell RH, Rikkers LF, Mulholland MW, eds. *Digestive Tract Surgery.* Philadelphia, PA: Lippincott-Raven; 1996:295–380.

3 Truncal Vagotomy with Antrectomy and Billroth I Reconstruction

Stanley W. Ashley and Thomas E. Clancy

INDICATIONS/CONTRAINDICATIONS

Vagotomy has been recognized as a means of reducing gastric acidity, and thus it has been used in treating gastroduodenal ulcers since the early years of the 20th century. The use of vagotomy for peptic ulcer disease was found to be associated with delayed gastric emptying, so a gastric drainage procedure was added. The combination of truncal vagotomy and antrectomy, whereby the gastrin-producing antrum is removed, was subsequently proposed. Alternatives to truncal vagotomy to spare the celiac and hepatic branches (proximal selective vagotomy) or with preservation of vagal innervations of the antrum (highly selective vagotomy) have been proposed to mitigate postvagotomy complications of dumping and diarrhea. Still, the loss of receptive relaxation and gastric accommodation with all procedures makes some drainage procedure desirable.

The past few decades have seen a dramatic decrease in the role of surgical management of uncomplicated peptic ulcer disease. While operative management was previously routine for gastric and duodenal ulcers, the use of acid-suppressing medications such as histamine-2 receptor antagonists and proton pump inhibitors, as well as the treatment of *Helicobacter pylori* infection, has made many such procedures rare. Surgical management of peptic ulcer disease is now predominantly limited to complications of the disease, such as hemorrhage, perforation, and obstruction. This approach largely avoids the use of acid-reducing operations. Still, acid-reducing procedures may play an important role in the management of complicated and refractory ulcer disease, particularly in patients who have failed acid-suppressing medications.

Truncal vagotomy remains an important option for complicated peptic ulcer disease, particularly in the acute setting with a medication-refractory patient. Antrectomy will remove approximately 35% of the stomach, including all of the nonparietal cell portion of the stomach. This will allow resection of a distal gastric or prepyloric ulcer. Given very effective antisecretory medications and antibiotics to treat *H. pylori,* truncal vagotomy and antrectomy is primarily useful in the setting of pyloric outlet obstruction with recurrent ulcer symptoms or peptic ulcer disease complicated by bleeding or perforation. Reconstruction of intestinal continuity can be performed via gastroduode-nostomy (Billroth I) or loop gastrojejunostomy (Billroth II).

The indications for truncal vagotomy, antrectomy, and Billroth I gastroduodenos-tomy are as follows:

- prepyloric ulcer
- gastric ulcer
- peptic ulcer disease with gastric outlet obstruction
- recurrent ulcer after treatment with antisecretory medications
- emergency treatment of complicated ulcer disease, in a patient who is refractory to antisecretory medications

 PREOPERATIVE PLANNING

Preoperative evaluation should include detailed imaging and laboratory data as well as endoscopic evaluation. In the case of complicated peptic ulcer disease, emergency sur-gery may not allow extensive preoperative workup. Preoperative laboratory indices should include hematocrit, bleeding parameters, basic chemistries, and tests of nutri-tional reserve given the risk of preoperative malnutrition and postoperative ileus com-plicating major gastrointestinal surgery.

Endoscopy is essential for the evaluation of the patient with bleeding secondary to peptic ulcer disease; endoscopic management is often sufficient to manage bleeding without surgery. Surgery is required for bleeding in the unstable patient, after extensive transfusion (over 6 units of blood), or for rebleeding after initial endoscopic manage-ment. Precise localization of the bleeding source is important.

Endoscopy is also important in the diagnosis of *H. pylori* infection. In patients with refractory peptic ulcer disease, endoscopy is important for biopsy to rule out occult gastric malignancy. Workup should include biopsies of the ulcer base and surrounding gastric mucosa. Endoscopy also has a role in the documentation of healing of gas-troduodenal ulcers after the initiation of antisecretory medications, as failure of ulcers to heal may portend occult malignancy.

Imaging to include a chest x-ray and CT scan of the abdomen is useful to detect potential metastatic disease when malignancy is considered.

 SURGICAL TECHNIQUE

Pertinent Anatomy

The vagal nerves, a plexus around the intraabdominal esophagus, will join to form two trunks at the esophageal hiatus. The anterior (left) vagus nerve is positioned along the anterior wall of the esophagus, while the posterior vagus is found between the postero-medial wall of the esophagus and the right crus of the diaphragm (Fig. 3.1).

Positioning

Patients are positioned in the supine position. As access to the upper stomach and distal esophagus is critical, an upper midline incision to the xiphoid process is typi-cally utilized. A bilateral subcostal incision, providing excellent exposure to the duo-denum, may compromise optimal exposure of the upper abdomen. The abdomen is prepped from the low chest to the pubis.

Mild reverse Trendelenburg position is useful, and a nasogastric tube not only decompresses the stomach but will also allow easier identification of the esophagus. Mobilization of the left lobe of the liver by dividing the triangular ligament is performed selectively; although this maneuver may aid exposure of the gastroesophageal junction

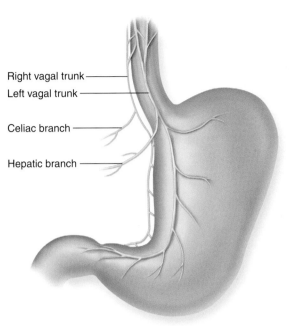

Figure 3.1 The vagal nerves from the intrathoracic esophagus form two major trunks before entering the abdomen at the esophageal hiatus.

Right vagal trunk

Left vagal trunk

Celiac branch

Hepatic branch

in some patients, a large or redundant left lateral segment may be held in place by the triangular ligament and exposure may be impeded by its division in some patients.

Technique

Vagotomy

Mobilization of the liver medially or superiorly may be necessary for optimal visualization of the gastroesophageal junction. The left triangular ligament of the liver can be divided with cautery to facilitate medial rotation of the left lateral segment of the liver.

The distal esophagus is exposed by incising the peritoneal covering of the gastroesophageal junction with cautery, incising the peritoneum from the lesser curvature to the cardiac notch at the greater curvature. Gentle blunt dissection is used to surround the esophagus. A Penrose drain is placed around the distal esophagus for retraction. Care should be taken to place the Penrose drain at a sufficient distance from the esophagus to include the vagal trunks. The posterior vagal trunk may be palpated during this maneuver as a tight cord. For complete vagotomy, the distal esophagus must be mobilized proximally and stripped of peritoneal attachments for approximately 5 cm.

The operator should note the clockwise rotation of vagal trunks as the vagi pass from the thoracic cavity into the abdominal cavity. Exposure of the anterior vagal trunk is facilitated by inferior–posterior traction on the Penrose drain. Similarly, the posterior vagus may run along the posterior-right side of the distal esophagus, and exposure is facilitated by retracting the Penrose drain into the wound and toward the left of the incision. A single anterior vagal trunk is usually identified in the anterior midportion of the esophagus, 2 to 4 cm above the gastroesophageal junction. It is not uncommon for vagal fibers to be distributed among two or three smaller cords at this level. These trunks are individually lifted up and 2- to 4-cm segments of each are separated from the surrounding tissues. The nerves are surrounded, clipped on two sides, and a 2-cm middle portion is excised and sent to pathology to confirm the presence of the nerve via frozen section. The posterior vagal trunk is usually identified along the right edge of the esophagus. If the anterior vagus has already been divided, the esophagus is more mobile. This mobility allows downward traction on the gastroesophageal junction, which allows the posterior vagus to "bowstring" and makes it easier to identify. A 2- to 4-cm segment is separated from the surrounding tissues, its margins marked with clips, resected, and sent to pathology for frozen section (Figs. 3.2 and 3.3).

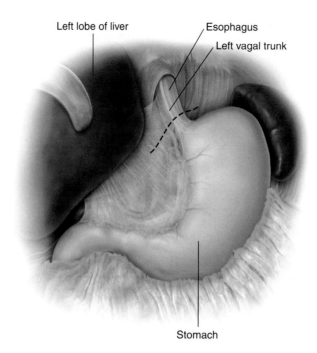

Left lobe of liver   Esophagus
                                      Left vagal trunk

Stomach

Figure 3.2 The peritoneum over the gastroesophageal junction is divided with cautery to expose the esophagus. The left lateral segment of the liver may require superior or medial retraction for exposure.

Antrectomy

After vagotomy is performed, antrectomy is a useful drainage procedure, particularly in the setting of duodenal or pyloric channel ulcer with gastric outlet obstruction. Antrectomy removes approximately 35% of the stomach to include the gastrin-producing mucosa. Useful landmarks include the incisura angularis on the lesser curvature and a point between the pylorus and the fundus on the greater curvature where the right and the left gastroepiploic vessels meet (watershed area).

The lesser sac is entered via the gastrocolic ligament, an avascular plane in the omentum. Dissection should begin at the mid-greater curvature and continue along the greater curvature of the stomach toward the pylorus. Adhesions between the posterior wall of the stomach and the pancreas are divided sharply. Near the pylorus, the right gastroepiploic vessels are divided and ligated. Dissection should be carried about 1 cm

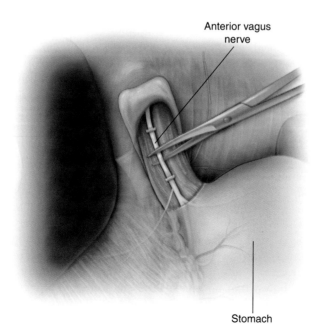

Anterior vagus
nerve

Stomach

Figure 3.3 Gentle traction to the stomach facilitates identification of the vagus nerves. Clips are applied to each trunk proximally and distally, with removal of a 2- to 3-cm segment between the clips.

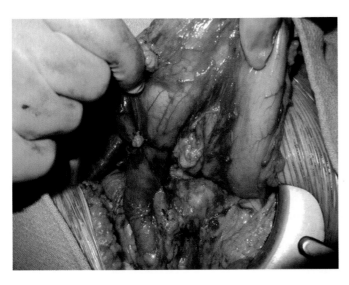

Figure 3.4 The stomach has been mobilized, with division of the gastrocolic ligament and right gastroepiploic vessels. The pancreas is visible at the base of the lesser sac.

past the pylorus, taking care to avoid injury to the pancreas. Along the lesser curvature between the incisura and the pylorus, tissues including distal branches of the left gastric artery are divided and ligated. The right gastric artery is similarly divided and ligated.

If a Billroth I anastomosis is planned, it is essential to mobilize the duodenum thoroughly with a generous Kocher maneuver. The peritoneum along the lateral duodenum should be divided with cautery. Dissection should begin near the porta hepatis, taking care to avoid injury to the common bile duct and portal vein. The Kocher maneuver should include the peritoneum along the inferior border of the third portion of the duodenum, separating the third portion of the duodenum from the transverse mesocolon to allow mobilization of the duodenum superiorly as well as laterally. If duodenal scarring prevents Billroth I anastomosis, a Kocher maneuver is not required.

A GIA linear stapler is used to divide the stomach at the estimated border of the antrum. The antrum is retracted anteriorly and to the patient's left side. The duodenum is divided with a TA stapler. Particular care must be taken with a thickened and inflamed duodenum in the setting of chronic scarring or perforation. For thick tissue, primary suture closure is preferable to stapled closure, and omental patch reinforcement of the duodenal stump may be helpful (Figs. 3.4–3.7).

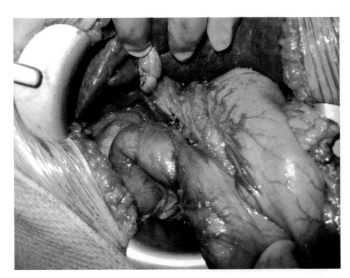

Figure 3.5 A full Kocher maneuver has been performed to mobilize the duodenum medically and superiorly.

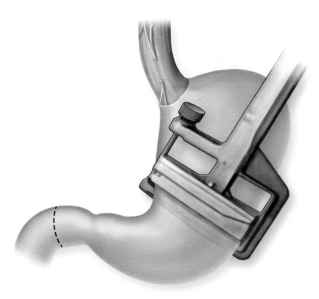

Figure 3.6 After entering the lesser sac, the stomach is divided proximally between the incisura and midway along the greater curvature to include the entire antrum.

Billroth I Gastroduodenostomy

Primary gastroduodenostomy, or Billroth I reconstruction, is preferable to allow preservation of antegrade flow. The gastroduodenostomy is created in two layers. A posterior row of interrupted seromuscular silk sutures are placed first in the Lembert manner between the duodenum and the stomach at the inferior/lateral border of the gastric staple line. The superior/medial portion of the duodenal staple line is removed with cautery, and the gastric staple line is opened a corresponding length. An inner layer of running 3-0 vicryl suture (or other absorbable suture) is placed, followed by an anterior outer row of interrupted 3-0 silk Lembert sutures. The junction of the anastomosis and the gastric staple line has been referred to as the "angle of sorrow" due to the complication of leakage at this intersection of suture/staple lines. This angle should be reinforced with additional 3-0 silk Lembert sutures.

Stapling techniques have been described for the gastroduodenostomy as well; the anvil of a 25-mm EEA stapler may be sewn into the duodenal stump with a purse-string suture. The circular stapler may be inserted through anterior gastrostomy, with the gastrotomy closed with a TA stapler (Figs. 3.8–3.10).

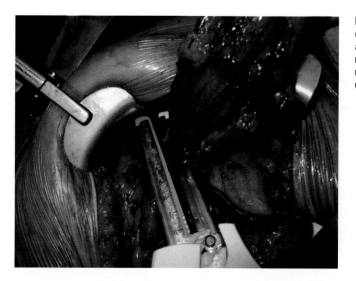

Figure 3.7 The stomach has been divided just proximal to the antrum, from the incisura to the mid-greater curvature. The duodenum is divided with a stapler 1 cm distal to the pylorus.

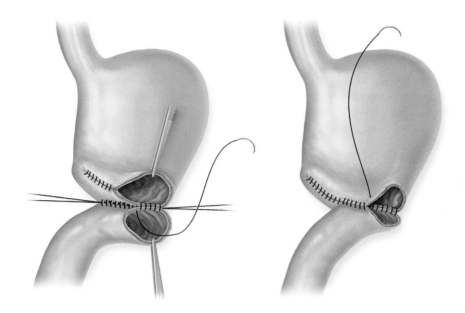

Figure 3.8 The gastroduodenostomy is created in two layers. The posterior layer is completed with 3-0 silk. An inner layer of running absorbable suture is placed, followed by an anterior row of interrupted 3-0 silk seromuscular sutures.

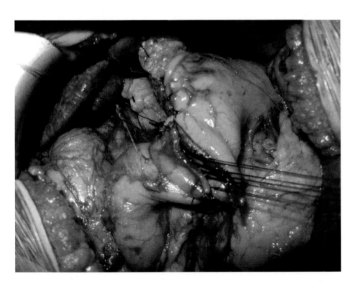

Figure 3.9 The Billroth I gastroduodenostomy is constructed first with a posterior row of interrupted seromuscular silk sutures. The gastric and duodenal staple lines have not yet been removed. The medial portion of the gastric staple line has been oversewn with seromuscular silk sutures.

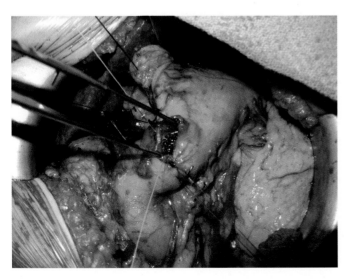

Figure 3.10 The Billroth I anastomosis is continued by removing the staple lines of the stomach and duodenum with cautery. An inner running layer of full-thickness 3-0 Vicryl suture is used in this case.

POSTOPERATIVE MANAGEMENT

Nasogastric suction is continued postoperatively until the volume of gastric effluent falls to less that 1,000 mL/24 hours and there is no clinical evidence of anastomotic leak. Typically patients will require nasogastric decompression for several days. Routine radiographic analysis via barium swallow is not necessary unless there is clinical suspicion for an anastomotic leak (Fig. 3.11).

 COMPLICATIONS

An unfortunate complication after vagotomy is recurrent ulceration due to persistent vagal innervations. While some recurrences can be managed medically, some will require reoperation, particularly in an acute presentation such as perforation. Dense adhesions to the left lobe of the liver can make reoperative vagotomy difficult, and the best approach for repeat truncal vagotomy is via transthoracic or thoracoscopic access.

Given the loss of vagally mediated receptive relaxation of the stomach, emptying of liquids is accelerated after vagotomy. Dumping, manifest as postprandial discomfort and dizziness, can be seen in 10% to 15% of patients after truncal vagotomy and antrectomy and can be disabling in 1% to 2% of patients. "Early" dumping may occur soon after a meal and include discomfort, dizziness, syncope, and palpitations. "Late" dumping occurs several hours postprandially and may include hypoglycemia. Dietary changes are effective in mitigating symptoms for most patients. Somatostatin analogues are also reported to have a beneficial effect on symptoms of dumping when administered prior to meals. Delayed gastric emptying after gastrojejunostomy is managed conservatively. Refractory delayed gastric emptying after Billroth I reconstruction is managed with gastrojejunostomy to the greater curvature of the stomach to avoid devascularization and duodenal stump leakage. Bleeding after partial gastrectomy is generally seen as intraluminal blood loss. An endoscopic approach with coagulation or epinephrine injection of the anastomosis is preferable to surgical exploration.

Alkaline reflux gastritis is common after partial gastrectomy, affecting 5% to 15% of patients. Reflux is common, although pain and nausea are less commonly seen. Endoscopy is important in the setting of postoperative epigastric discomfort to rule out recurrent ulceration. Endoscopy may show bile reflux into the stomach, as well as gastritis. HIDA scan (99mTc hepatic iminodiacetic acid scan) can also be used to establish the diagnosis. Medical management, including antacids, bile acid chelators, and dietary

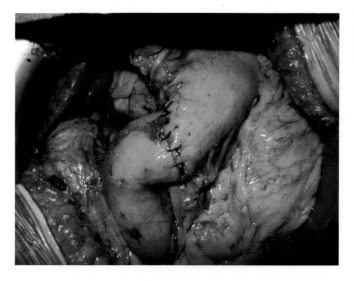

Figure 3.11 The Billroth I anastomosis is completed with an anterior row interrupted seromuscular 3-0 silk sutures.

changes, is not typically beneficial and surgical management with Roux-en-y gastrojejunostomy is often indicated

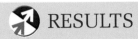

RESULTS

Truncal vagotomy with antrectomy is highly effective in reducing both basal and stimulated acid secretion in the stomach, as well as highly effective in reducing ulcer recurrence. Recurrence rates of 1% to 2% have been reported after truncal vagotomy and antrectomy, even prior to the use of treatment for *H. pylori.*

CONCLUSIONS

Truncal vagotomy and antrectomy is an effective means of treating refractory symptoms of peptic ulcer disease, particularly with pyloric channel ulcers, gastric outlet obstruction, or in the acute setting in a patient with ulcer disease while on antisecretory medications. In the setting of highly effective antisecretory therapy and the recognition and treatment of *H. pylori* colonization, surgical therapy is rarely required as an acid-reducing intervention. However, these procedures remain an important tool for the gastrointestinal surgeon treating refractory ulcer disease or faced with emergency complications of peptic ulcer disease such as perforation, bleeding, or obstruction.

Recommended References and Readings

Eagon JC, Meidema BW, Kelly KA. Postgastrectomy syndromes. *Surg Clin North Am.* 1992;72:445.

El-Omar E, Penman I, Dorrian CA, et al. Eradication of *Helicobacter pylori* infection lowers gastrin mediated acid secretion by two thirds in patients with duodenal ulcer. *Gut.* 1993;34:1060–1065.

Fiser WB, Wellborn JC, Thompson BW, et al. Age and morbidity of vagotomy with antrectomy or pyloroplasty. *Am J Surg.* 1982; 144:694.

Kanaya S, Gomi T, Momoi H, et al. Delta-shaped anastomosis in totally laparoscopic Billroth I gastrectomy: new technique of intraabdominal gastroduodenostomy. *J Am Coll Surg.* 2002;195: 28–287.

Laine L, Peterson WL. Bleeding peptic ulcer. *N Eng J Med.* 1994; 331:717–727.

Ng EK, Lam YH, Sung JJ, et al. Eradication of *Helicobacter pylori* prevents recurrence of ulcer after simple closure of duodenal ulcer perforation: randomized controlled trial. *Ann Surg.* 2000; 231:153.

Schwesinger WH, Page CP, Sirineck KR, et al. Operations for peptic ulcer disease: paradigm lost. *J Gastrointest Surg.* 2001;5:1038.

Smith BR, Stablie BE. Emerging trends in peptic ulcer disease and damage control surgery in the *H. Pylori* era. *Am Surg.* 2005;71: 797.

Taylor TV, Bunn AA, MacLeod DA, et al. Anterior lesser curve seromyotomy and posterior truncal vagotomy in the treatment of chronic duodenal ulcer. *Lancet.* 1982;2:846.

Welch CE, Rodkey GV, Gryska PV. A thousand operations for ulcer disease. *Ann Surg.* 1984;204(4):454–467.

Zinner MJ. *Atlas of Gastric Surgery.* New York: Churchill Livingstone Inc.; 1992.

4 Laparoscopic Truncal Vagotomy with Antrectomy and Billroth I Reconstruction

Aurora D. Pryor

 ## INDICATIONS/CONTRAINDICATIONS

Peptic Ulcer Disease

Surgical management of peptic ulcer disease has metamorphosed with the advent of proton pump inhibitor (PPI) therapy and elucidation of the role of *Helicobacter pylori* in gastric pathology. While gastric resections for ulcer disease were formerly a mainstay in the practice of general surgery, such procedures are now rare. Most patients are treated with 6 weeks of PPI therapy and eradication of *H. pylori.* This combination of therapies is effective in treating the majority of ulcers. However, indications do remain for surgical therapy for ulcer disease. The major indication is failure of medical management presenting as either intractable ulceration after a 3-month medical trial or issues such as perforation or bleeding while on therapy. Ulcers can also present acutely as a complication of nonsteroidal anti-inflammatory drug use. Long-term complications of ulcers, such as gastric outlet obstruction or malignancy, remain reasons for surgery as well. An additional relative indication for surgery is a patient with complicated ulcer disease and poor access to care or unlikely follow-up.

The choice of surgical procedure is based on the indication. Simple Graham (omental) patch closure can be performed for pyloric channel or duodenal perforation. Vagotomy and pyloroplasty offers a definitive approach to a bleeding pyloric channel or duodenal ulcer. Wedge gastrectomy results in excision of perforated gastric ulcers, while providing adequate tissue to evaluate for underlying malignancy. Antrectomy, usually in conjunction with vagotomy, is most commonly used for patients with gastric outlet obstruction from chronic ulcer disease. Vagotomy and antrectomy can also be used for definitive management of a perforated pyloric channel ulcer in a stable patient with minimal soilage.

Vagotomy is performed to minimize acid production in patients undergoing surgery for peptic ulcer disease. It works by blocking acetylcholine-mediated acid release as well as preventing antral interneuron release of gastrin-releasing peptide which in turn stimulates antral G-cell gastric release. However, histamine and nonvagal-mediated gastrin release still occur following vagotomy. Truncal vagotomy gained popularity in the 1940s in the management of gastric acid production to limit ulcer formation. It was performed in conjunction with a drainage procedure to minimize complications of delayed gastric emptying that were witnessed in up to one-third of patients following vagotomy alone. Selective and highly selective vagotomy came into favor to maximize the benefits of diminished acid production without causing gastric dysmotility. With the success of PPI therapy, even these selective procedures have fallen out of favor. Most patients requiring surgery for ulcer disease today require either antrectomy for obstruction or duodenal access and therefore pyloroplasty closure. In these patients, concomitant truncal vagotomy can obviate the need for and expense of postoperative PPI with minimal added risk.

Gastrointestinal Stromal Tumors

Gastrointestinal stromal tumors (GISTs) are mesenchymal neoplasms originating from the cells of Cajal. Sixty percent of these tumors are found in the stomach. The diagnosis is suspected with any submucosal mass and confirmed in most cases with reactivity to KIT (CD117) and/or DOG1. Many GISTs are incidentally found, but some present as a source of bleeding due to rupture. The malignant potential increases with both size and mitotic index, with tumors <2 cm in diameter and with ≤5 mitoses per 50 HPF considered very low risk. Surgery is the mainstay of treatment for localized GISTs amenable to resection.

Surgical resection for GISTs involves complete margin-negative resection with an intact pseudocapsule. Lymphadenectomy is not required. Although most of these lesions may be treated with wedge resection, occasionally antrectomy is required.

Pancreatic rests and adenomas may present preoperatively as suspected GISTs. Although they have low malignant potential, they are usually managed as if GISTs unless a benign diagnosis can be confirmed.

Carcinoids

Gastric neuroendocrine tumors are an unusual cause of gastric pathology. These lesions can be benign carcinoid tumors or neuroendocrine carcinomas. This determination can usually be made on the basis of hematoxylin- and eosin-stained biopsies. Some carcinoid lesions may be associated with atrophic gastritis, pernicious anemia, or elevated gastrin levels. Most small lesions confirmed to be benign can be removed with endoscopic or laparoscopic wedge techniques. Some advocate surveillance for benign lesions 10 to 20 mm or smaller. Many suggest that multifocal carcinoids should be resected with antrectomy. Neuroendocrine carcinomas should be managed with more radical resection, often total gastrectomy with lymphadenectomy.

Adenocarcinoma

Gastric adenocarcinoma is rarely confined to just the distal stomach in Europe or the Americas. The surgical approach is geared at obtaining an R0 resection, with negative margins and no evidence of residual disease whenever possible. In the United States and Europe, D1 lymphadenectomy involving just the perigastric nodes is standard. More extensive D2 lymphadenectomy adding nodal tissue surrounding the left gastric, splenic, and hepatic arteries as well as the celiac axis, although beneficial in Japan, has been associated with increased morbidity and mortality in Western trials. Removal of at least 15 lymph nodes is important for staging information.

Outcomes after laparoscopic versus open gastric resection are oncologically equivalent based on several studies in the setting of experienced laparoscopic surgeons and low-risk patients (ASA < 3). There are benefits with length of stay, resumption of oral intake, blood loss, and analgesia use as well.

On the basis of results of a landmark 2006 study by Cunningham and colleagues, patients with gastric or gastroesophageal adenocarcinoma should receive preoperative chemotherapy to improve progression-free and overall survival.

For patients with advanced disease, palliative resection, even involving total gastrectomy, has improved outcomes compared with surgical bypass. This includes both quality of life and possibly survival benefits.

 # PREOPERATIVE PLANNING

Chronic ulcer disease patients require a trial of medical therapy prior to surgery. Most patients are expected to complete two 6-week courses of PPI therapy as well as eradication of *H. pylori* with proven failure. No specific bowel prep is required.

For patients with acute complications of ulcer disease, such as bleeding or perforation, preoperative resuscitation is important. These patients should have a urinary catheter placed. Blood or fluids should be given as necessary to assure adequate perfusion. In the setting of perforation, broad-spectrum antibiotics are also advised. A nasogastric tube may be placed to facilitate gastric decompression, but it should be removed before stapling.

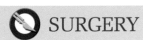 # SURGERY

Positioning

The setup for laparoscopic antrectomy in our practice has the patient placed supine with the arms extended out at the sides (Fig. 4.1). The surgeon stands at the patient's right, with the assistant on the left. Monitors are placed over the patient's shoulders.

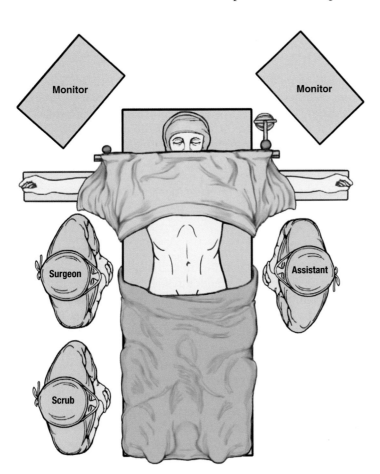

Figure 4.1 OR setup for laparoscopic gastrectomy. The patient is placed supine on the table with arms extended. The surgeon stands to the patient's right and the assistant is on the left.

Figure 4.2 Port placement for laparoscopic gastrectomy. The ports are placed higher for proximal pathology or lower (*arrows*) for more distal lesions.

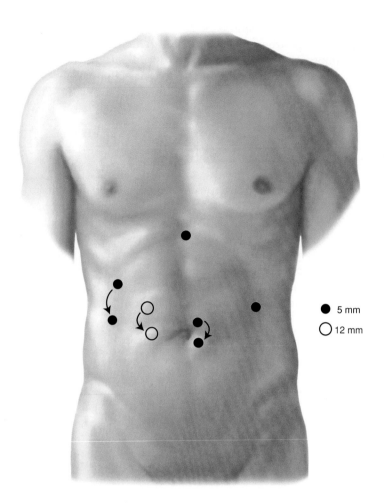

An endoscope should be readily available to help with identification of pathology or to test for leak at the completion of the procedure. Ports are placed to allow good access to the hiatus and distal stomach (Fig. 4.2). The procedure is performed in reverse Trendelenburg position. A liver retractor is helpful for proximal gastric and hiatal exposure. This is placed through a subxiphoid port.

 SURGICAL TECHNIQUE

Distal Gastrectomy

Distal gastrectomy may be performed for ulcer disease, benign lesions as well as cancer. If the resection is being performed for adenocarcinoma, the resection should include the greater omentum, duodenal bulb, and surrounding nodal tissue. The technical ease of antrectomy is greatly improved with modern vessel sealing technology. These devices can divide vessels up to 7 mm in diameter without requiring skeletonization or clips.

The variability of distal gastrectomy is greatly dependent on the planned reconstruction. The procedure can be completed with a gastroduodenostomy (Billroth I anastomosis), loop gastrojejunostomy (Billroth II anastomosis), or with Roux-en-Y reconstruction (Fig. 4.3). Billroth I reconstruction is the most anatomic and is preferred in our practice when technically possible. It also minimizes postoperative complications such as duodenal stump leak, afferent loop syndrome, and marginal ulceration. This approach will be the focus of this chapter. The anastomosis may be placed in a

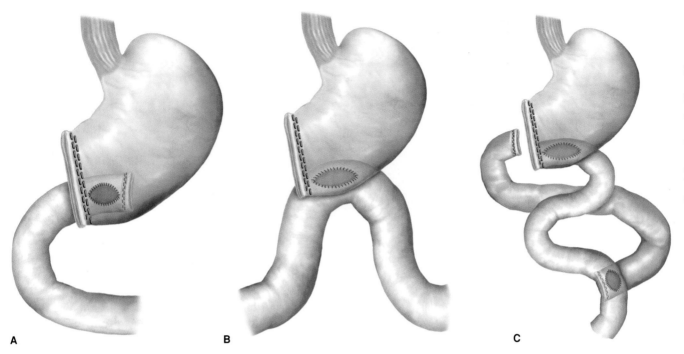

A   B   C

Figure 4.3 Alternatives for reconstruction after distal gastrectomy. (**A**) Billroth I gastroduodenostomy. (**B**) Billroth II loop gastrojejunostomy, or (**C**) Roux-en-Y reconstruction.

variety of locations, but the distal posterior gastric wall is usually preferred to facilitate gastric emptying.

- The procedure should begin with duodenal mobilization (Kocher maneuver, Fig. 4.4). The more extensive this mobilization, the easier the reach for the eventual anastomosis.
- Omental mobilization is next if the procedure is performed for cancer. This begins with separating the omentum off of the transverse colon and carrying this mobilization up to the stomach.
- The transection line on the stomach is then identified. Antrectomy is usually performed proximal to the crow's foot, such as insertion of vessels onto the lesser curvature and at a point corresponding to the transition between the right and left gastroepiploic vessels on the greater curvature. The line between these points will include the entire antrum.
- The gastroepiploic vessels are divided along the greater curvature at the transection plane and the lesser sac window is confirmed (Fig. 4.5). After removing any nasogastric tube, the stomach is divided with staples (Fig. 4.6). In our practice we prefer a bioabsorbable buttress material and 4.8-mm staple leg lengths for this division (Duet, Covidien, North Haven, CT). Other staple options can be used per surgeon preference. The transection is continued toward the lesser curvature.

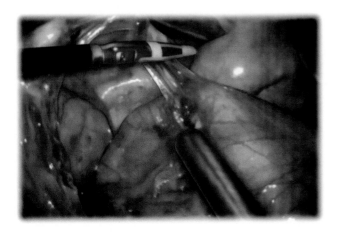

Figure 4.4 Laparoscopic Kocher maneuver.

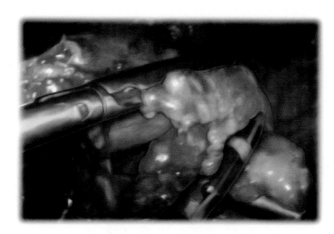

Figure 4.5 Mobilizing the antrum for resection.

- After fully dividing the stomach, the tissue along the lesser curvature is separated with a bipolar sealing device, care being taken to keep the nodal tissue with the specimen when operating for cancer.
- The distal stomach then functions as a handle to assist with pyloric and duodenal mobilization. It is reflected to the patient's right to facilitate exposure. Surrounding nodal tissue is kept with the specimen.
- The right gastric and right gastroepiploic vessels may be divided with vessel sealing. Alternatively, staples may be used.
- The duodenum is then divided with 2.5-mm staples (Fig. 4.7). Staple line reinforcement or oversewing of this staple line should be considered if the duodenum will not be used for reconstruction.
- The specimen is then placed in a retrieval bag for removal at the completion of the procedure.

Vagotomy

Exposure for vagotomy mimics hiatal exposure for other procedures involving the gastroesophageal junction.

- The lesser omentum is incised with an electrosurgical instrument and the hiatus is exposed.
- This dissection is carried anterior to the esophagus to mobilize the gastroesophageal junction.
- The anterior vagus nerve is identified overlying the esophagus, toward the patient's left. It can usually be palpated and separated easily from the esophagus with careful dissection.
- Traditionally, clips have been placed proximally and distally on the vagus nerve to mark the vagotomy. This may be performed at the surgeon's discretion.

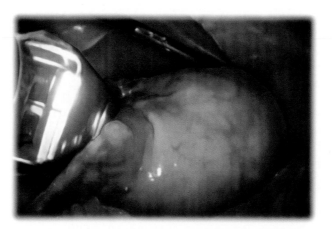

Figure 4.6 Dividing the stomach.

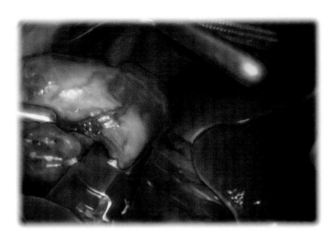

Figure 4.7 Dividing the duodenum with staples.

- The nerve is divided with scissors, bipolar sealing, or ultrasonic dissection (Fig. 4.8). It is then removed from the operative field and labeled.
- A plane is then created posterior to the esophagus, adjacent to the right crus.
- The esophagus is retracted anteriorly and to the patient's left to facilitate adequate visualization.
- The posterior vagus nerve can usually be identified running between the esophagus and the right crux. It can be dissected off the esophagus with gentle dissection.
- The nerve should be divided as high in the chest as possible to assure that the criminal nerve of Grassi is divided. Clips are again used at the surgeon's discretion (Fig. 4.9).
- The nerve is then removed from the operative field and labeled.
- The specimens should be sent to pathology for confirmation of peripheral nerve on frozen section. Anterior and posterior nerve candidates should be carefully labeled. While waiting for results of the frozen section, reconstruction may be performed.

Billroth I Reconstruction

If the scarring near the duodenum is minimal and the resection confined to the antrum, Billroth I reconstruction is reasonably straightforward. Gastroduodenostomy can be completed with linear staples, circular staples, or a hand-sewn anastomosis. In our practice a linear stapled anastomosis is preferred.

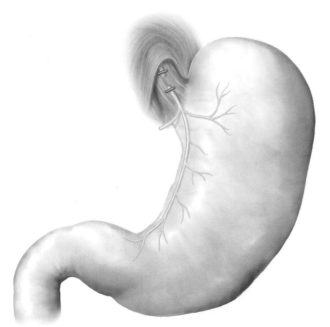

Figure 4.8 Completing the anterior vagotomy.

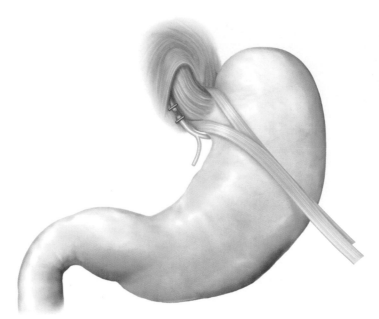

Figure 4.9 Posterior vagotomy. It is essential to get high on the esophagus (at least 5 cm) to include the criminal nerve of Grassi in the vagotomy. The exposure is similar to that used for a hiatal hernia repair.

- To complete this anastomosis, a gastrotomy is placed on the posterior stomach near the inferior edge of the staple line (Fig. 4.10).
- A duodenotomy is created on the anterior surface of the duodenum with adequate distance to the duodenal staple line to accommodate a linear stapled anastomosis (at least 3 cm) (Fig. 4.11).
- The 3.5-mm leg-length endoscopic linear stapler is then placed into the duodenotomy and brought toward the stomach, advancing the anterior staple anvil leg into the gastrotomy.
- The stapler is then fired (Fig. 4.12).
- A suture is placed on the posterior gastric wall and duodenum at the end of the staple line to diminish any tension.
- The remaining enterotomy is closed with sutures in a running fashion. To facilitate this, we place a post suture at the distal end of the anastomosis, incorporating both full thickness stomach and duodenum (Fig. 4.13).
- We then start with a longer (25 cm) suture at the other end of the anastomosis and run with a single suture to the original post (Fig. 4.14). This completes a single-layer anastomosis (Fig. 4.15).
- An endoscope is placed transorally to evaluate the anastomosis for bleeding and leak. The anastomosis is submerged while the endoscope is used for insufflation.
- A second layer of sutures is placed only if the leak test is positive. Interrupted sutures may be placed to contain any area of air leak.

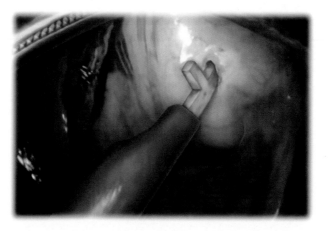

Figure 4.10 Creating a gastrotomy on the posterior stomach near the inferior border of the staple line.

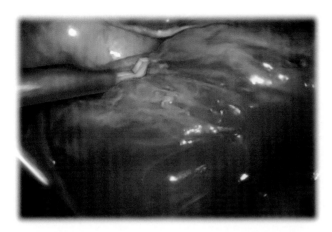

Figure 4.11 Creating a duodenotomy with adequate space to allow for passage of the stapler proximally.

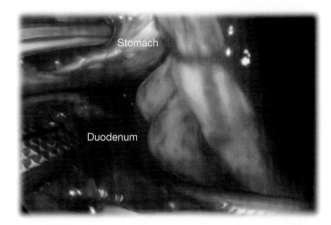

Figure 4.12 Creating the gastroduodenostomy with a linear stapler.

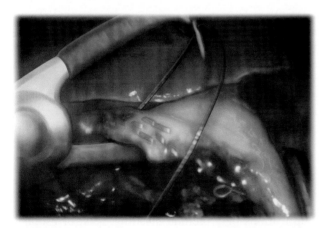

Figure 4.13 Placing a post stitch across the posterior portion of the gastroduodenostomy staple line.

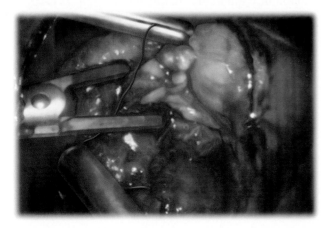

Figure 4.14 Suturing the common enterotomy on a gastroduodenostomy.

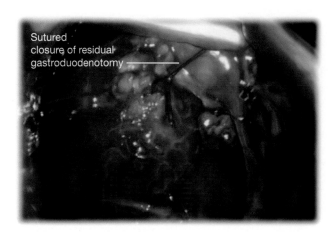

Sutured closure of residual gastroduodenotomy

Figure 4.15 Completing the gastroduodenostomy.

Use of Endoscopic Adjuncts

Some surgeons have found that endoscopic visualization is helpful during transgastric resections. We have found it difficult to keep the field of view level and appropriately oriented when using the endoscope exclusively. We feel the endoscope is helpful for confirming pathology and assuring adequacy of final closure with a negative leak test.

 POSTOPERATIVE MANAGEMENT

For most gastric resections, we do not place drains or nasogastric tubes. Exceptions to this are for high-risk patients (malnutrition, chemotherapy, chronic gastric outlet obstruction) or high-risk anastomoses (poor tissue, tension). In straightforward procedures, if the patients look and feel good on the morning of postoperative day 1, a liquid diet is implemented. Diet is advanced to semisolid foods at 2 weeks. If there are clinical signs of difficulty such as fever or tachycardia, or other reasons for clinical suspicion, a water-soluble contrast upper GI is obtained. Patients are discharged as early as postoperative day 1.

 COMPLICATIONS

Procedure-related perioperative complications may include bleeding, leak, or esophageal injury, although these are not commonly reported. Complications of open gastrectomy are seen in the laparoscopic population as well. These include alkaline reflux gastritis in 1% to 2%, gastroparesis in 2% (particularly if resection is accompanied by vagotomy), dumping syndrome, and postvagotomy diarrhea in 2% to 4%.

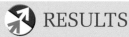 RESULTS

Although few large laparoscopic series exist, most patients do well after laparoscopic antrectomy. Truncal vagotomy and antrectomy is curative for 99% of ulcer disease patients. Outcome for other pathology depends on the adequacy of the resection for cure. Recurrence is unlikely for low-grade GISTs and benign carcinoids. For results in cancer, see Table 4.1.

TABLE 4.1		Laparoscopic-Assisted Distal Gastrectomy (LADG) for Early Gastric Cancer				
Year	N	Procedure	Extent of Resection	Complications	Follow-up (mo)	Recurrence
2002	14	LADG	D1	Pancreatic injury, 1 delayed gastric emptying, 1	24 ± 9.6	None
2001	7	LADG	D1	None	17	None
2003	76	LADG	D1	Anastomotic leakage, 3 Abscess, 5 Postoperative bleeding, 1	29	None
2002	116	LADG	D1	Pneumonia, 1 Anastomotic leakage, 1 Pancreatic injury, 1 Anastomotic stenosis, 1	45	None
2003	43	LADG	D1	Anastomotic leakage, 6 Wound infection, 2 Intraoperative hemorrhage, 2 Anastomotic ulcer, 1	37 ± 7	One systemic recurrence

From: Fischer JF and Bland KI, editors. *Mastery of Surgery*. 5th ed. Volume I. Philadelphia, PA: Lippincott, Williams and Wilkins.

CONCLUSIONS

- Antrectomy is appropriate for a variety of gastric pathologies.
- If antrectomy is performed for ulcer disease, it is due to acute complications or medical failure.
- Truncal vagotomy is added when performing antrectomy for ulcer disease.
- Laparoscopic antrectomy can be facilitated with bipolar sealing and linear stapling.
- Reconstruction after antrectomy can be with gastroduodenostomy, loop gastrojejunostomy, or Roux-en-Y gastrojejunostomy.
- For patients without duodenal scarring, gastroduodenostomy is straightforward and the most anatomic anastomosis.
- Gastroduodenostomy can be performed with linear staplers, with suture closure of the remaining gastroduodenostomy.
- Outcomes following laparoscopic antrectomy +/– truncal vagotomy are excellent, with minimal recurrence for benign pathologies.

Recommended References and Readings

Balfe P, O'Brian S, Daly P, et al. Management of gastric lymphoma. *Surg J R Coll Surg E*. 2008;6(5):262–265.

Cunningham D, Allum WH, Stenning SP, et al. Perioperative chemotherapy versus surgery alone for resectable gastroesophageal cancer. *N Engl J Med*. 2006;355(1):11–20.

Cuschieri A. Laparoscopic gastric resection. *Surg Clin North Am*. 2000;80:1269.

Debas HT. Surgical management of peptic ulcer disease [Review]. *J Assoc Acad Minor Phys*. 1992;3(4):137–141.

Gladdy RA, Strong VE, Coit D, et al. Defining surgical indications for type I gastric carcinoid tumor. *Ann Surg Oncol*. 2009;16(11):3154–3160.

Hoshino M, Omura N, Yano F, et al. Usefulness of laparoscope-assisted antrectomy for gastric carcinoids with hypergastrinemia. *Hepatogastroenterology*. 2010;57(98):379–382.

Jaffe BM, Florman SS. Postgastrectomy and postvagotomy syndromes. In: Fischer JF, Bland KI, ed. *Mastery of Surgery*. 5th ed. Volume I. Philadelphia, PA: Lippincott, Williams and Wilkins; 2006:938–955.

Kim HH, Hyung WJ, Cho GS, et al. Morbidity and mortality of laparoscopic gastrectomy versus open gastrectomy for gastric cancer. An interim report—a phase III multicenter, prospective randomized trial (KLASS Trial). *Ann Surg*. 2010;251(3):417–420.

Kodera Y, Fujiwara M, Ohashi N, et al. Laparoscopic surgery for gastric cancer: a collective review with meta-analysis of randomized trials [Review]. *J Am Coll Surg*. 2010;211(5):677–686.

Massironi S, Sciola V, Spampatti M-P, et al. Gastric carcinoids: between underestimation and overtreatment. *World J Gastroenterol*. 2009;15(18):2177–2183.

Pisters P, Patel WT, Shreyaskumar R. Gastrointestinal stromal tumors: current management [Review]. *J Surg Oncol*. 2010;102(5):530–538.

Sexton JA, Pierce RA, Halpin VJ, et al. Laparoscopic gastric resection for gastrointestinal stromal tumors. *Surg Endosc*. 2008;22(12):2583–2587.

Wong J, Jackson P. Gastric Cancer Surgery: An American Perspective on the Current Options and Standards. *Current Treatment Options in Oncology*, DOI 10.1007/s11864-010-0136-y. Online first on January 28, 2011.

Zullo A, Hassan C, Cristofari F, et al. Effects of helicobacter pylori eradication on early stage gastric mucosa associated lymphoid tissue lymphoma. [Review] *Clin Gastroenterol Hepatol*. 2010; 8(2):105–110.

Part I: Procedures for Ulcer Disease

5 Truncal Vagotomy with Antrectomy and Billroth II Reconstruction

Michael W. Mulholland

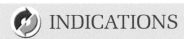 INDICATIONS

Truncal vagotomy and antrectomy is usually performed in the treatment of complications of peptic ulcer disease. Indications include perforation, hemorrhage, and obstruction. The elucidation of the pathogenic role of *Helicobacter pylori* in the development of peptic ulceration has decreased the need for operative treatment of peptic ulceration. In addition, the wide availability of proton pump inhibitors and histamine-2 receptor blockers has further diminished the need for truncal vagotomy, an operation designed to permanently suppress gastric acid production.

When truncal vagotomy and antrectomy is used, the first goal is safety from immediate surgical complications and avoidance of long-term undesirable side effects. The second goal is repair of associated anatomic defects, such as pyloric obstruction.

PREOPERATIVE PLANNING

Preparation for elective antrectomy should seek to optimize physiologic status. Electrolyte imbalances, common with gastric outlet obstruction, should be corrected. Retained food and particulate matter may also accumulate within an obstructed stomach. These materials can cause bacterial overgrowth and should be evacuated preoperatively. Scrupulous attention to general nutrition, anemia, and associated comorbid conditions is also required preoperatively.

Vagal Anatomy

The vagal nerves form a plexus which surrounds the intrathoracic esophagus. The nerve trunks coalesce within the thorax before entering the abdomen through the esophageal hiatus. The anterior (left) vagus nerve is positioned in immediate contact with anterior wall of the esophagus. The posterior vagal trunk has greater variability but is usually positioned between the posterior-medial wall of the esophagus and the right diaphragmatic crus. The anterior vagus nerve forms a hepatic division which separates from the anterior trunk at the level of the esophageal junction and passes between the avascular leaves of the gastrohepatic ligament. Fibers within the hepatic division innervate the gallbladder, biliary ducts, and liver.

The posterior vagal trunk gives rise to a celiac division which crosses the right diaphragmatic crus in parallel to the left gastric artery. The celiac division is usually

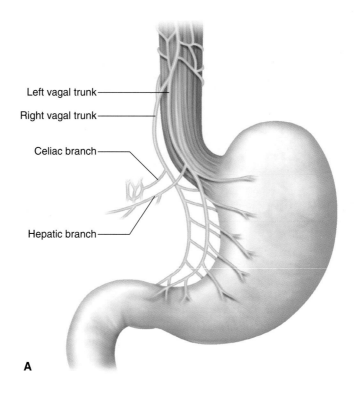

A

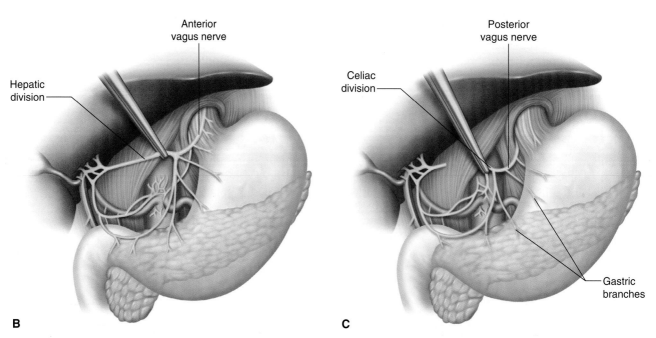

B   C

Figure 5.1 Vagal anatomy.

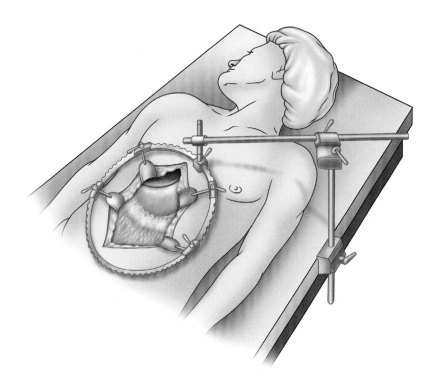

Figure 5.2 Topographic anatomy of the stomach.

larger than the hepatic division. Branches of the celiac division pass through the celiac ganglion. The anterior and posterior gastric divisions of the vagal trunks parallel the lesser curvature of the stomach and are contained within the gastrohepatic omentum. They run approximately 0.5 to 1 cm from the wall of the stomach along the lesser curvature. Small gastric branches terminate within the gastric fundus, body, and antrum (Fig. 5.1).

Position

The patient is positioned supine on the operating table. A vertical midline incision extending from the xyphoid inferiorly provides exposure of the upper abdomen for truncal vagotomy performed via laparotomy. Exposure is provided by a self-retaining retractor. The costal margins should be retracted superiorly and elevated. A moderate amount of reverse Trendelenburg position is often helpful in shifting the omentum and other abdominal contents inferiorly and in improving exposure of the upper abdomen (Fig. 5.2).

Truncal Vagotomy

Exposure of the intra-abdominal esophagus can usually be obtained without mobilization of the left lateral segment of the liver. If the left lateral segment of the liver is hypertrophic or enlarged due to fatty infiltration, mobilization of this segment can sometimes improve exposure of the intra-abdominal esophagus. To do this, the surgeon places the right hand under the left lateral segment, palm upward, and retracts the liver inferiorly. The left triangular ligament is often thin and translucent. The fingers of the surgeon's hands are usually visible through the peritoneum (Fig. 5.3).

The left triangular ligament can be divided without cautery using this exposure. As the line of division proceeds medially, care must be taken to expose the anterior and posterior leaves of the triangular ligament separately. The peritoneal layers and the tissue between them may be divided individually using electrocautery. The inferior phrenic vein is often close to the posterior peritoneal edge of the triangular ligament,

Figure 5.3 Mobilization of the left lateral segment of the liver.

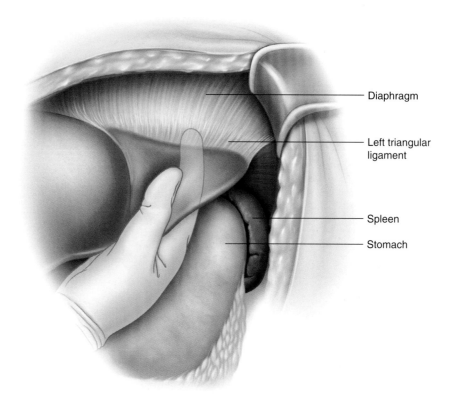

Diaphragm

Left triangular ligament

Spleen

Stomach

and care must be taken not to injure this vessel. This can be avoided by proper exposure. Mobilization of the left triangular ligament need not extend beyond the midline (Fig. 5.4).

With the left lateral segment of the liver retracted and protected, the anterior surface of the intra-abdominal esophagus can be appreciated visually and also by palpation of a previously placed nasogastric tube. The peritoneum overlying the esophagogastric

Figure 5.4 Division of the triangular ligament.

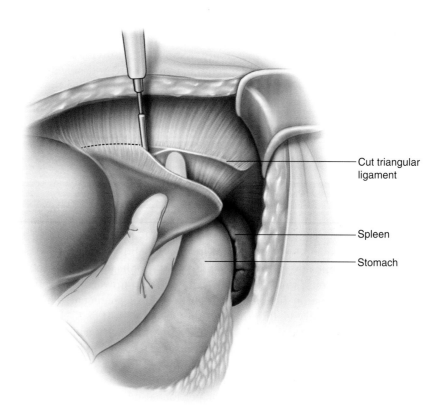

Cut triangular ligament

Spleen

Stomach

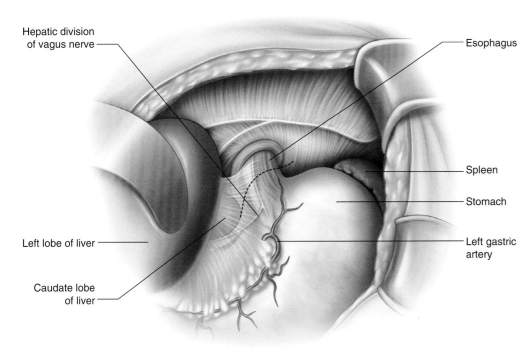

Figure 5.5 Exposure of the esophagogastric junction.

Hepatic division
of vagus nerve

Esophagus

Spleen

Stomach

Left gastric
artery

Left lobe of liver

Caudate lobe
of liver

junction is divided transversely using electrocautery. In doing so, the hepatic branch of the anterior vagus nerve is sometimes visible in the leaves of the gastrohepatic ligament and should be preserved (Fig. 5.5).

After division of the peritoneum, the anterior vagus nerve can usually be seen on the anterior surface of the esophagus. The nerve can also be palpated with an index finger passed along the anterior surface of the esophagus. Retraction of the stomach caudally aids in the palpation of the vagal trunk by placing it on gentle tension (Fig. 5.6).

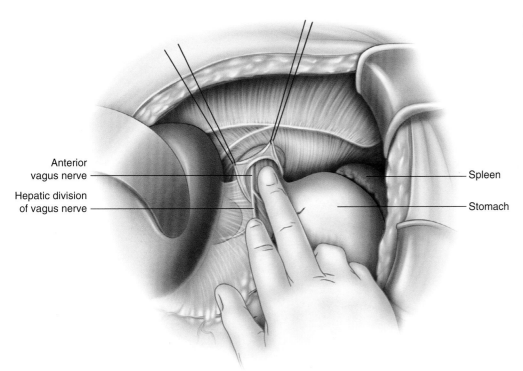

Figure 5.6 Exposure of anterior vagus nerve.

Anterior
vagus nerve

Hepatic division
of vagus nerve

Spleen

Stomach

Figure 5.7 Isolation of the anterior
vagal trunk.

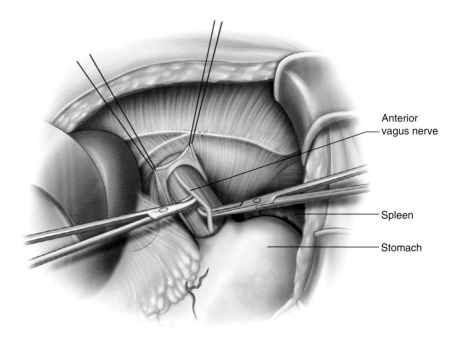

The anterior vagal trunk is elevated from the anterior wall of the esophagus using
a nerve hook or right angle. The nerve should be sharply dissected from the underlying
esophageal musculature (Fig. 5.7).

The anterior vagus nerve is ligated both proximally and distally using metallic
surgical clips. A segment between the clips is excised and sent for permanent pathologic examination (Fig. 5.8).

With the esophagus retracted to the patient's left, the operating surgeon then
exposes the right diaphragmatic crus. The posterior vagal nerve can be identified
visually or by palpation in the space between the posterior medial wall of the esophagus and the right crus. The position of the posterior vagal nerve can also be verified

Figure 5.8 Ligation of the nerve
trunk.

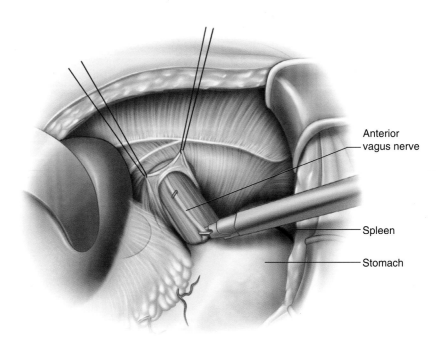

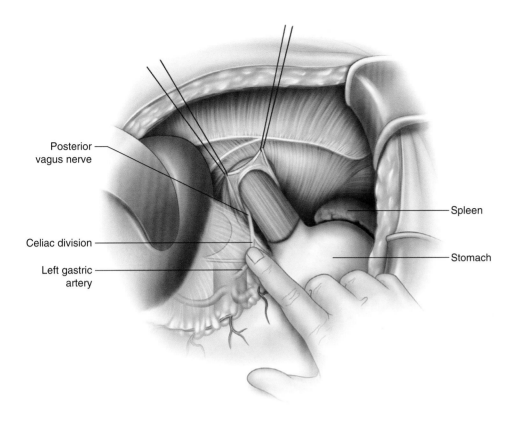

Figure 5.9 Exposure of the posterior vagal trunk.

Posterior vagus nerve

Celiac division

Left gastric artery

Spleen

Stomach

by retraction of the celiac division; this maneuver places the posterior vagus nerve under some tension and accentuates its position. Because the celiac division of the posterior vagus nerve lies in proximity to the left gastric artery, this pulse can also be used as a landmark (Fig. 5.9).

The posterior vagus nerve is elevated from the surrounding tissue using a nerve hook or right angle clamp (Fig. 5.10).

A segment of the posterior trunk is excised after ligation by surgical clips (Fig. 5.11).

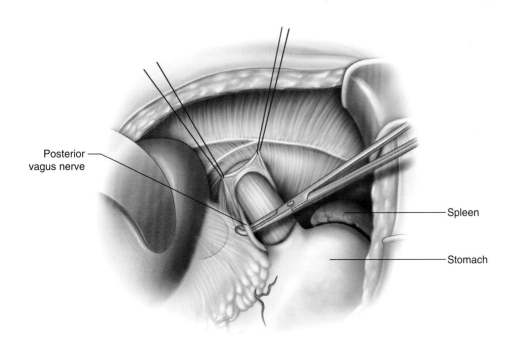

Figure 5.10 Isolation of the posterior vagal trunk.

Posterior vagus nerve

Spleen

Stomach

Figure 5.11 Nerve division.

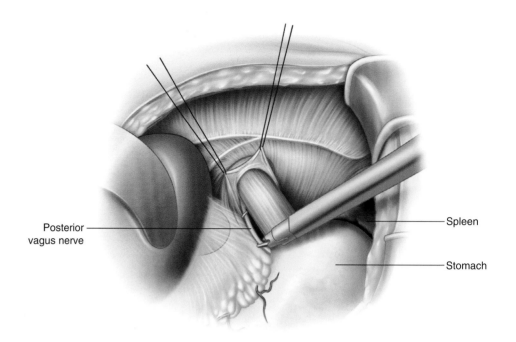

Posterior
vagus nerve

Spleen

Stomach

Antrectomy

When operating for either benign or malignant disease, it is useful to examine the posterior wall of the stomach for possible inflammatory or neoplastic involvement of associated retrogastric strictures. This can be accomplished after entry into the lesser sac. The lesser sac is entered by dividing the attachment of the greater omentum to the transverse colon. An avascular plane can be developed immediately adjacent to the superior aspect of the transverse colon. This is best accomplished by retracting the omentum superiorly and retracting the corresponding segment of transverse colon inferiorly. While care must be taken not to injure the middle colic vessels, the omentum can be separated from the transverse mesenteric layers using electrocautery (Fig. 5.12).

Alternatively, the retrogastric space can also be obtained by division of the avascular portion of the gastrohepatic omentum. Through this exposure, the posterior wall of the stomach and associated retrogastric strictures can be assessed (Fig. 5.13).

In treatment of neoplastic disease, the omentum may be resected en bloc with the distal stomach. Alternatively, for benign gastric diseases omental resection is not always necessary. The gastroepiploic vessels can be preserved. A line of dissection can be developed paralleling the left gastroepiploic vessel. Small blood vessels in this area can be taken between clamps and tied. In addition a number of alternative energy sources can be used during both open and laparoscopic operations to divide these vessels without suturing or ligatures (Fig. 5.14).

Antrectomy usually involves resection of approximately 50% of the distal gastric tissue. Preparation for a 50% gastric resection involves the division of the gastrocolic ligament to a point approximately half way between the pylorus and the esophagogastric junction along the greater curvature. This point corresponds to the transition between the right and left gastroepiploic vessels. The gastric wall should be clear of fat and areolar tissue for a short distance in preparation for subsequent resection and then anastomosis (Fig. 5.15).

The right gastroepiploic vessels are exposed by retracting the stomach superiorly. The right gastroepiploic artery is divided close to its origin from the gastroduodenal artery. Fine areolar tissue between the posterior antropyloric region and the anterior surface of the pancreas can be divided sharply (Fig. 5.16).

Part I: Procedures for Ulcer Disease

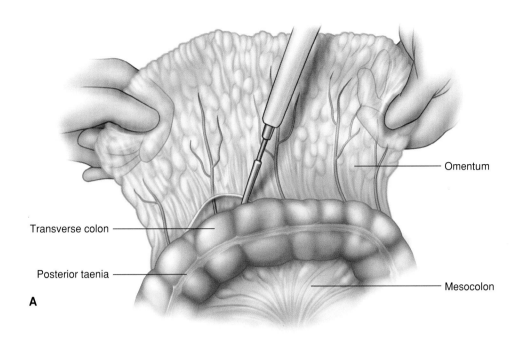

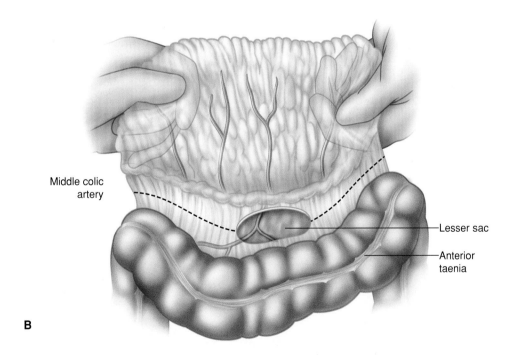

Figure 5.12 Entry into the lesser sac. (**A**) The omentum is retracted superiorly and the transverse colon inferiorly. (**B**) An avascular plane above the transverse colon provides entry into the lesser sac.

The right gastric artery and its corresponding vein are often quite small. The right gastric vessels will be identified at the superior border of the proximal duodenum. The vessel should be divided close to the duodenal wall. Care must be taken to avoid injury to the common hepatic artery or common bile duct. Inflammation or tumor may obscure the anatomy in the region of the first portion of the duodenum (Fig. 5.17).

The area along the lesser curvature is used for division and anastomosis. Branches of the left gastric artery supply the lesser curvature. These are often represented as paired vessels to the anterior and posterior surfaces. These vessels should be ligated separately. Connective tissue and fat between these arterial branches and the gastric wall should be cleaned in preparation for subsequent anastomosis (Fig. 5.18).

The proximal duodenum is then divided using a GIA stapler. This provides closure at both ends and is convenient. The double staple closure of the divided duodenum

Figure 5.13 Incision of gastrohepatic ligament.

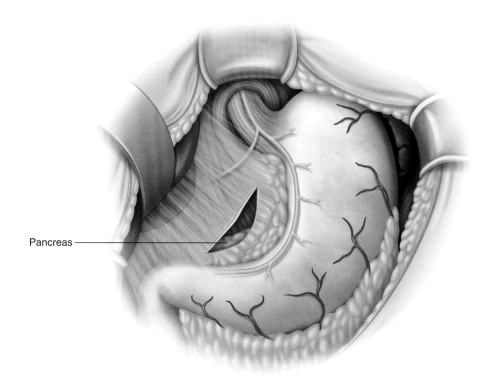

Pancreas ———

Figure 5.14 Division of gastrocolic omentum.

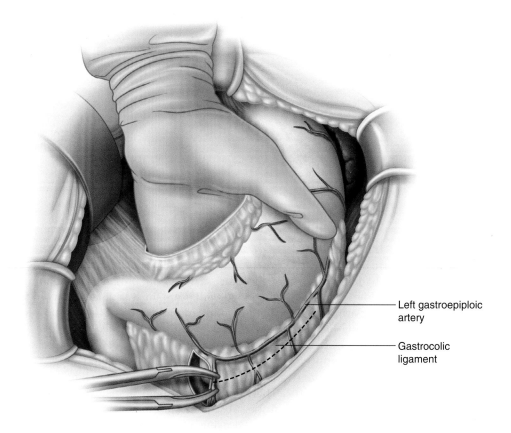

———— Left gastroepiploic artery

———— Gastrocolic ligament

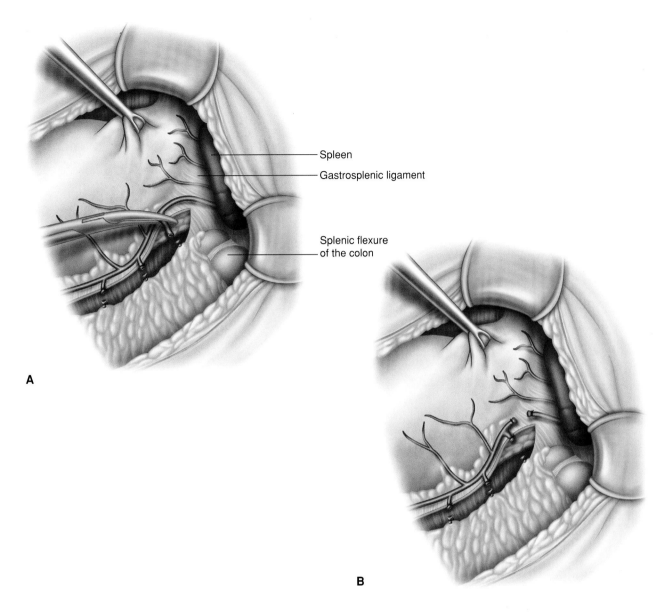

Spleen
Gastrosplenic ligament
Splenic flexure
of the colon

A

B

Figure 5.15 Preparation of greater curvature for hemigastrectomy. (**A**) Vessels entering the greater curvature of the stomach are individually ligated. (**B**) The dissection continues to the level of the short gastric vessels in the gastrosplenic ligament.

does not require suture reinforcement, although this can be done at the surgeon's preference using interrupted 3-0 nonabsorbable sutures (Fig. 5.19).

A TA-type stapler can be used to close the gastric remnant with a double row of staples. An occlusive clamp can be placed distally to prevent spillage of gastric contents during resection. Alternatively, this area may be divided with the application of a GIA-type stapling device (Fig. 5.20).

Billroth II gastrojejunostomy is illustrated as one of the means of restoration of gastrointestinal continuity. Billroth II reconstruction is most appropriate when the duodenum is not amenable to safe, tension-free anastomosis as a Billroth I reconstruction due to chronic scarring, inflammation, or inadequate length. A portion of the gastric wall is oversewn with interrupted sutures. A loop of proximal jejunum is brought through an incision in the transverse mesocolon to lie in tension-free apposition to the stomach. Interrupted nonabsorbable sutures are placed in a seromuscular fashion from the posterior gastric wall to the antimesenteric border of the jejunum. Using electrocautery, an incision is made in both organs of equal length. Gastrotomy is performed by partial excision of the stapled gastric closure. The posterior mucosal suture is created using continuous absorbable suture (Fig. 5.21).

Figure 5.16 Division of right gastroepiploic vessels.

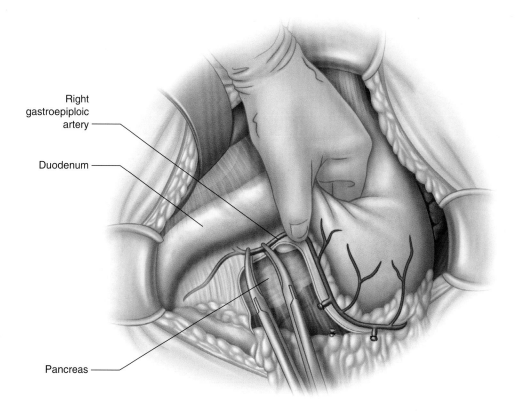

Right
gastroepiploic
artery

Duodenum

Pancreas

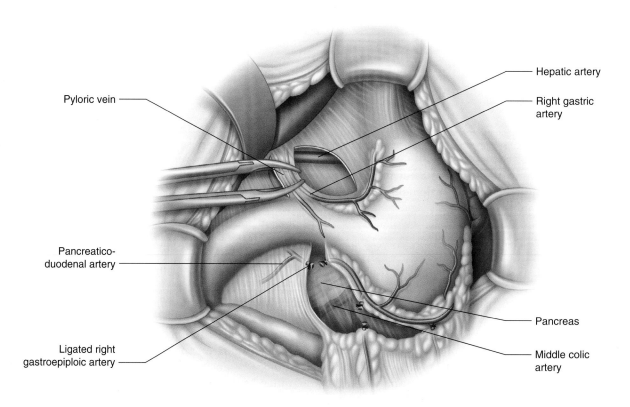

Pyloric vein

Hepatic artery

Right gastric
artery

Pancreatico-
duodenal artery

Ligated right
gastroepiploic artery

Pancreas

Middle colic
artery

Figure 5.17 Ligation of right gastric vessels.

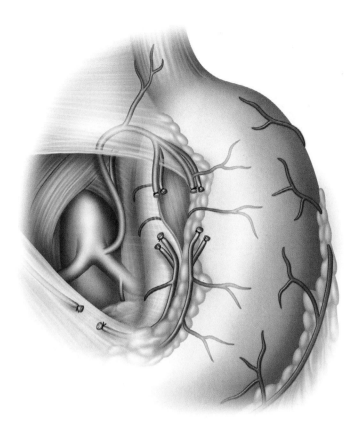

Figure 5.18 Dissection of lesser curvature.

This mucosal suture is continued along the length of the anterior aspect of the anastomosis. A layer of 3-0 nonabsorbable sutures is then placed in completion of the anterior anastomosis. Corner stitches must include the anterior gastric wall, posterior gastric wall, and the jejunum.

The gastrojejunal anastomosis is reduced inferior to the transverse mesentery. The anastomosis is secured in this position by sutures placed from the mesenteric defect to the gastric wall (Fig. 5.22).

Figure 5.19 Division of the duodenum.

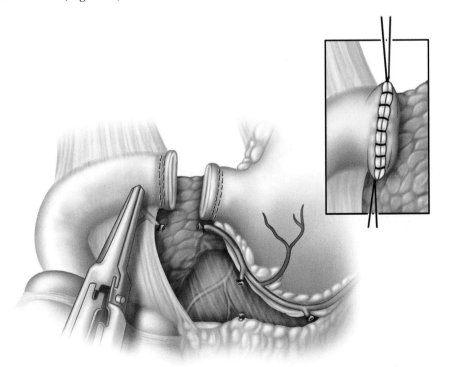

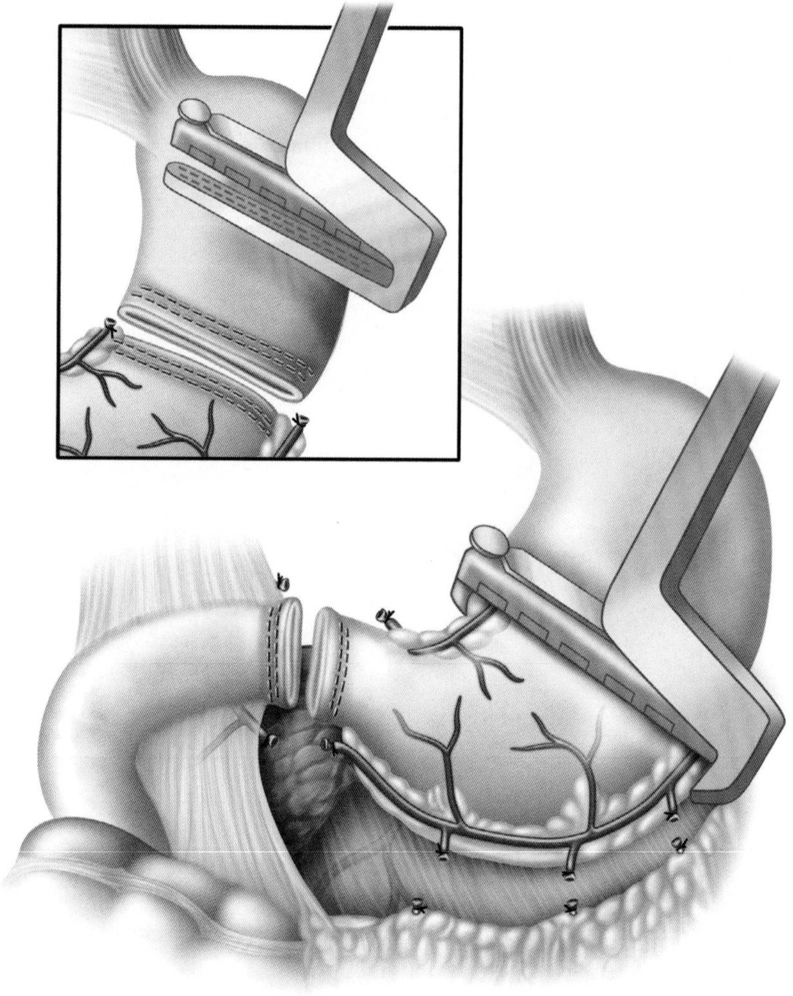

Figure 5.20 Division of the proximal stomach.

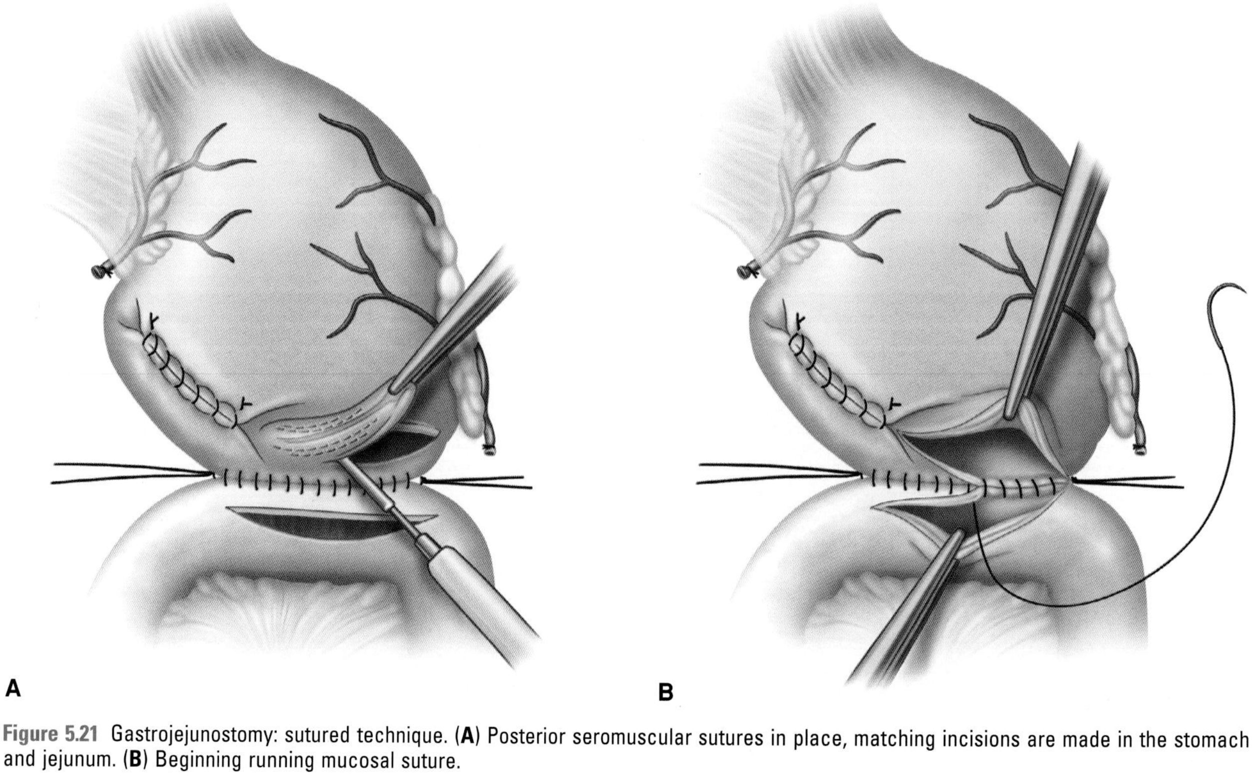

A

B

Figure 5.21 Gastrojejunostomy: sutured technique. (**A**) Posterior seromuscular sutures in place, matching incisions are made in the stomach and jejunum. (**B**) Beginning running mucosal suture.

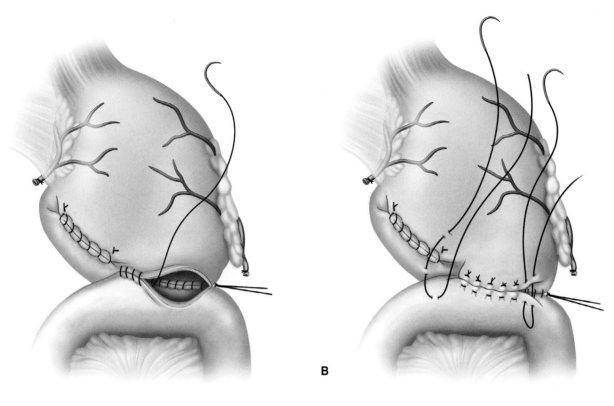

A

B

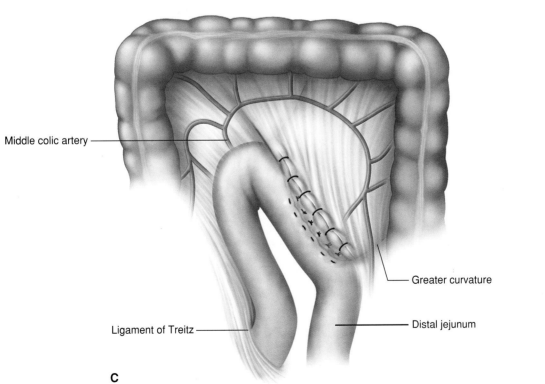

Middle colic artery

Greater curvature

Ligament of Treitz

Distal jejunum

C

Figure 5.22 Anterior anastomosis. (**A**) Completion of running suture. (**B**) Anterior interrupted seromuscular suture line. (**C**) Delivery of gastrojejunal anastomosis inferior to the transverse mesentery and suture of the mesentery to the gastric surface.

→ POSTOPERATIVE MANAGEMENT

Nasogastric decompression is required for variable periods postoperatively. Gastric ileus or dysmotility is usually brief after elective operation; return of gastric emptying may be more prolonged if gastric outlet obstruction was present preoperatively. Atelectasis is more common after upper abdominal operations. Pulmonary hygiene and incentive spirometry are mandatory following antrectomy. If antrectomy has been performed for hemorrhage or in the setting of systemic hypotension, stress gastritis is a potential postoperative complication. The development of stress gastritis is critically dependent upon the presence of low intragastric pH; acid production suppression with proton pump inhibitors or histamine-2 receptor antagonists should be used as prophylaxis, in addition to attention to nutrition and restoration of normal mucosal perfusion.

Recommended References and Readings

Boey J, Lee NW, Koo J, et al. Immediate definitive surgery for perforated duodenal ulcers: a prospective controlled trial. *Ann Surg.* 1982;196:338.

Boey J, Wong J, Ong GB. A prospective study of operative risk factors in perforated duodenal ulcers. *Ann Surg.* 1982;195:265.

Imhof M, Schroders C, Ohmann C, et al. Impact of early operation on the mortality from bleeding peptic ulcer—ten years' experience. *Dig Surg.* 1998;15:308–314.

Kujath P, Schwandner O, Bruch H-P. Morbidity and mortality of perforated peptic gastroduodenal ulcer following emergency surgery. *Langenbecks Arch Surg.* 2002;387:298–302.

Millat B, Fingerhut A, Borie F. Surgical treatment of complicated duodenal ulcers: controlled trials. *World J Surg.* 2000;24:299–306.

Vaira D, Menegatti M, Miglioli M. What is the role of *Helicobacter pylori* in complicated peptic ulcer disease? *Gastroenterology.* 1997;113:S78–S84.

6 Laparoscopic Truncal Vagotomy with Antrectomy and Billroth II Reconstruction

Kfir Ben-David and George A. Sarosi Jr

 ## INDICATIONS/CONTRAINDICATIONS

Recent advancements in pharmaceutical therapy and endoscopic treatments have significantly decreased the incidence of gastric surgery for peptic ulcer disease (PUD). With the advent of proton pump inhibitors, histamine receptor blockers, and multidrug therapy treatment for *Helicobacter pylori,* previously common operations for PUD have become very infrequent. Consequently, medical progress and new surgical innovations have completely transformed our approach to patients with benign gastric and PUD in need of surgical treatment. With the use of flexible endoscopy and minimally invasive surgical approaches the diagnosis and surgical treatment of PUD has resulted in less invasive surgical treatments resulting in shorter hospital stay, less overall cost, and quicker return to base-line activity while being able to maintain the same surgical technique without patient compromise.

The laparoscopic approach to PUD with truncal vagotomy, antrectomy, and Billroth II reconstruction is theoretically possible in nearly all patients with benign surgical disease who have failed medical and endoscopic treatments. Many minimally invasive gastrointestinal surgeons feel that PUD should be preferentially treated via a laparoscopic approach since it is associated with less intraoperative blood loss, earlier return of bowel function, less usage of analgesics, and a shorter postoperative hospital stay. Despite these strong case series favoring a laparoscopic surgical approach, there is a relative paucity of randomized clinical trials addressing this issue, likely due to the decreasing incidence of PUD and the infrequent need for elective surgical treatment. However, a number of patient characteristics represent relative indications and contraindications to the laparoscopic approach.

Even though the natural course of PUD is changing and intractable disease and pyloric obstruction as an indication for surgery is decreasing, the incidence of bleeding and perforation remains constant. Treatment of *H. pylori* and cessation of nonsteroidal anti-inflammatory drugs is imperative prior to any surgical procedure for PUD. Although there have been a number of case reports describing laparoscopic surgical treatment with antrectomy, vagotomy, and Billroth II reconstruction for acutely perforated or bleeding PUD, many of these procedures were performed by very skilled laparoscopic surgeons. Furthermore, prior upper abdominal midline incisions and previous gastric and/or esophageal surgery are a relative contraindication to a laparoscopic truncal vagotomy, antrectomy, and Billroth II reconstruction. Mesh placement in the upper midline makes laparoscopic resection and reconstruction much more difficult. Liver cirrhosis and portal hypertension are also a contraindication to laparoscopic truncal vagotomy, antrectomy, and Billroth II reconstruction because of the risk of bleeding from gastric and esophageal varices. However, with increased experience utilizing laparoscopic approaches to gastric resection and reconstruction, patients with advanced age and its associated chronic medical conditions are not generally contraindications.

PREOPERATIVE PLANNING

Most of the preoperative evaluation is directed toward ensuring that the patient is adequately prepared for anesthesia. As a result, a careful assessment of the patient's fitness to undergo general anesthesia represents a major portion of the preoperative assessment. Because truncal vagotomy, antrectomy, and Billroth II reconstruction will almost always be performed under elective circumstances, chronic medical conditions such as cardiopulmonary disease and diabetes mellitus should be optimally managed prior to operation. The combination of careful history and documentation indicating the appropriate treatment of *H. pylori* and cessation of any nonsteroidal anti-inflammatory drugs usage is necessary to decrease the incidence of recurrent PUD. Additionally, a preoperative endoscopic evaluation of the gastric and duodenal mucosa is essential to rule out any abnormal pathology prior to surgical resection. Routine biopsy of nonhealing gastric ulcers is also imperative to exclude malignant disease. These can also be tattooed intraluminally preoperatively to help with intraoperative identification.

Confirmation of the correct diagnosis, ulcer location, previous surgical history, comorbidities, and patient's nutritional status are all important factors when treating patients with PUD with laparoscopic truncal vagotomy, antrectomy, and Billroth II reconstruction. Operative preparation should include a first- or second-generation cephalosporin in patients without achlorhydria or gastric outlet obstruction. Otherwise, a broader-spectrum antibiotic may be necessary for these patients. The intravenous antibiotic administration needs to be completed prior to skin incision and be discontinued 24 hours postoperatively. Prophylaxis for deep vein thrombosis can be achieved by the subcutaneous administration of heparin and the use of pneumatic compression devices prior to anesthetic induction, during the case and postoperatively.

SURGERY

After general anesthesia is administered, a bladder catheter is placed along with an orogastric or a nasogastric tube depending on the surgeon's preference. Although a nasogastric tube is often maintained postoperatively, routine gastric decompression has not been shown to affect outcomes in postgastrectomy patients. Depending on the surgical approach, the patient can be placed in supine or lithotomy position. For minimally invasive gastric resection approaches, our preferred method is to have the patient in a supine position allowing the operating surgeon to be on the right side of the patient while the assistant is on the contralateral side. The patient is secured to the table with two safety straps, a foot board, and all of their bony prominences are well padded. This positioning allows the patient to be securely placed in steep reverse Trendelenburg when performing the gastric resection and reconstruction. Lower and upper body warmer devices are applied to the patient throughout the case to help maintaining core body temperature.

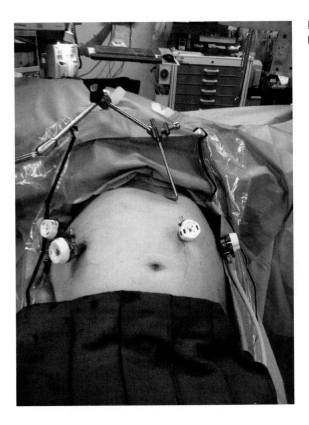

Figure 6.1 Trocar and liver retractor placement.

The peritoneal cavity is accessed via a 5-mm port under direct visualization in the left subcostal region using a 5-mm 0° scope. The 5-mm 0° scope is then switched out to a 5-mm 30° scope. Three additional trocars are placed under direct visualization. A 5-mm trocar is placed in the supraumbilical region just left of the midline approximately 18–22 cm from the xiphoid process. A 12-mm trocar is placed on the contralateral side and a 5-mm trocar is placed in the right subcostal margin opposite the initial access trocar for the surgeon's right and left hand instruments, respectively. A 5-mm incision is also created in the subxiphoid region to allow for the placement of the Nathanson liver retractor (Fig. 6.1). This retractor is used to elevate the lateral segment of the left lobe of the liver and expose the gastroesophageal junction and anterior portion of the stomach.

The gastrocolic omentum is dissected from the stomach permitting entry into the lesser sac. This is performed by cephalad retraction of the greater omentum while incising the avascular plane above the transverse colon (Fig. 6.2). The dissection continues at the pylorus with ligation of the right gastroepiploic artery using a laparoscopic vascular stapler inserted through the 12-mm trocar (Fig. 6.3). This dissection proceeds along the greater curvature of the stomach and ends halfway between the pylorus and the gastroesophageal junction. This maneuver spares the left gastroepiploic vessels and the short gastric vessels. If there is any concern as to the level of division of the stomach to achieve adequate margins an intraoperative endoscopy can help determine the site of gastric resection. The posterior wall of the stomach is separated from the anterior pancreas and base of the transverse mesocolon by blunt dissection and sharp division of connective tissue attachments which can be very inflamed and dense in some patients. The duodenum is carefully kocherized, and in patients with pyloric inflammation, care must be taken to avoid injury to the bowel, common hepatic artery, common bile duct, and portal vein. The right gastric vessels are similarly ligated close to the stomach using a laparoscopic vascular stapling device or ultrasonic shears (Fig. 6.4).

The gastrohepatic ligament is incised, and the lesser curvature is dissected. The right crus is identified and dissected along the medial border in a cephalad fashion up to the diaphragm and circumferentially to the left crus. Using a pars flaccida technique,

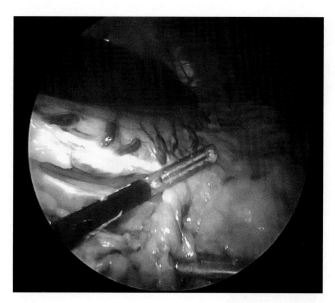

Figure 6.2 Gastrocolic omentum dissection.

a Penrose is placed around the GE junction through the retroesophageal space. The phrenoesophageal ligament is divided as the stomach is retracted in a caudal posterior fashion. Meticulous and direct dissection will prevent injury to the spleen, short gastric vessels, esophagus, or stomach while performing this maneuver. A minimum of 5 cm of the esophagus is mobilized to allow adequate space to identify and ligate the vagus nerves. This dissection exposes the distal esophagus along with the anterior and the posterior trunks of the vagus nerves. Each nerve is individually identified, freely dissected from the esophagus, and excised. Approximately 1 cm of fiber from the anterior and posterior trunk of the vagus nerves is excised and sent to pathology for histologic confirmation (Fig. 6.5).

The proximal duodenum is divided with care with a 60-mm endoscopic linear stapler to avoid injury to the common hepatic artery, common bile duct, and portal vein (Fig. 6.6). The duodenal staple line can be reinforced with interrupted imbricated sutures or stapler buttressing at the discretion of the surgeon. Once the proximal duodenum is divided the distal stomach is rotated toward the patient's left side to help assist with the proximal transection of the stomach. Similarly, the proximal end of the stomach is divided with multiple linear stapling devices from the lesser to the greater

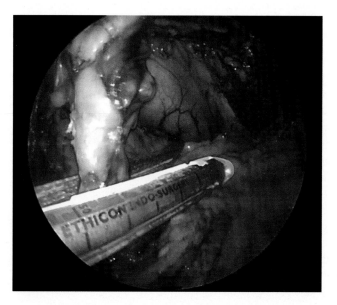

Figure 6.3 Ligation of right gastroepiploic vessels.

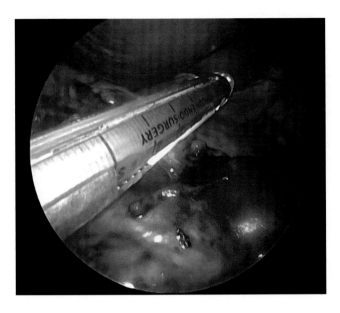

Figure 6.4 Division of right gastric vessels.

curvature via the right-sided 12-mm trocar (Fig. 6.7). The resected stomach is moved to the right upper quadrant and is removed via an endoscopic specimen bag. In order to reduce problems with loss of pneumoperitoneum from the extraction site the specimen is not removed until the remainder of the case is completed.

The laparoscopic Billroth II reconstruction can be performed by various surgical techniques. The authors prefer a retrocolic, sutured, and linear stapled gastrojejunostomy. This portion of the operation requires the patient to be in and out of reverse Trendelenburg position to accommodate appropriate positioning for the reconstruction. A proximal jejunal loop 30 to 40 cm distal to the ligament of Treitz is delivered through an incision in the transverse mesocolon (Fig. 6.8). The jejunum is brought up in cephalad fashion via the transverse mesocolon defect to the newly created gastric pouch in an isoperistaltic manner (Fig. 6.9). The antimesenteric surface of the jejunum is apposed to the posterior gastric wall starting from the greater to the lesser curvature of the stomach with a nonabsorbable suture in a continuous fashion (Fig. 6.10). Matching gastrotomy and enterotomy are performed with electrocautery or ultrasonic shears. The laparoscopic stapler's cartridge and anvil limbs are inserted into the gastrotomy and enterotomy incisions, respectively (Fig. 6.11). After the stapler is fired, the device is withdrawn and the staple line is inspected for hemostasis. The common gastrotomy and enterotomy defect is closed with the application of a laparoscopic stapling device

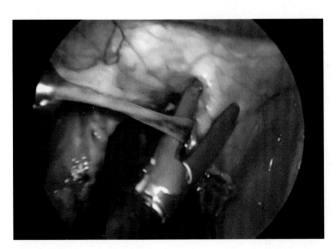

Figure 6.5 Excision of Vagus Nerve.

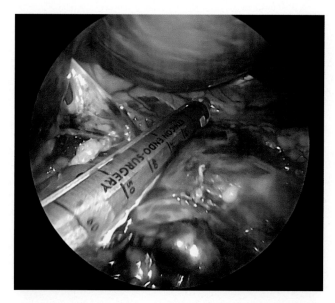

Figure 6.6 Division of proximal duodenum.

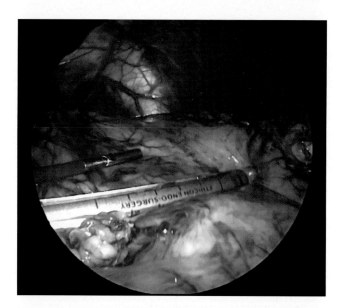

Figure 6.7 Gastric resection using linear stapler.

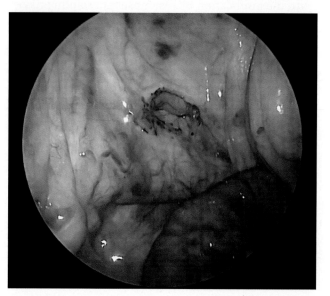

Figure 6.8 Transverse mesocolon window.

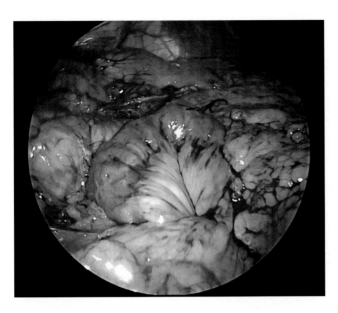

Figure 6.9 Jejunum via transverse mesocolon defect in an isoperistaltic manner.

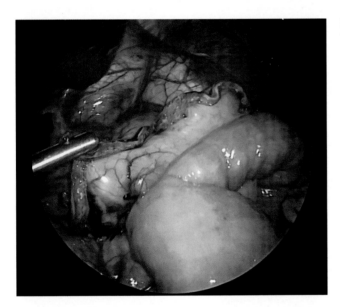

Figure 6.10 Jejunum is apposed to the posterior gastric wall.

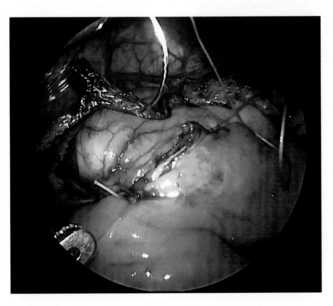

Figure 6.11 Closure of common gastrotomy and enterotomy defect.

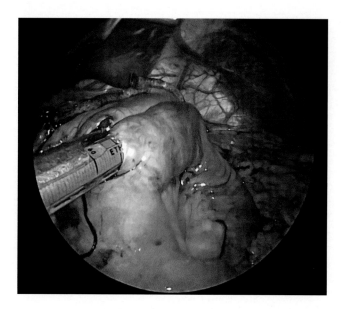

Figure 6.12 Linear stapler's cartridge and anvil limbs are inserted into the gastrostomy and enterotomy.

or with a continuous absorbable suture (Fig. 6.12). The entire staple line and/or suture line is inverted in a running fashion using a nonabsorbable suture (Figs. 6.13 and 6.14). The transverse mesocolon defect is reapproximated using nonabsorbable interrupted sutures. The jejunal loop is also sutured in an interrupted fashion to the transverse mesocolon defect to prevent potential bowel herniation through this defect (Fig. 6.15). A flexible endoscope is frequently used in these cases to determine the adequacy of the gastric inlet and/or outlet, visualization of the intraluminal staple line, and evaluation of the integrity of the anastomosis under saline irrigation (Fig. 6.16). Finally, the resected stomach is placed in an endoscopic specimen bag and retrieved via the 12-mm trocar. The 12-mm trocar fascial incision site is closed. The remaining 5-mm trocars and Nathanson liver retractor are removed under direct visualization. Local anesthetic is administered to all incision sites. The subcutaneous tissue and skin are reapproximated with absorbable subcuticular suture and Dermabond dressing, respectively.

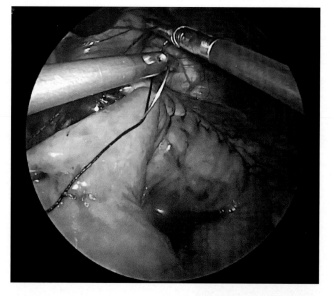

Figure 6.13 Inversion of stapled and suture line.

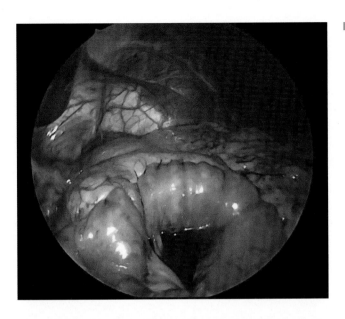

Figure 6.14 Completed anastomosis.

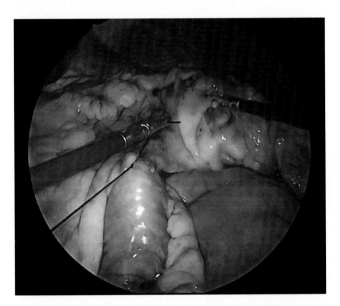

Figure 6.15 Jejunal loop sutured to the transverse mesocolon defect.

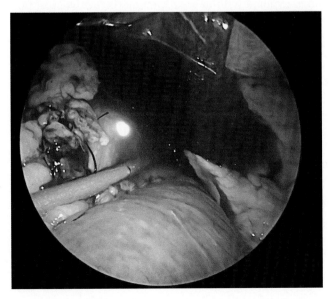

Figure 6.16 Endoscopic evaluation of anastomosis.

POSTOPERATIVE MANAGEMENT

All patients are admitted to our surgical floor and are encouraged to ambulate on the same day of surgery. Deep venous thrombosis prophylaxis is continued during their hospitalization with subcutaneous heparin injections and sequential compression devices while in bed. The patient's urinary catheter and antibiotics are both discontinued on postoperative day 1. Pain is controlled with intravenous narcotic medication for the first 24 hours followed by oral analgesic medication. The majority of the patients are started on a clear liquid diet on the first postoperative morning. In patients without adynamic small intestinal ileus their diet is quickly advanced as tolerated. Most patients are discharged home on postoperative day 3 and instructed to eat 4 to 6 small meals a day. Prior to discharge, all patients are evaluated by our registered dietitian and are instructed about a postgastrectomy diet. All patients return for their routine postoperative visit 2 weeks following hospital discharge to ensure appropriate healing of their incisions and adequate nutritional intake.

 COMPLICATIONS

As with most laparoscopic operations, the patient's postoperative course is usually benign but any deviation from the normal course requires further investigation as with all other surgical patients. With meticulous and hemostatic dissection, bleeding after laparoscopic surgery is fairly uncommon but can occur from the trocar site insertions, multiple vessel ligations, transected stomach, or intraluminal anastomosis. These are often identified intraoperatively by careful inspection at the completion of the case with the aid of the laparoscope and a flexible endoscope.

A number of postgastrectomy syndromes have been described following gastric operations performed for PUD and gastric neoplasms, regardless of the surgical approach, which can be disabling in 1% to 2% of patients. The two most frequent manifestations are dumping and alkaline reflux gastritis. Although the precise cause of dumping syndrome is not known, it is believed to be related to the rapid passage of ingested food into the proximal small bowel. Approximately 10% to 15% of patients who have had a truncal vagotomy, antrectomy, and Billroth II reconstruction will experience mild dumping symptoms of postprandial nausea, epigastric pain, diarrhea, and palpitations. Minor dietary alterations and passage of time will improve the symptoms for most patients. In the most severe of cases, low-dose subcutaneous octreotide, a somatostatin analogue, can be administered to help with early and late dumping symptoms.

Alkaline reflux gastritis is often associated with nausea and emesis, evidence of bile reflux in the stomach, and histological evidence of gastritis. Patients who present with this syndrome must undergo endoscopic examination to exclude recurrent ulcer. Unfortunately the only proven treatment is the conversion of gastrojejunostomy to Roux-en-Y configuration to prevent reflux of intestinal contents and bile.

Despite these well-described postoperative complications, ulcer recurrence rate is the lowest for patients with truncal vagotomy and antrectomy regardless of surgical technique. With the laparoscopic approach, the patient's ability to return to normal daily activities and work, incidence of wound infections, hospital analgesic use, and hospital length of stay are all improved when compared to open truncal vagotomy, antrectomy, and Billroth II reconstruction.

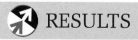 RESULTS

Although there are few large series reporting the outcomes after laparoscopic vagotomy and antrectomy for intractable or obstructing peptic ulcers, experience from the use of open vagotomy and antrectomy suggests that excellent long-term outcomes can be achieved. Multiple authors have reported ulcer recurrence rates of 1% to 2% percent after antrectomy and vagotomy. Rivera and colleagues in a series of 14 patients who underwent laparoscopic gastrectomy for ulcer disease reported a conversion rate of 5%, a mean operative length of 165 minutes with a mean estimated blood loss of 84cc. Time to resumption of diet was 3 days and mean length of stay was 4 days. Complications were seen in 14% percent of patients. Goh and colleagues reported the outcomes of 63 laparoscopic gastric resections for ulcer disease. They noted a conversion rate of 5% with a mean operative length of 215 minutes. The mean time to resumption of liquid diet was 3 days, solid diet 5 days, and mean length of stay was 8 days. Complications were observed in 13% of patients. The mean time to return to usual activities was 17 days.

CONCLUSIONS

Laparoscopic truncal vagotomy with antrectomy and Billroth II reconstruction is a technically challenging but feasible operation in the patient with intractable peptic ulcer or gastric outlet obstruction secondary to PUD. In skilled hands it can be performed with outcomes comparable to open truncal vagotomy and antrectomy and offers the potential to reduce postoperative hospitalization and recovery time.

Recommended References and Readings

Goh P, Tekant Y, Isaac J, et al. The technique of laparoscopic Billroth II gastrectomy. *Surg Laparosc Endosc.* 1992;2:258–260.

Goh P, Tekant Y, Kum CK, et al. Totally intra-abdominal laparoscopic Billroth II gastrectomy. *Surg Endosc.* 1992;6:160.

Gomez-Ferrer F, Balique JG, Azagra S, et al. Laparoscopic surgery for duodenal ulcer: first results of a multicentre study applying a personal procedure. *Br J Surg.* 1996;83:547–550.

Kang KC, Cho GS, Han SU, et al. Comparison of Billroth I and Billroth II reconstructions after laparoscopy-assisted distal gastrectomy: a retrospective analysis of large-scale multicenter results from Korea. *Surg Endosc.* 2010;25:1953–1961.

Lee WJ, Wang W, Chen TC, et al. Totally laparoscopic radical BII gastrectomy for the treatment of gastric cancer: a comparison with open surgery. *Surg Laparosc Endosc Percutan Tech.* 2008; 18:369–374.

Lointier P, Leroux S, Ferrier C, et al. A technique of laparoscopic gastrectomy and Billroth II gastrojejunostomy. *J Laparoendosc Surg.* 1993;3:353–364.

Oh SJ, Hong JJ, Oh CA, et al. Stapling technique for performing Billroth II anastomosis after distal gastrectomy. *J Gastrointest Surg.* 2010;16:1244–1246.

Rivera RE, Eagon JC, Soper NJ, et al. Experience with laparoscopic gastric resection: results and outcomes for 37 cases. *Surg Endosc.* 2005;19:1622–1626.

Ryu KW, Kim YW, Lee JH, et al. Surgical complications and the risk factors of laparoscopy-assisted distal gastrectomy in early gastric cancer. *Ann Surg Oncol.* 2008;15:1625–1631.

Saccomani GE, Percivale A, Stella M, et al. Laparoscopic Billroth II gastrectomy for completely stricturing duodenal ulcer: technical details. *Scand J Surg.* 2003;92:200–202.

Soper NJ, Brunt LM, Brewer JD, et al. Laparoscopic Billroth II gastrectomy in the canine model. *Surg Endosc.* 1994;8:1395–1398.

7 Truncal Vagotomy with Antrectomy and Roux-En-Y Reconstruction

Kevin E. Behrns and Angel M. Caban

 ## INDICATIONS/CONTRAINDICATIONS

The introduction and evolution of acid-suppressive medications and the discovery of *Helicobacter pylori* as the cause of peptic ulcer disease have decreased markedly the number of patients who require elective surgical therapy. However, even though surgical therapy is indicated only in refractory cases of ulcer disease, it is essential that practicing general surgeons understand the pathophysiology and surgical options for the treatment of peptic ulcer disease. The early and important contributions of Dr. Lester Dragstedt identified the vagus nerve as an important stimulus to acid secretion. His experimental work provided the rationale for vagotomy as a mechanism to eliminate the direct cholinergic stimulus for acid secretion to the parietal cells. His work set the stage for the development of three variations of surgical vagal stimulus interruption: truncal vagotomy, selective vagotomy, and highly selective vagotomy. Since truncal vagotomy markedly alters gastric motility patterns, a gastric drainage or emptying procedure should be performed in conjunction with truncal vagotomy. Several surgical options for gastric drainage exist, but this chapter will focus on truncal vagotomy with antrectomy and Roux-en-Y reconstruction. It should be recognized that this operation was developed experimentally by Cesar Roux as a model of gastrojejunal anastomotic ulcer and, therefore, should be used only in refractory cases of ulcer disease. In fact, many surgeons preferably perform a gastroduodenostomy (Billroth I) or a gastrojejunostomy (Billroth II) for reconstruction after antrectomy because these operations represent more physiologic reconstructions of gastroenteric continuity.

Despite the limited application of this procedure, the indications for surgical intervention have not changed; surgery is often needed for intractable ulcers, bleeding, perforation, or obstruction. Importantly, the rate of emergency operations for complicated peptic ulcer disease has not changed since the introduction of acid-suppressive medications and antibiotics. Thus, emergent surgical therapy for complicated ulcer disease remains constant and requires that the general surgeon be up-to-date regarding new advances in surgical treatment. However, the emergent management of complicated peptic ulcer disease is beyond the scope of this work. The aims of this chapter are to describe the modern surgical approach to truncal vagotomy and antrectomy with Roux-en-Y reconstruction with emphasis on the indications, techniques, and postoperative outcomes. It is important to realize that the treatment of peptic ulcer disease is often individualized on the basis of the location of the ulcer, the inflammatory response, and the mode of presentation.

PREOPERATIVE PLANNING

Truncal vagotomy and antrectomy with Roux-en-Y reconstruction is most often performed in an elective setting for recalcitrant peptic ulcer disease, and hence, a complete upper gastrointestinal tract evaluation should be completed. The evaluation should include an upper flexible endoscopy to identify the location of the ulceration, to rule out malignancy, and to test for *H. pylori*. In patients with prior upper gastrointestinal surgery a barium contrast study or computed tomography with oral contrast may be useful in delineating surgical anatomy. Serum gastrin level should also be obtained in patients with recurrent ulcers that are refractory to medical therapy and salicylate concentration should be determined for patients on nonsteroidal anti-inflammatory medications. Additional blood tests to assess the patient's overall health and nutritional status may include serum electrolytes, a complete blood count, and nutritional markers such as albumin or pre-albumin.

A thorough history and physical examination is essential to assess the patient's suitability for operative therapy with special emphasis on the history of previous surgery since most of these operations are now accomplished laparoscopically. A discussion with the patient regarding the benefits, risks, and long-term side effects of the operation is imperative. This conversation should include discussion of possible conversion to an open procedure, inadvertent or missed injuries, and postgastrectomy syndromes requiring lifestyle and dietary modifications.

SURGERY

In our practice the majority of the elective gastric resections are performed by a laparoscopic approach. Therefore, the laparoscopic approach will be presented in detail, but ultimately, the same operative steps are generally true for an open approach. In the unusual instance when the laparoscopic approach to this procedure is employed in patients presenting with bleeding or perforation, a low threshold for conversion to an open procedure should exist since visualization of important structures will be impaired in these cases.

Positioning

The patient is placed in the supine position and secured to the operative table on which a foot-board is applied to prevent patient slippage as a substantial portion of the procedure is performed in steep reverse Trendelenburg. The patient's arms are usually abducted though they may be tucked at the patient's side depending on the surgeon's and the anesthesiologist's preference. Typical trocar placement for upper gastrointestinal surgery is used as depicted in Figure 7.1. When an open approach is used, an upper midline incision from the xiphoid process to the umbilicus is often sufficient. Alternatively, a bilateral subcostal incision can be used for excellent exposure to the upper abdomen. However, if the patient has had previous abdominal surgery, adhesiolysis in the lower abdomen may prove difficult with the bilateral subcostal incision. Therefore, we prefer a midline incision.

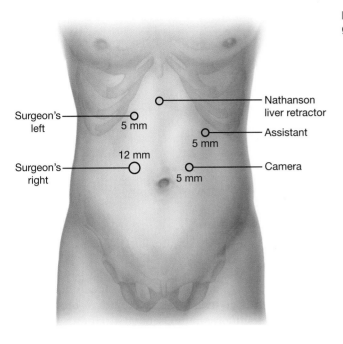

Part I: Procedures for Ulcer Disease

Figure 7.1 Port placement for upper gastrointestinal surgery.

Operative Technique

Following proper positioning, establishment of pneumoperitoneum, and port placement the operative approach is as follows:

- Dissection begins at the esophageal hiatus. The gastrohepatic ligament is incised until the right crus of the diaphragm is well visualized from apex to insertion (Fig. 7.2).
- The phrenoesophageal ligament is divided from right to left anterior to the esophagus, until the left crus is visualized.
- Circumferential dissection of the esophagus is performed to free approximately 4 cm of esophagus. The right and left vagus nerves are identified along the esophagus. The right vagus nerve is typically a relatively large cord-like structure and readily identified in the periesophageal tissue directly adjacent to the posterior surface of the esophagus. The more diminutive left vagus nerve is often directly applied on the anterior surface of the esophagus and less easily identified (Fig. 7.3).
- Each nerve is then clipped and divided using a 5 mm clip applier and laparoscopic scissor. Approximately 1 cm of the nerve is removed and sent to pathology for histologic confirmation. To ensure complete vagotomy, 4 cm of the esophagus should be skeletonized of nerve-like tissue with particular attention to a criminal nerve of Grassi, which is the first branch of the right vagus nerve.

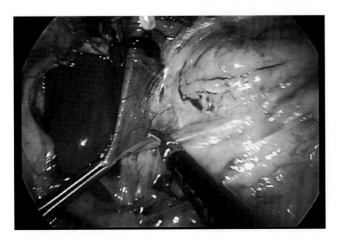

Figure 7.2 Dissection of the right crus of the diaphragm.

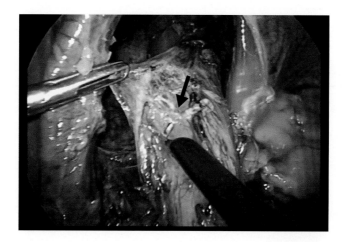

Figure 7.3 The anterior vagus nerve is mobilized from the esophagus (*arrow*). The nerve is then clipped and divided using a clip applier and laparoscopic scissors.

- To perform the antrectomy the lesser sac is entered by dividing the gastrocolic omentum with a laparoscopic energy device. Once in the lesser sac, the omentum and the retrogastric attachments are divided toward the pylorus until the origin of the right gastroepiploic vessel is seen (Fig. 7.4). Circumferential dissection around this vascular pedicle is performed, and the pedicle is divided with a laparoscopic 60 mm linear stapler with a vascular load (2.5 mm staples) (Fig. 7.5).
- Division of the gastrocolic omentum is continued orally until the selected point of gastric transection (Fig. 7.6). For antrectomy, approximately one-third of the stomach is removed.
- Along the lesser curvature of the stomach, the right gastric artery is identified and divided using a clip applier and laparoscopic scissors or a stapling device as desired. Small arteries may also be divided with a laparoscopic energy device (Fig. 7.7).
- A tunnel posterior to the first portion of the duodenum is created. In the presence of chronic inflammation this can be difficult and time consuming (Fig. 7.8). However, careful identification of surrounding structures will guide a safe dissection. Certainly, the location of the common hepatic artery and common bile duct should be known prior to division of the duodenum.
- The duodenum can be divided just distal to the pylorus with a laparoscopic 60 mm linear stapler with 3.5 mm staples (blue load) (Fig. 7.9). The staple line should be examined carefully for defects; if integrity of the staple line is in question or significant inflammation or thickening is present, the staple line should be reinforced with suture.
- The stomach is divided proximally to complete antrectomy, using a linear 60 mm stapler with 3.5 mm staples (Fig. 7.10).

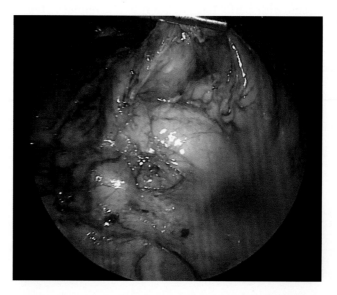

Figure 7.4 After dividing the gastrocolic omentum and entering the lesser sac, the origin of the right gastroepiploic vessels can be found near the pylorus.

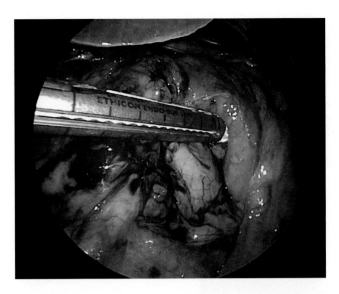

Figure 7.5 Division of the right gastroepiploic pedicle is performed with a laparoscopic linear stapler.

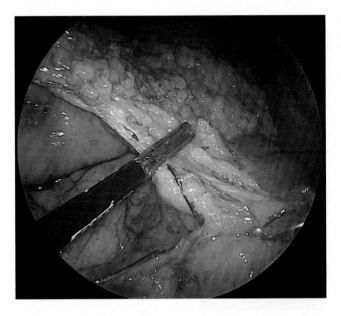

Figure 7.6 Cephalad division of the gastrocolic omentum using a laparoscopic energy device. Transections are continued proximally until the selected point of gastric transection.

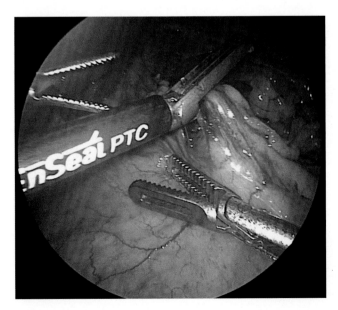

Figure 7.7 Division of the right gastric artery using a laparoscopic energy device.

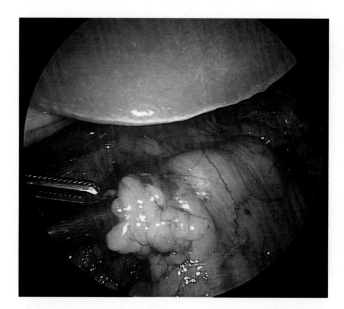

Figure 7.8 A tunnel posterior to the first portion of the duodenum is created to accommodate the laparoscopic stapler.

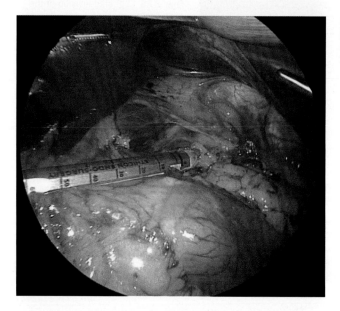

Figure 7.9 The duodenum is divided just distal to the pylorus with a laparoscopic 60 mm linear stapler with 3.5 mm staples (blue load).

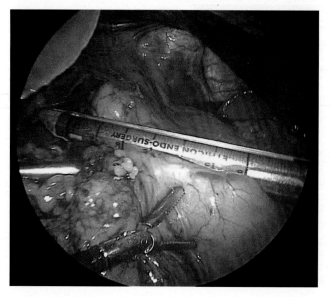

Figure 7.10 The proximal stomach is divided to complete the antrectomy. Approximately one-third of the stomach is removed.

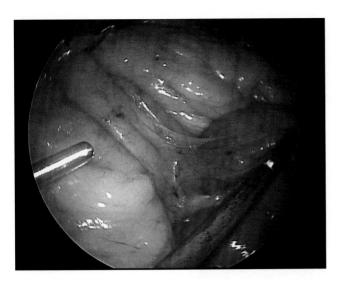

Figure 7.11 View of the ligament of Treitz.

- The specimen is placed in a plastic bag in the right upper quadrant for later retrieval.
- The Roux limb is then created. The operating table is returned to a neutral position. The transverse colon is elevated and the ligament of Treitz is identified (Fig. 7.11). The bowel is run distally for approximately 30 cm where the jejunum is divided using a linear stapler with 2.5 or 3.5 mm staples (white or blue load depending on bowel thickness) (Fig. 7.12).
- The mesentery is divided using an energy device down to its base. Alternatively, a linear stapler with 2 mm staples (gray load) can be used to divide the mesentery (Fig. 7.13).
- A 40 to 50 cm Roux limb is then created and a side-to-side jejunojejunostomy is created using a linear stapler for the posterior and anterior rows, respectively (Fig. 7.14).
- The mesenteric defect is closed using a running 2-0 silk to prevent formation of internal hernia (Fig. 7.15).

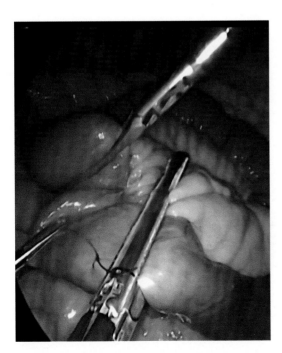

Figure 7.12 The jejunum is divided approximately 30 cm distally to the ligament of Treitz. Prior to division, the biliopancreatic limb was marked with an absorbable suture to provide limb identification and orientation.

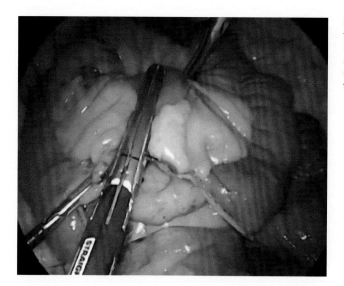

Figure 7.13 The small bowel mesentery is divided down to its base using a laparoscopic stapler with 2 mm staples. Alternatively, a laparoscopic energy device can be used to divide the mesentery safely.

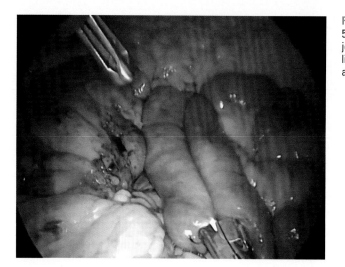

Figure 7.14 After creating a 40 to 50 cm Roux limb, a side-to-side jejunojejunostomy is created using a linear stapler for the posterior and anterior rows, respectively.

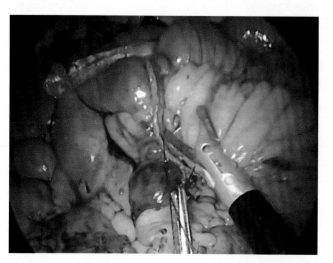

Figure 7.15 The mesenteric defect is closed using a running 2-0 silk to prevent formation of internal hernia.

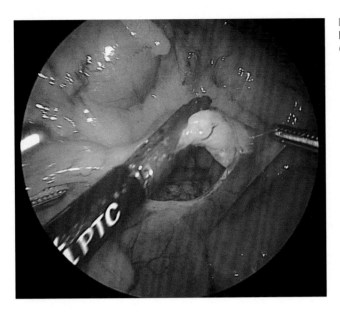

Figure 7.16 Creation of the mesocolonic window to the left of the middle colic artery.

- The transverse colon is again elevated and a mesocolic window is created to the left of the middle colic artery (Fig. 7.16). The Roux limb is advanced through this window taking great care not to twist the mesentery and compromise the blood supply.
- We will describe two approaches to create gastrojejunal anastomosis. First the linear stapler technique will be described, and second, the circular stapler (end-to-end anastomosis [EEA]) technique will be outlined.
- Linear stapler technique:
  - Once the Roux limb is placed in the desired orientation, a running 2-0 silk posterior seromuscular suture line is placed between the Roux limb and the posterior wall of the distal stomach (Fig. 7.17).
  - Enterotomies in the stomach and small bowel are made to accommodate the 60 mm linear stapler with a blue load, and the side-to-side anastomosis is created (Fig. 7.18). The anterior layers of the stomach and jejunum are closed using a running 2-0 absorbable suture (Fig. 7.19).
  - The two-layer anastomosis is then completed anteriorly using a running 2-0 silk in the seromuscular layer (Fig. 7.20).

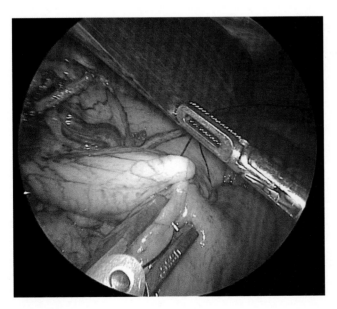

Figure 7.17 Once the Roux limb is placed in the desired orientation, a running 2-0 silk posterior seromuscular suture line is placed between the Roux limb and the posterior wall of the distal stomach.

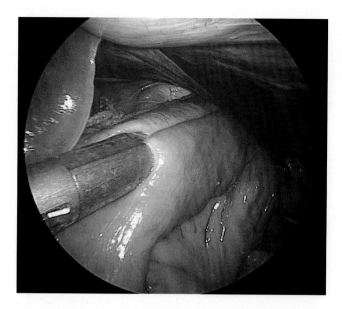

Figure 7.18 Enterotomies in the stomach and small bowel are made to accommodate the 60 mm linear stapler with a blue load (3.5 mm staples), and the side-to-side gastro-jejunal anastomosis is created.

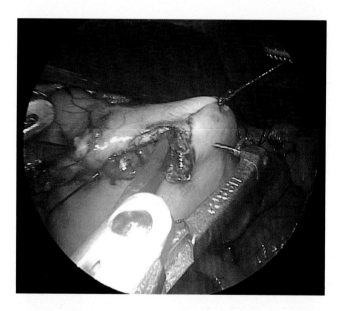

Figure 7.19 The anterior layers of the stomach and jejunum are closed using a running 2-0 absorbable suture.

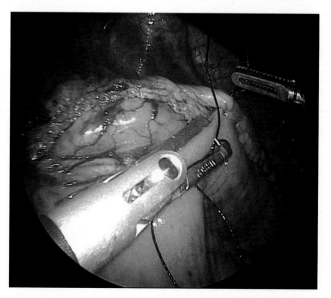

Figure 7.20 The two-layer anastomosis is then completed anteriorly using a running 2-0 silk in the seromuscular layer.

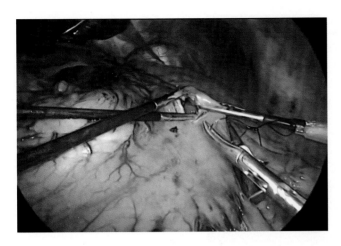

Figure 7.21 A distal anterior gastrostomy is performed to place the anvil inside the stomach. The anvil is then spiked through the posterior wall of the stomach in a location favorable for gastrojejunostomy. We use a 25 mm EEA stapler with 4.8 mm staples.

- ▣ Circular stapler technique:
  - ▣ This approach uses a 25 mm EEA stapler with 4.8 mm staples. A distal anterior gastrostomy is performed to place the anvil inside the stomach (Fig. 7.21). The anvil is then spiked through the posterior wall of the stomach in a location favorable for gastrojejunostomy.
  - ▣ The anterior gastrostomy is then closed using either sutures or the linear stapler with 3.5 mm staples (Fig. 7.22).
  - ▣ The Roux limb is then opened by removing the end staple line to accommodate the placement of the EEA stapler into the jejunum. The EEA stapler is advanced through the abdominal wall and inserted inside the Roux limb. The sharp post on the EEA stapler is delivered through the wall of the Roux limb 4 to 5 cm from the free margin. The stapler post and the anvil are mated, and the anastomosis is created by firing the stapler (Figs. 7.23–7.26).
  - ▣ The redundant portion of the Roux limb is excised using a linear stapler with 2.5 mm staples (Fig. 7.27).
  - ▣ It is our practice to perform an endoscopic air leak test after creation of gastrojejunostomy.
  - ▣ The stomach is secured to the mesocolic window using interrupted 2-0 silk sutures to prevent herniation (Fig. 7.28).
  - ▣ The specimen is retrieved and the wounds are closed using the surgeon's preferred method.

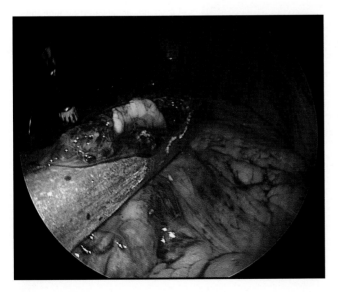

Figure 7.22 The anterior gastrostomy is then closed using either sutures or the linear stapler with 3.5 mm staples.

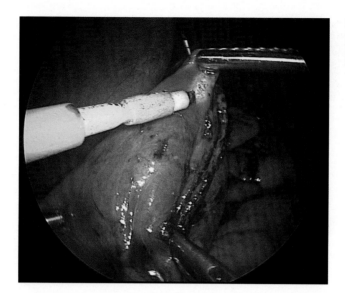

Figure 7.23 The Roux limb is then opened by removing the end staple line to accommodate the placement of the EEA stapler into the jejunum.

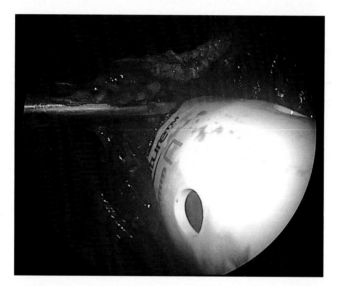

Figure 7.24 The EEA stapler is advanced through the abdominal wall and inserted inside the Roux limb.

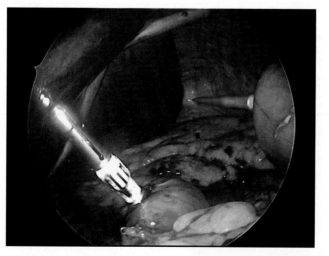

Figure 7.25 The sharp post on the EEA stapler is delivered through the wall of the Roux limb 4 to 5 cm from the free margin.

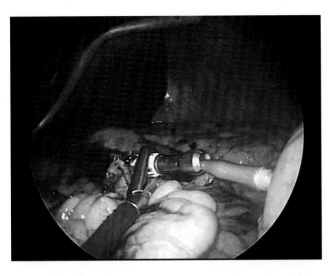

Figure 7.26 The stapler post and the anvil are mated and the anastomosis is created by firing the stapler.

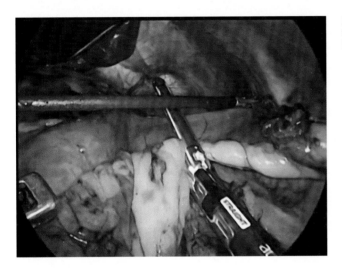

Figure 7.27 The redundant portion of the Roux limb is excised using a linear stapler with 2.5 mm staples.

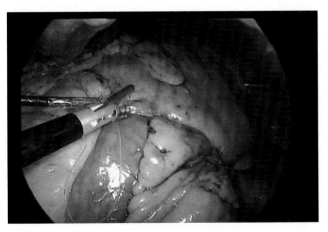

Figure 7.28 The stomach is secured to the mesocolic window using interrupted 2-0 silk sutures to prevent herniation.

POSTOPERATIVE MANAGEMENT

The postoperative period for patients undergoing elective laparoscopic surgery for peptic ulcer disease is usually uneventful. On postoperative day 0, analgesia is provided with a patient-controlled anesthesia (PCA) pump. Ambulation and hourly incentive spirometer use are strictly enforced. The patient remains nothing per os (NPO), but nasogastric decompression is infrequently used.

On postoperative day 1 a liquid diet is introduced, IV fluids are discontinued and the urinary bladder catheter is removed. Nutritional counseling for a postgastrectomy diet is provided, and the patient is prepared for discharge on postoperative day 2.

Patients presenting with acute perforation or bleeding tend to have developed an inflammatory response and likely will require a longer hospital stay and closer monitoring.

 COMPLICATIONS

Early complications after gastric surgery include bleeding, infection, unrecognized intra-abdominal injuries, and anastomotic leaks. The reported complication rates are quite variable but overall morbidity is 5% to 10% for the early complications (Table 7.1). Approximately 25% of the patients will develop symptoms associated with physiologic derangements after vagotomy and antrectomy. These disorders are collectively referred to as *postgastrectomy syndromes.*

- *Dumping syndrome* is an amalgamation of symptoms that occurs after rapid emptying of hyperosmolar chime into the Roux limb, particularly carbohydrates. It exists in an *early phase* and a far less common *late phase.* The early phase of dumping usually occurs after 20 to 30 minutes following food ingestion, whereas the late form appears 2 to 3 hours after food consumption. Collective symptoms include epigastric distention, nausea, vomiting, palpitations, diaphoresis, dizziness, and flushing. In most patients mere avoidance of the offending nutrients results in symptom relief. In addition, frequent small meals low in carbohydrates is often helpful.
- *Postvagotomy diarrhea* is experienced by approximately 30% of the patients after truncal vagotomy. For the majority of these patients, the symptoms are self-limiting after 3 to 4 months and less than 1% will experience disabling diarrhea. Nonsurgical treatment including dietary and lifestyle modifications usually is sufficient for improvement and resolution. In more severe cases, antidiarrheals, octreotide, or cholestyramine to bind bile salts may be needed.
- *Delayed gastric emptying* or *gastric atony* is a multifactorial symptom complex that presents frequently after gastric resection with or without vagotomy. The most common

TABLE 7.1

Early Complications	Frequency (%)
Bleeding	1–10
Wound infection (open)	3–5
Pneumonia	5–10
Gastric stasis	4–5
Obstruction	1
Anastomotic leaks	1–4
Bowel perforation	1–3
Deep venous thrombosis	1–2
Cerebrovascular accident	<1

symptoms are early satiety, nausea, vomiting, and/or epigastric pain. Gastric atony can be diagnosed clinically, but radiologic, endoscopic, and scintigraphic studies can be used to confirm the clinical suspicion. The physician must consider other medical causes of gastroparesis, including diabetes mellitus, electrolyte imbalance, drug toxicity, and neuromuscular disorders. In addition, mechanical causes of gastric outlet obstruction such as anastomotic stricture, postoperative adhesions, Roux stasis, or internal herniation must be ruled out. As with postvagotomy diarrhea, the treatment is usually nonsurgical with diet and lifestyle modifications. Prokinetic agents such as metoclopramide or erythromycin can be used, but a significant clinical response is uncommon. In severe cases, a near total gastrectomy with Roux-en-Y reconstruction is an acceptable surgical option.

- *Roux stasis syndrome* has a similar clinical presentation to gastric atony. The etiology is not completely understood but is likely associated with alterations in jejunal motility. Construction of a Roux limb of more than 40 cm has been found to increase the incidence of Roux stasis syndrome and should be prevented when possible. Surgical treatment is reserved for those patients who do not respond to medical management and lifestyle changes. Reconstruction and shortening of the Roux limb to less than 40 cm is the surgical option of choice for these patients.
- *Recurrent ulcers* can be seen in approximately 1% to 2% of the patients undergoing truncal vagotomy and antrectomy. Incomplete transection or erroneously identifying the vagus nerve below its first hepatic or celiac branch can significantly jeopardize the outcome of the surgery. The rate of recurrent ulceration may be in direct proportion to the accuracy of identification and division of the vagus nerves. Additional technical factors that may lead to recurrent ulceration include retained gastric antrum and inadequate resection of the antrum.

RESULTS

Truncal vagotomy and antrectomy is infrequently performed due to improvements in medical management of ulcer disease, but when used for complicated cases it offers a 90% reduction in acid production. The mortality rate is approximately 1% to 2% with an overall complication rate of 5% to 10% (Table 7.2). With recent advances in surgical technology, the vast majority of these operations can now be performed laparoscopically; thus, decreasing surgical morbidity and improving patient satisfaction.

CONCLUSIONS

Truncal vagotomy with antrectomy is infrequently indicated in the treatment of peptic ulcer disease. However, this operation is reasonable for recurrent peptic ulcer disease. When possible, more physiologic operations such as Billroth I gastroduodenostomy or Billroth II gastrojejunostomy should be performed. Even though the indications for this operation have waned, the appropriate preoperative evaluation, technical performance, and postoperative management involved in this operation should be in the repertoire of all general surgeons.

TABLE 7.2

Truncal Vagotomy + Antrectomy	Results (%)
Morbidity	5–10
Mortality	1–2
Acid reduction	85–90
Ulcer reduction	1–2

Recommended References and Readings

Chang TM, Chen TH, Tsou SS, et al. Differences in gastric emptying between highly selective vagotomy and posterior truncal vagotomy combined with anterior seromyotomy. *J Gastrointest Surg.* 1999;3:533–536.

De la Fuente S, Khuri S, Schifftner T, et al. Comparative analysis of vagotomy and drainage vs vagotomy and resection procedures for bleeding peptic ulcer disease. *J Am Coll Surg.* 2006;202:78–86.

Dragstedt LR. Vagotomy for gastroduodenal ulcer. *Ann Surg.* 1945; 122:973–989.

Fischer JF, Johannigman J. *Surgical complications.* In: Schwartz S, ed. *Principles of Surgery.* McGraw-Hill; 1999:470–471.

Forstner-Barthell AW, Murr MM, Nitecki S, et al. Near-total completion gastrectomy for severe postvagotomy gastric stasis: Analysis of early and long-term results in 62 patients. *J Gastrointest Surg.* 1999;3:15–21, discussion 21–23.

Fujita T, Katai H, Morita S, et al. Short-term outcomes of roux en Y stapled anastomosis after distal gastrectomy for gastric adenocarcinoma. *J Gastrointest Surg.* 2010;14:289–294.

Herrington J, Jr, Davidson J, III, Shumway S. Proximal gastric vagotomy. *Ann Surg.* 1986;204:108–113.

Huscher C, Mingoli A, Sgarzini G, et al. Laparoscopic vs open gastrectomy for distal gastric cancer. *Ann Surg.* 2005;241:232–237.

Jiang X, Hiki N, Nunobe S, et al. Postoperative outcomes and complications after laparoscopy-assisted pylorus-preserving gastrectomy for early gastric cancer. *Ann Surg.* 2011;253:928–933.

Koo J, Lam SK, Chan P, et al. Proximal gastric vagotomy, truncal vagotomy with drainage, and truncal vagotomy with antrectomy for chronic duodenal ulcer. A prospective, randomized controlled trial. *Ann Surg.* 1983;197:265–271.

Lai LH, Sung JJ. Helicobacter pylori and benign upper digestive disease. *Best Pract Res Clin Gastroenterol.* 2007;21:261–279.

Martin RF. Surgical management of ulcer disease. *Surg Clin North Am.* 2005;85:907–929, vi.

Memon M, Ed C, Subramanya M, et al. Meta-analysis of D1 vs D2 gastrectomy for gastric adenocarcinoma. *Ann Surg.* 2011;253: 900–911.

Mercer DW, Robinson EK. Stomach. In: Townsend. *Sabiston Textbook of Surgery.* 18th ed. Philadelphia, PA: WB Saunders; 2007.

Mine S, Sano T, Tsutsumi K, et al. Large-scale investigation into dumping syndrome after gastrectomy for gastric cancer. *J Am Coll Surg.* 2010;211:628–636.

Tu BL, Kelly KA. Surgical treatment of Roux stasis syndrome. *J Gastrointest Surg.* 1999;3:613–617.

Roux C. L'esophago-jejune-gastrome. Nouvelle op'eration pour retricissement infranchissable de L'esophage. *Semaine Med.* 1907; 27:37.

Speicher JE, Thirlby RC, Burggraaf J, et al. Results of completion gastrectomies in 44 patients with postsurgical gastric atony. *J Gastrointest Surg.* 2009;13:874–880.

Turnage RH, Sarosi G, Cryer B, et al. Evaluation and management of patients with recurrent peptic ulcer disease after acid-reducing operations: a systematic review. *J Gastrointest Surg.* 2003;7:606–626.

Viste A, Haugstvedt T, Eide G, et al. Postoperative complications and mortality after surgery for gastric cancer. *Ann Surg.* 1988;207: 7–13.

8 Proximal Gastric Vagotomy

Michael S. Nussbaum and Mark Alan Dobbertien

Introduction

Open proximal gastric vagotomy (PGV), as practiced now for over 40 years and known by other pseudonyms as highly selective vagotomy and parietal cell vagotomy, is a proven effective operation for the definitive surgical management of many complicated gastroduodenal ulcer disease patients and should be part of the armamentarium of all surgeons who care for such patients worldwide. This refined vagotomy operation has the basic surgical tenets of interrupting the vagal innervation to the parietal cell mass in the cardia, fundus, and body of the stomach (responsible for acid secretion) while maintaining the vagal innervation to the antrum and pylorus as well as to the branches of the celiac and hepatic plexus, thus minimizing motility and secretory disturbances in the stomach and the gastrointestinal tract. The effectiveness of PGV in lowering acid secretion has resulted in long-term cure of ulcer in over 90% of the patients and has had the added benefit of virtually eliminating the untoward side effects of less selective uses of vagotomy and drainage procedures or limited gastrectomy (antrectomy) such as dumping, stasis, bile reflux, and diarrhea. Although the PGV operation has been reported to be only performed once, on average, in training by graduating residents and is more technically demanding and time consuming (about 120 minutes average) than truncal vagotomy, the procedure can be performed safely and efficiently when done correctly and mastered. The many advantages of this procedure certainly outweigh the above disadvantages and they should not be considered a cogent rationale to abandon the procedure when performing definitive ulcer surgery.

In this chapter, the indications for the operation will be outlined and the preoperative, operative, and postoperative management for patients undergoing PGV will be presented along with the expected results and complications associated with open PGV.

INDICATIONS

PGV is indicated in patients with chronic duodenal ulcers who have failed the currently available maximal medical management regime. It is also sometimes the procedure of choice in stable patients who are not ulcer naïve and have a perforated or bleeding duodenal ulcer and are able to tolerate a definitive operative ulcer procedure once a Graham patch (or accepted alternative) or artery ligation has been performed. In addition,

PGV can be used in active ulcer patients receiving medical management who need aortic surgery or organ transplantation to prevent serious, life-threatening ulcer complications such as bleeding or perforation. PGV alone should not be used in patients with pyloric or prepyloric ulcers or for gastric outlet obstruction as the recurrence rate and failure rate are 31% and 55%, respectively, unless a drainage procedure is added to PGV. The indication for PGV in type I gastric ulcer in addition to wedge resection or submucosal resection remains controversial.

PREOPERATIVE PLANNING

Proper preoperative evaluation and management of patients necessitating either elective or emergency surgery using PGV should not be underestimated. Any lack of attention to detail may result in untoward morbidity and mortality. In all cases, a detailed history and physical examination is required as is a review of up-to-date laboratory and imaging data. A preoperative assessment of the patient's cardiopulmonary risk factors, ASA PA class, APACHE score as well as entering data in the American College of Surgeons National Surgical Quality Improvement Program (ACS NSQIP) data base (if available) may assist in the proper management of patients needing elective and emergency PGV. Of particular importance is a detailed review of the individual patient's ulcer diathesis history, endoscopic findings, pathology, and treatment up to that point. The emergency surgical management of duodenal ulcer complications, such as perforation and bleeding, is often predicated on the previous history of ulcer care prior to their presentation. After the above review and assessment, therapies and technical considerations are manipulated to minimize cardiopulmonary morbidity and mortality, venous thromboembolism (VTE), and surgical site infection. In order to minimize perioperative myocardial infarction, patients with intermediate to high-risk scores are treated with beta blockers without intrinsic sympathomimetic activity (unless contraindicated), and this has resulted in a greater than 50% relative reduction in postoperative cardiac events. High-risk pulmonary patients would benefit from incentive spirometry, selective nasogastric tube use, and short-term neuroaxis blockage via epidural anesthetic techniques. Evidence shows that patient-related risk factors, such as chronic obstructive pulmonary disease, age older than 60 years, ASA class of II or higher, functional dependence, congestive heart failure, prolonged surgery, and abdominal surgery, increase the risk for postoperative pulmonary complications. All patients should receive VTE prophylaxis with either unfractionated or low-molecular weight heparin plus sequential compression devices may be used in addition to anticoagulation in the high-risk surgical patient and in those who have a contraindication to anticoagulation prophylaxis. Caution is advised in using low-molecular weight heparin in patients with renal insufficiency or failure, and it either must be dose-adjusted or unfractionated heparin must be used as a substitute. For most cases of uncomplicated gastroduodenal ulcer surgery, no prophylactic antibiotics are recommended. However, in complicated patients or patients where the gastrointestinal tract will be opened, a first-generation cephalosporin (i.e., cefazolin) should be administered within 1 hour of the surgical incision to reduce the likelihood of a postoperative surgical site infection.

SURGICAL TECHNIQUES

Positioning, Anesthesia, and Skin Preparation

The patient is positioned on the operating table in the supine position. At least one arm should be tucked in most instances to provide more room for the operating team and any mechanical retractors. Care must be taken to ensure that the patient is properly off-loaded to prevent nerve injury in both the upper and lower extremity and to prevent back pain in the lordotic areas of the lumbar and cervical spine. A footboard should be used so that the patient will not move during the procedure when reverse Trendelen-burg positioning may cause shifting of the patient on the operating table. Patients should be secured to the operating table using a safety strap. The patient should have a large bore intravenous line and, in the high-risk patient, may need central venous pressure monitoring as well as invasive blood pressure monitoring with an arterial line. A urinary catheter is placed for urine output monitoring and a nasogastric tube is placed once the patient has undergone rapid sequence intubation and the endotracheal tube has been secured. The nasogastric tube is helpful for decompression of the stomach as well as for identifying the esophagus at the diaphragmatic hiatus and as a retraction device on the greater curve of the stomach. Patients should be offered perioperative thoracic epidural analgesia which should be placed prior to the induction of general anesthesia. All patients undergoing PGV should be considered to have a full stomach and therefore require rapid sequence intubation techniques. Muscle relaxation is neces-sary for open PGV. The patient's abdomen and lower chest is clipped in the operating room and the patient's skin is prepared with chlorhexidine-alcohol, which has recently been shown to be superior to povidone-iodine in preventing postoperative surgical site infection. Sterile draping should include the lower chest well above the xiphisternum.

Incision, Exposure, Exploration, and Definitive Management of Bleeding and Perforation

An upper midline, epigastric incision is recommended when performing open PGV and provides excellent overall exposure. Infrequently, the incision needs to be carried below the umbilicus. An alternative chevron incision may be used, but the disadvantages of muscle transection seem to outweigh the exposure benefits in most cases. Care must be taken to avoid injuring the periosteum of the xiphoid process in order to prevent the rare but under-reported incidence of heterotopic ossification of the abdominal wound. The xiphoid, in most instances, does not need to be excised. Once the skin has been incised, blunt bilateral force is used to transect the subcutaneous tissue in a bloodless field, and this technique reliably identifies the midline fascia and linea alba in situa-tions when previous laparotomies have not been performed. The midline fascia is incised precisely in the midline to avoid disruption of the confluence of the anterior and posterior rectus sheaths. The properitoneal fat is sharply transected and the peri-toneum is opened to the full extent of the wound, avoiding any adhesions when present. The ligamentum teres hepatis does not need to be transected in most cases and may be used to patch a perforated duodenal ulcer when omentum is not readily available. Full abdominal exploration is mandatory in order to assess the suspected pathology as well as identify any other unsuspected pathology, unless mitigating circumstances would call for a truncated exploration, such as dense adhesions, when the risk of enterotomy may outweigh the benefits of exploration. Any peritoneal soiling is quickly addressed with suction, irrigation, and control of ongoing spillage from the perforated viscous. The left triangular ligament may be incised to provide right upward mobilization of the lateral segment of the left lobe of the liver for better exposure of the esophageal hiatus. A laparotomy sponge is placed lateral and posterior to the spleen to release any tension on the gastrosplenic ligament, thus minimizing the risk of splenic injury. A self-retaining retractor is next implemented and attached to the operating table. A Thompson or Bookwalter retractor is preferred over a Balfour retractor in most cases. In order to provide the best exposure and retraction, the liver needs to be retracted superiorly and to the right and the parieties need to be placed on tension inferiorly and mediolaterally. The upper abdominal retractors should be placed with the patient in Trendelenburg position. Once the retractors are in place, reversing the Trendelenburg position will provide optimal exposure of the upper abdomen. All of the many important surgical aspects of PGV and the emergency management of perforation and bleeding will be able to be addressed without any further manipulation of the retractor system. In clinical scenarios of duodenal ulcer hemorrhage, an anterior longitudinal gastroduodenostomy across the pylorus is performed and the bleeding artery is ligated, making sure to control the transverse pancreatic artery with a U stitch. After controlling the arterial hemorrhage the duodenotomy is closed horizontally in a Heineke–Mikulicz fashion. A perforated duodenal ulcer should be patched with well vascularized omentum when available and should not be closed primarily especially if the closure would create narrowing of the duodenum. Closure and patching is an acceptable modification of Graham's technique, when the ulcer is small and would not result in significant stricturing. The PGV can be added to both of these procedures when indicated. A chronically scarred and obstructed duodenum should be managed either by resection or by PGV with gastrojejunostomy to alleviate the obstruction and to minimize recurrent duodenal ulcer.

Proximal Gastric Vagotomy

PGV requires a surgeon with a tremendous requisite knowledge of vagal and foregut anatomy and a meticulous technical skill-set for best results. The procedure should be able to be performed in less than 2 hours and consists of four (or five) important steps for optimal denervation (completeness of vagotomy), preservation of antral-pyloric mobility, and prevention of ulcer recurrence. The procedural steps involved in PGV are that of anterior lesser omental dissection, posterior lesser omental dissection, distal esophageal dissection, lesser curvature closure, and possibly consideration of extended PGV in the area along the greater curvature across the incisura described by Rosati in order to bring cure rates as high as 98%. The steps in the operation are not necessarily done sequentially and may be altered depending on local conditions for a given patient.

Distal Esophageal Dissection

The PGV is usually begun at the level of the esophageal hiatus and the distal esophagus (Fig. 8.1). The distal esophageal dissection and proximal lesser curvature dissection along the cardia and fundus can be very challenging to surgeons who are unfamiliar with the anatomy of the right and left vagus nerve as they descend in the posterior mediastinum (right) and through the esophageal hiatus. The dissection plane is not limited in scope and should be envisioned as a 360-degree operating plane around the distal 5 to 10 cm of esophagus and the proximal dome of the stomach's cardia and fundus. The left and right vagus nerves form a plexus over the posterior mediastinal esophagus and eventually unite to form the trunks of the anterior and posterior vagus at the level of the distal esophagus before dividing into divisions at or near the esophageal hiatus, but certainly above the angle of His. For this reason, it is recommended to begin this portion of the procedure at the angle of His by encircling the esophagus at

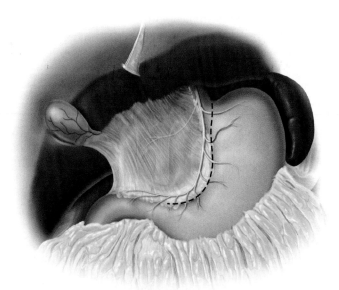

Figure 8.1 Anterior view of the stomach demonstrating the anterior nerve of Laterjet. The dotted line represents the line of dissection. The dissection is begun at the esophagogastric junction and the vagus nerves are isolated prior to the lesser curvature dissection.

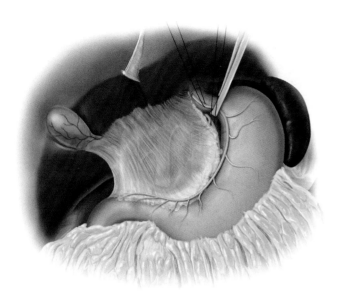

Figure 8.2 The lower esophagus is exposed and the gastroesophageal junction is encircled with a Penrose drain and retracted inferolaterally. The anterior and posterior nerves of Laterjet are secured with stays for proper identification, preservation, and retraction.

the cardioesophageal junction with a Penrose drain so that downward traction can be applied on the junction tenting the nerves for easy identification. In addition, starting the dissection at this point provides the best window for free mobilization of the esophagus and proximal stomach from the vagi, which are usually not as intimate with the esophageal musculature at this anatomical area. The encircling of the esophagus at the angle of His is accomplished by incising the peritoneum in this area and at the phrenicoesophageal ligament overlying the right crus of the diaphragm passing a blunt instrument from left to right, thus encircling the esophagus at the cardioesophageal junction (Fig. 8.2). Next, the anterior and posterior vagal trunks are encircled with umbilical tapes or vessel loops. The anterior nerve is usually intimately draped obliquely across the distal anterior esophagus and should be mobilized to the right of the esophagus. Occasionally, two divisions are seen before forming the anterior nerve of Laterjet. The hepatic branch can be seen in the lesser omentum running toward the caudate lobe of the liver. The larger posterior nerve is usually not intimate with the muscular wall of the esophagus as it enters the abdomen and is located typically at 8 o'clock on the esophagus close to the right crus of the diaphragm. The celiac nerve, a division of the posterior vagus, runs in the lesser omentum toward the left gastric artery, a branch of the celiac trunk. The phrenicoesophageal ligament is then incised completely and the distal esophagus is mobilized proximally into the mediastinum for approximately 5 to 7 cm to ensure complete esophagogastric vagotomy.

Anterior Lesser Omental Dissection

Once the vagal trunks are isolated and separated from the esophagogastric region, attention should be directed to the anterior lesser omentum. In order to provide distraction between the lesser omental contents and the lesser curvature of the stomach, an incision is made in the pars flaccida to provide superior retraction on the lesser omentum. This technique also provides a window into the upper recess of the lesser sac and exposure to the right crus of the diaphragm where the posterior vagus nerve is usually identified posterior and medial to the esophagus. The stomach is retracted inferiorly, either with direct anterior greater curvature retraction or by incising the gastrocolic omentum distal to the gastroepiploic vessels and dividing some anterior epiploic vessels such that combined anterior and posterior gastric wall inferior retraction can be applied. The anterior nerve of Laterjet is identified 1 to 2 cm from the lesser curve and must always be visualized directly during the procedure to avoid injury. Distraction of the lesser omentum helps prevent injury to the nerve. Location of the anterior nerve of Laterjet's oblique ending in the crow's foot with its three typical end branches is another important landmark

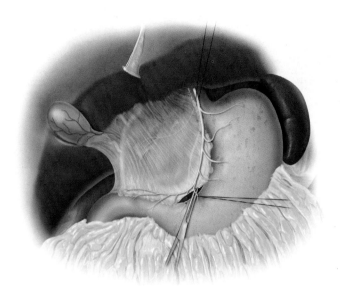

Figure 8.3 The anterior lesser curvature dissection is begun 5 to 7 cm proximal to the pylorus, and each gastric vagal branch from the anterior nerve of Laterjet and their accompanying vessels are isolated, ligated, and divided. Occasionally, when the crow's foot is proximal on the antrum, the heel of the crow's foot may be used as a starting point.

as is the 5- to 7-cm mark proximal to the pylorus on the lesser curvature (Fig. 8.3). In some patients the crow's foot is relatively proximal on the antrum and may not represent the best starting position to begin the lesser curvature devascularization and end gastric branch vagotomy. In such situations, either the heel of the crow's foot (most proximal neurovascular bundle of the crow's foot) should be transected in order to achieve complete parietal cell vagotomy without compromising antral motility. In general, the anterior lesser omental dissection begins about 5 to 7 cm from the pylorus. The peritoneum overlying the anterior leaf of the lesser omentum is then scored sharply from the distal dissection margin at the antral–body junction as close to the serosa of the anterior lesser curvature of the stomach as possible without injuring the stomach. The peritoneum is scored all the way from the incisura along the lesser curve across the cardioesophageal junction below the esophageal fat pad and across the angle of His. For surgeons who routinely incise the gastrocolic ligament, the posterior peritoneum corresponding to the above mentioned anterior peritoneum may be scored as well once all gastropancreatic adhesions are cleared and the stomach is retracted anteriorly and superiorly. Certainly, releasing both sleeves of the peritoneum will increase the distance between the nerves of Laterjet and the lesser curvature of the stomach reducing the likelihood of nerve injury and converting a parietal cell vagotomy to a total gastric vagotomy, defeating the benefits of the procedure and requiring a drainage procedure for salvage. Care must be taken in not applying too much tension on the lesser omental structures as this could cause avulsion of the end gastric branches of the ascending and descending left gastric artery. Once the peritoneum has been scored, the surgeon should be cognizant of the concave and, reciprocally, convex nature of the relationships between the lesser curvature of the stomach and the perpendicular neurovascular end gastric branches. This important relationship can be manipulated either by proper movement of surgical ligation and division devices or by rolling the lesser curvature of the stomach more anteriorly and inferiorly as the lesser omental dissection proceeds more posteriorly. In either case, ligation and division of the neurovascular bundles should be done as close to the stomach as possible without injuring the gastric wall. Both techniques can be used in tandem during the lesser curvature devascularization and vagotomy if the surgeon chooses so. It is best to divide the perpendicular neurovascular bundles as they enter the lesser curvature with a 2-0 or 3-0 silk suture using a fine right angle clamp and tying the pedicles in continuity, limiting the possibility of injury to the surrounding structures and blood loss from inappropriate tension on these fine neurovascular bundles that clamps may precipitate. An alternative approach is to use an energy source to provide ligation and division. The ultrasonic shears, Ligasure, or Enseal devices may be used to facilitate this dissection, and all these devices have been used safely and

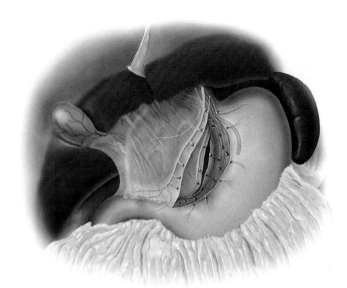

Figure 8.4 The lesser curvature dissection consists of three layers of nerves and vessels—an anterior, posterior, and unpredictable middle layer—all of which must be divided to ensure a complete proximal gastric vagotomy. The nasogastric tube is important for both gastric decompression and inferior gastric retraction.

effectively in minimally invasive vagotomy procedures. Either way, care must always be taken to avoid injury to the anterior nerve of Laterjet and the lesser curvature of the stomach. The anterior gastric nerve transection should continue to the prior proximal dissection at the cardioesophageal junction to ensure that the anterior and posterior nerves of Laterjet and the hepatic and celiac branches are identified before beginning the posterior lesser omental dissection. Care must be taken not to apply too much tension on the vagal trunks which could produce neuropraxia, or worse, traction neurolysis.

Posterior Lesser Omental Dissection

Before beginning the posterior lesser omental dissection, it is important to realize that there are numerous and variable small gastric vagal branches from both the anterior and posterior nerves of Laterjet that innervate the stomach's lesser curve and arise in the midportion of the gastrohepatic sleeve of mesentery (Fig. 8.4). It is imperative that these branches be ligated and divided with precision as most of the times they are not accompanied by a gastric end artery. This middle sleeve of mesentery should be ligated and divided in continuity and carried out from anterior to posterior and from inferior to superior extending up to the cardioesophageal junction. This procedure is best performed close to the lesser curve of the stomach and can be facilitated by rolling the lesser curve anteriorly and inferiorly. At this point, the posterior sleeve of the mesentery with its posterior nerve of Laterjet and the gastric branches of the descending branch of the left gastric artery to the posterior wall of the lesser curvature of the stomach should be easily identified. Dissecting the midportion of the mesentery en bloc with the posterior lesser omental dissection is not recommended. In obese patients, the midportion of the mesentery should be dissected in multiple layers to ensure completeness of the vagotomy. The posterior lesser omental dissection should be performed as described for the anterior lesser omental dissection. Finger dissection and pinching of the posterior lesser omentum is occasionally helpful and can disperse the omental adipose tissue from the surrounding neurovascular pedicles ensuring that the posterior nerve of Laterjet is not injured. The dissection is carried out from distal to proximal on the posterior lesser curvature up to the cardioesophageal junction dissection. The two sleeves of mesentery should be inspected to ensure that the anterior and posterior nerves of Laterjet have been preserved and inserted adequately on the anterior and posterior aspect of the antrum 5 to 6 cm from the pylorus. The distal margin of neuro/devascularization on the antrum should be re-inspected for adequacy of vagotomy and all remaining vagus nerve tissue in this area should be divided (Fig. 8.5).

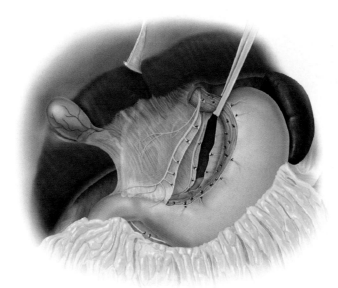

Figure 8.5 The completed proximal gastric vagotomy. All vagus fibers to the distal 5 to 10 cm of the esophagus are divided sharply making sure to divide the criminal nerve of Grassi in the gastropancreatic fold.

Finally, with minimal traction on the anterior nerve of Laterjet and inferolateral traction on the cardioesophageal junction, all structures to the left of the vagus entering the esophagus or stomach are ligated. Next, the same traction is applied to the posterior nerve of Laterjet and all the neurovascular structures to the left of the nerve are transected. The criminal nerve of Grassi, a branch of the posterior vagus, is identified and transected in the gastropancreatic fold as it makes its way to the fundus posteriorly. The esophagus is re-inspected ensuring that no gastric branches are imbedded in the esophageal musculature and no piercing mucosa are left untransected. Gentle blunt dissection with a finger or sharp dissection may be used to complete the esophageal portion of the vagotomy.

Lesser Curvature Closure

The open mesenteric surface of the lesser curvature of the stomach is closed by placing Lembert sutures using interrupted 2-0 or 3-0 silk (Figs. 8.6 and 8.7). This technique may prevent neural regeneration of the vagal fibers, potentially implicated in some incomplete vagotomies. In addition, this seromuscular closure of the lesser curvature of the stomach may avoid the potential complications of ischemic necrosis or perforation of

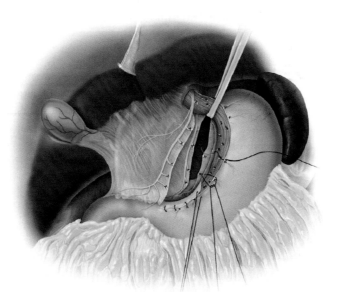

Figure 8.6 Lesser curvature closure is accomplished by approximation of the anterior and posterior seromusculature layers over the area of lesser curvature bare muscle in order to prevent free perforation from ischemic necrosis or from salient full thickness injury.

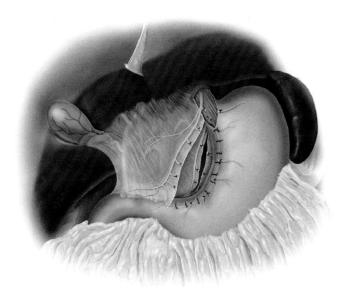

Figure 8.7 The completed seromuscular closure of the lesser curvature.

the lesser curvature of the stomach. Although these complications are exceedingly rare, a greater than 70% mortality rate has been reported in some series that experienced lesser curvature perforation as a complication. The likelihood of lesser curvature ischemic necrosis would be extremely rare, given the extensive submucosal blood supply, and therefore, these perforations are likely a result of unrecognized iatrogenic injury to the gastric wall during dissection. Crural repair can be carried out at this point when hiatal hernia is present, and fundoplication may be indicated when significant gastroesophageal reflux is documented preoperatively.

Extended PGV

When ulcer recurrence would be an untenable consequence for certain patients undergoing PGV, an extended PGV may be performed and has been reported to decrease ulcer recurrence rates to 2% versus 10% reported in most series. The "seven areas of vagotomy" described by Nyhus and his colleagues at the University of Illinois may serve as an anatomical template for surgeons performing PGV and extended PGV and may reduce the incidence of incomplete vagotomy (Fig. 8.8). Rosati et al. have recommended

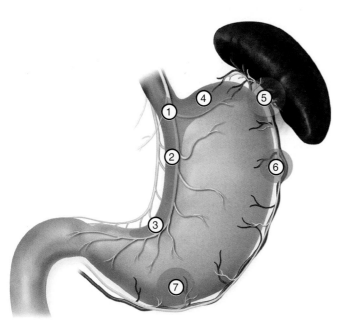

Figure 8.8 The seven areas of vagotomy are (1) periesophageal, (2) lesser curve, (3) crow's foot, (4) gastropancreatic fold, (5) short gastric, (6) left gastroepiploic, and (7) right gastroepiploic. Areas 3, 4, 6, and 7 are routinely divided during extended PGV while area 5 is always preserved to preserve blood supply to the proximal stomach.

that the preganglionic vagal fibers along the greater curvature across the incisura of the stomach (area 7) be divided to provide a more complete vagotomy. This additional procedure can be done with impunity for patients requiring PGV especially with regard to gastric blood supply and potential ischemic necrosis by avoiding disrupting the main right gastroepiploic vessels located near the gastric wall. The nerve fibers and end vascular gastric branches should be ligated and divided in continuity, avoiding injury to the gastroepiploic vessels. Energy devices for ligation and division may be used as an alternative to ligation in-continuity techniques.

Abdominal Closure

The abdomen is closed once the PGV is completed and the instrument, sponge, and needle counts are correct. Copious warm isotonic saline or antibiotic lavage can be performed and the effluent should be grossly clear. All surgical sites are inspected for hemostasis and potential injury to the nerves of Laterjet or the abdominal hollow or solid viscera. All viscera are then placed back in their anatomical locations and the omentum is preserved anteriorly. A film of hyaluronic acid and carboxymethylcellulose may be added prior to fascial closure in an attempt to decrease adhesion formation to the anterior abdominal wall as well as to decrease the complexity of potential reoperative surgery. Closure of the midline fascia should be done with a running monofilament suture. The skin can either be stapled or closed with a running subcuticular absorbable suture.

 POSTOPERATIVE MANAGEMENT

Postoperatively, the routine use of a nasogastric tube is not necessary and may cause morbidity in patients with underlying pulmonary disorders. VTE prophylaxis should be continued throughout the hospitalization unless contraindicated. Pain control should be provided via the epidural catheter that was placed prior to induction, either continuously or via patient-controlled measures. If epidural analgesia is not used then a patient-controlled analgesia device should be used. Early feeding is recommended starting with clear liquids and subsequently with a postgastrectomy diet. Acid reduction therapy is not required after PGV unless it is an integral part of therapy for *Helicobacter pylori* eradication. Resumption of all preoperative medications indicated for significant medical comorbidities should be started as soon as possible. Good pulmonary toilet and early ambulation is recommended. Close clinical observation for the development of complications is mandatory. Patients are typically discharged within 3 to 5 days after an uncomplicated procedure.

 EXPECTED RESULTS AND COMPLICATIONS

Open PGV will yield excellent results with few complications for ulcer patients when the procedure is performed for the proper indications by a surgeon with the requisite skill and knowledge outlined above. The attractive features of PGV are its low morbidity and mortality along with the almost total absence of undesirable side effects of dumping, diarrhea, alkaline reflux, weight loss, and nutritional problems. The most consistent criticism of open PGV has been the variable rate of ulcer recurrence from 2% to 30% reported in the literature. The average recurrence rate should be between 2% and 8% in most centers. This variation is often due to technical factors and surgeon variability as well as their ability to complete the PGV effectively. In addition, distal migration of parietal cells into the antrum may also result in recurrence. For most part, the recurrences of the ulcer diathesis can be managed medically; however, in cases where surgery is necessary, truncal vagotomy with antrectomy with either Billroth I or II reconstruction is recommended. Mortality rates below 0.3% are reported. Dumping and diarrhea have been reported in 3% to 5% of patients but is usually transient. After the operation, the patients may feel some early satiety and upper-abdominal fullness, but these symptoms disappear within a few weeks. Stasis is rare (0.7%) and may be due to either unrecognized pyloric obstruction or complete or near complete antral vagotomy. Jensen demonstrated that the upper 2 to 5 cm of antrum may be denervated without leading to stasis. Stasis that cannot be managed medically often requires reoperation and resection or gastroenterostomy.

✦ CONCLUSIONS

Open PGV is a proven safe and effective operation for the definitive treatment of patients with medically refractory and complicated gastroduodenal ulcer disease in certain clinical settings. Although new paradigms exist today that have revolutionized the treatment of patients with peptic ulcer disease, there still remains a need for occasional definitive ulcer surgery. PGV offers many advantages over truncal vagotomy and antrectomy. It is ironic that the near-ideal surgical procedure finally evolved for the operative treatment of peptic ulcer as the need for such treatment was diminishing.

Recommended References and Readings

Amdrup E, Jensen H-E. Selective vagotomy of the parietal cell mass preserving innervation of the undrained antrum-A preliminary report of results with duodenal ulcer. *Gastroenterology.* 1970; 59:522–527.

Donahue PE, Griffith C, Richter HM. A 50-year perspective upon selective gastric vagotomy. *Am J Surg.* 1996;172:9–12.

Goligher JC. A technique for highly selective (parietal cell or proximal gastric) vagotomy for duodenal ulcer. *Br J Surg.* 1974;61:337–345.

Harkins HN, Stavney LS, Griffith CA, et al. Selective gastric vagotomy. *Ann Surg.* 1963;158:448–460.

Herrington JL, Davidson J. Proximal gastric vagotomy for duodenal ulcer: 7-15 year follow-up. Role of the operation in the treatment of benign gastric ulcer. *Contemp Surg.* 1988;32:17–22.

Herrington JL, Sawyers JL, Scott HW. A twenty-five years experience with vagotomy-antrectomy. *Arch Surg.* 1973;106:469–474.

Johnston D, Wilkinson AR. Highly selective vagotomy without drainage procedure in the treatment of duodenal ulcer. *Br J Surg.* 1970;57:289–296.

Jordan PH. Technique of parietal cell vagotomy. *Surg Rounds.* 1990; September: 17–28.

Jordan PH, Thornby J. Twenty years after parietal cell vagotomy or selective vagotomy antrectomy for treatment of duodenal ulcer final report. *Ann Surg.* 1994;220:283–296.

Katkouda N, Mouiel J. Minimally invasive approaches to ulcer therapy. In: Peters JH, DeMeester TR, eds. *Minimally Invasive Surgery of the Foregut.* 1st ed. London: Churchill Livingstone; 1995:215–229.

Kelly KA, Teotia SS. Proximal gastric vagotomy. In: Fischer JE, ed. *Mastery of Surgery.* 5th ed. Philadelphia, PA: Lippincott Williams and Wilkens; 2007:872–876.

Napolitano L. Refractory peptic ulcer disease. *Gastroenterol Clin N Am.* 2009;38:267–288.

Paul S, Soybel DI, Zinner MJ. Stomach and duodenum; operative procedures. In: Zinner MJ, Ashley SW, eds. *Maingot's Abdominal Operations.* 11th ed. Europe: McGraw-Hill; 2006: 377–416.

Scott-Connor CEH, Dawson DL. Truncal vagotomy and pyloroplasty and highly selective vagotomy. In: Scott-Connor CEH, Dawson DL, eds. *Operative Anatomy.* 3rd ed. Philadelphia, PA: Wolters Kluwer; 2009:380–389.

9 Laparoscopic Proximal Gastric Vagotomy

Namir Katkhouda and Joerg Zehetner

INDICATIONS/CONTRAINDICATIONS

The objective of the procedure is to divide all vagal nerve fibers innervating acid-producing cells of the stomach while preserving the terminal branches of the main vagal trunks and the nerves of Latarjet, thereby maintaining adequate antral motility. The success of the operation depends on meticulous technique because leaving a single fundic nerve branch intact will allow continued acid secretion in the corresponding gastric secretory zone, leading to early recurrence.

In the elective setting the current indications for the surgical treatment of duodenal ulcer disease are as follows:

- Patients in whom the disease is resistant to medical treatment despite medical therapy for at least 2 years and/or two or more documented recurrences after thorough medical treatment.
- Patients who cannot be followed regularly because of geographic or socioeconomic reasons or who cannot afford medication.
- Patients with complications such as perforation or hemorrhage.

Contraindications for the laparoscopic approach are previous operations on the stomach or upper abdomen with major adhesions and portal hypertension, especially in combination with coagulopathy. Other contraindications are patients with untreated *Helicobacter pylori* infection or patients on nonsteroidal anti-inflammatory drugs before presentation.

PREOPERATIVE PLANNING

The preoperative evaluation of the patient includes evaluation of the general medical status, the operative risk factors, comorbidities, and endoscopic and secretory investigation of the peptic ulcer disease.

The endoscopic examination of the upper gastrointestinal tract is done routinely and allows direct inspection of the diseased area. The duodenal ulcer is typically a linear defect without associated stenosis or hemorrhage. It allows biopsies to rule out possible

H. pylori infection as well as other rare diseases which are associated with duodenal ulcers (Crohn's disease). Other diseases such as esophageal cancer or gastroesophageal reflux disease can be ruled out, as these are diseases with similar symptoms to ulcer disease.

The secretory tests include measurements of basal acid output and peak acid output after stimulation with pentagastrin. These tests are necessary to evaluate the degree of acid hypersecretion in patients who are intractable to medical treatment. The serum gastrin level should always be assessed to exclude gastrinoma.

A radiographic videoesophagram and upper gastrointestinal study can be added if the endoscopy cannot assess a possible postpyloric stenosis.

 # SURGERY

As with all laparoscopic procedures, this procedure requires general anesthesia and endotracheal intubation. A nasogastric tube is necessary to deflate the stomach before establishing pneumoperitoneum. A urinary catheter is not routinely placed.

Positioning

The patient is positioned in an inverted Y position with the operating surgeon between the legs (French position). The video monitor is positioned above the head and slightly toward the left shoulder of the patient. If the video tower does not provide a flexible screen, the video endoscopic tower is placed on the left of the patient and a second monitor on the right of the patient. The second (camera) assistant stands to the right of the patient and the first assistant and the scrub nurse stand to the left of the patient. The trunk of the patient is elevated 15 degrees in a reverse Trendelenburg position.

Trocar placement

After establishing the pneumoperitoneum with a Veress needle and an optical trocar or with the Hassan technique, first a 12-mm trocar is inserted in the midline approximately one-third of the distance between the umbilicus and the xiphoid process.

A second 12-mm trocar is placed in the left subcostal position in the midclavicular line as a primary working port. Three additional 5-mm or 10-mm trocars are used:

- One in the subxyphoid position used to make a subcutaneous tract for the introduction of the Nathanson Hook Liver Retractor (Automated Medical Products Corporation, Sewaren, NJ). This retractor is secured to the right bed post using an Iron Intern (Automated Medical Products Corporation, Sewaren, NJ).
- Two retracting ports are placed in the right and left subcostal margins.

Technique

In addition to the standard laparoscopic instruments we recommend the following instruments:

- Clip appliers
- Two laparoscopic needle holders
- An L-shaped hook coagulator
- Absorbable monofilament sutures
- Endoloops with preformed Roeder knot
- Application system for fibrin sealant spray
- Ultrasonically activated coagulating shears

There are two major techniques of laparoscopic proximal gastric (highly selective) vagotomy (PGV) for the surgical treatment of chronic duodenal ulcer disease.

Laparoscopic PGV

The procedure begins by the elevation of the left lobe of the liver using a fan retractor or a liver retractor which is inserted via a 5-mm port next to the xyphoid. The surgeon should be certain that the operation is feasible and that the liver can be retracted so that the operative area is visible. Endoscopic babcock-type clamps provide lateral traction on the greater curvature of the stomach and the lesser omentum is carefully inspected to identify three landmarks: First, the avascular aspect of the lesser omentum, which is crossed by the hepatic branch of the anterior vagus nerve; second, the terminal branch of the anterior vagal nerve (nerve of Latarjet), which runs parallel to the lesser curvature; and third, the terminal "crow's foot."

With ultrasonic shears the anterior leaf of the omentum is incised between the nerve and the stomach proximal to the crow's foot, parallel to the nerve trunk. The lesser omentum is retracted using atraumatic graspers to ensure that the ultrasonic shears divide only the branches of the vagus nerve and not the trunk of the nerve of Latarjet. The identification of individual neurovascular bundles is not necessary. It is important that the blunt jaws of the shears are applied and coapted beyond the vessel to avoid a partial welding that might lead to hemorrhage. Division of the nerves begins at the "crow's foot" of the nerve of Latarjet. The two most distal branches of the nerve are left intact to be sure that antral and pyloric innervation is preserved. After four to five applications of the shears the dissection then proceeds proximally to include the esophageal branches of the anterior vagus nerve. The fat pad of the cardia containing the anterior nerve trunk is then raised upward and to the right to divide the "criminal" nerves of Grassi near the angle of His. The division of these aberrant branches is of paramount importance to ensure complete vagotomy of the posterior fundus.

The dissection returns to the distal stomach, to retract now the opened anterior leaf of the lesser omentum to expose the posterior vagal branches. The posterior leaf is incised between the stomach and the posterior nerve of Latarjet to open the lesser sac. With the ultrasonic shears all branches of the posterior vagus nerve proximal to the crow's foot are divided. Using the magnification of the laparoscope, the distal esophagus should be cleared of all nerve fibers for a length of 6 to 8 cm while the two trunks and their terminal gastric branches are preserved.

Alternatively to the technique described with the ultrasonic shears, the anterior and posterior vagal branches can be divided between endoscopic clips with a scissor or with the hook electrocautery (Fig. 9.1).

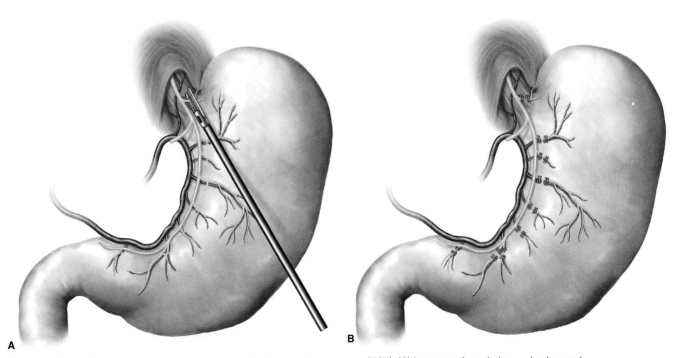

A   **B**

Figure 9.1 The technique of neurovascular ligation in highly selective vagotomy (HSV): **(A)** laparoscopic technique using harmonic shears, **(B)** laparoscopic technique using clips.

Laparoscopic Posterior Truncal Vagotomy with Anterior Seromyotomy (Taylor procedure)

This operation is an alternative approach to the previously described technique and was popularized by Taylor and redefined laparoscopically by Katkhouda. The operation has three steps: the hiatal dissection, the posterior truncal vagotomy, and the anterior seromyotomy.

Hiatal Dissection

With a liver retractor or with a probe over the subxiphoid trocar the left lobe of the liver is retracted. The lesser sac is entered through an opening in the pars flaccida. Dissection is continued with ultrasonic sheers, or alternatively the hook cautery, until the muscular portion of the right crus is reached. If left gastric veins are encountered, they may be divided between clips as necessary. Injury to the hepatic branch of the vagus nerve should be avoided if possible, although there is no evidence that division will result in clinically significant postoperative complications.

Posterior Truncal Vagotomy

There are two major landmarks for the posterior truncal vagotomy, which are the caudate lobe and the right crus (Fig. 9.2). With a right-sided forceps the right crus is grasped and held to the right while the ultrasonic shears or the hook coagulator is used to open the pre-esophageal peritoneum. The abdominal esophagus is retracted to the left, which allows visualization of the areolar tissue. The posterior vagus nerve is identified by its white color. With a grasper the nerve is retracted and adhesions coagulated and divided. The nerve is transected between two clips or with the ultrasonic shears and a segment of the nerve is removed for histopathology.

Figure 9.2 Posterior truncal vagotomy (important landmarks).

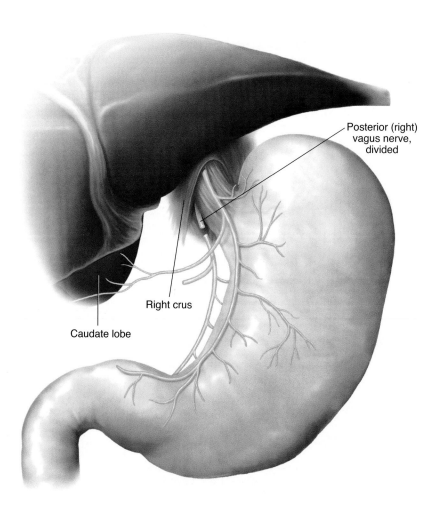

Posterior (right) vagus nerve, divided

Right crus

Caudate lobe

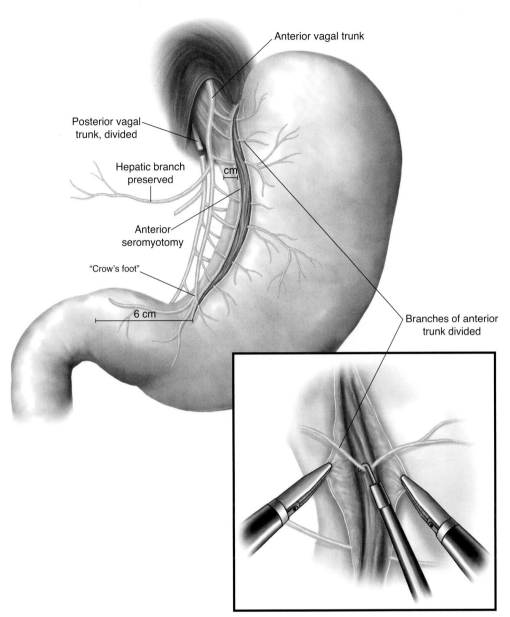

Figure 9.3 Anterior lesser curve seromyotomy.

Anterior vagal trunk

Posterior vagal trunk, divided

Hepatic branch preserved

cm

Anterior seromyotomy

"Crow's foot"

6 cm

Branches of anterior trunk divided

Anterior Seromyotomy

With two graspers the stomach is spread and the anterior aspect is inspected. With the tip of the electrocautery the line of incision is marked, starting from the gastroesophageal junction parallel to and 1.5 cm from the lesser curvature down to 5 to 7 cm from the pylorus at the level of the crow's foot. The two most distal branches of the nerve are left intact to be sure that the antral and pyloric innervation is preserved. The seromyotomy is then performed with the hook coagulator (monopolar current, blending coagulation, average intensity) along the previously marked line (Fig. 9.3). The hook incises the serosal layer, the oblique layer, and the circular muscular layer. The two borders are grasped and spread apart, which breaks the remaining deep circular fibers. Once the fibers are divided, the mucosa can be easily identified by its typical blue color as it bulges out of the incision. It is very important that the incision is anatomically accurate and hemostasis ensured, and on completion the incision appears 7 to 8 mm in width in the gastric wall. Air is injected through the nasogastric tube to make sure there are no mucosal leaks. Alternatively, the leak test can be performed with methylene blue injected through the nasogastric tube or with an endoscope. The seromyotomy is closed with an overlapping running suture and knotted on both ends (Fig. 9.4). By covering the seromyotomy in a nonanatomic fashion

Figure 9.4 Suture for seromyotomy.

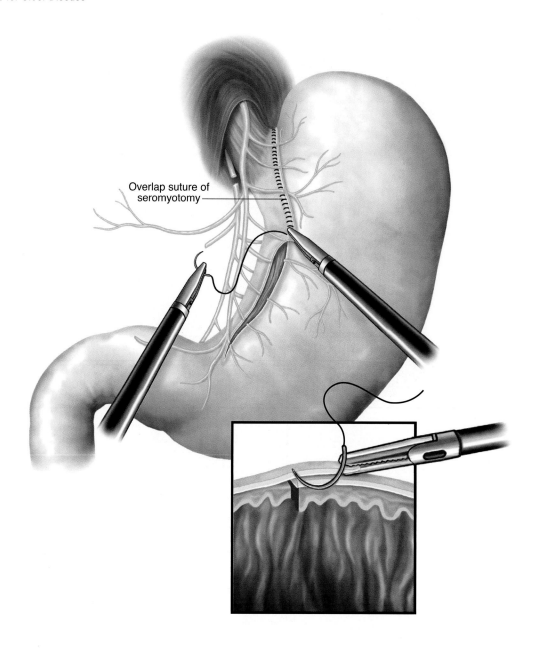

Overlap suture of
seromyotomy

(overlay), postoperative adhesions are prevented; it provides good hemostasis, and nerve regeneration is prevented by the disturbed architecture of the gastric layers.

Other Notes:

The nasogastric tube may be removed at the end of the procedure.

No drainage is placed. Dilation of the pylorus can be performed in the same setting or in a postoperative procedure. A dilation balloon is introduced with a flexible endoscope and moved into the pylorus, inflated to a pressure of 45 psi, and kept in the pylorus for 10 minutes. The success of this procedure is uncertain and might need repetitive sessions to achieve the ideal results.

 POSTOPERATIVE MANAGEMENT

The patient is encouraged to ambulate and resume a soft diet on the evening of the operation. Ideally this operation is performed as an outpatient procedure. PPI or H_2 blockers are continued for at least 4 weeks.

COMPLICATIONS

There is a possibility of leaks from the seromyotomy but this has never been experienced by the authors. In the series published by the senior author of this technical review there was no mortality and a low morbidity of 6.6% (mostly pseudo-obstruction with food postoperatively).

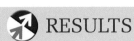 RESULTS

The success of the operation can be measured 4 weeks after surgery with pH monitoring. The mean acid reduction is 82%, and in a published series all patients showed healed ulcers on endoscopy. In 3.5% of patients a recurrent ulcer was found on long-term follow-up.

CONCLUSION

The indication for surgery is rare nowadays since the introduction of PPI and H_2 blockers and the successful medical therapy for the eradication of *H. Pylori.* In certain refractory patients this operation is still considered to be the therapy of choice as gastric resection should not be performed for benign cases such as duodenal ulcers, unless a stricture makes it necessary to perform a subtotal gastrectomy.

Recommended References and Readings

Dallemagne B, Weerts JM, Jehaes C, et al. Laparoscopic highly selective vagotomy. *Br J Surg.* 1994;81: 554–556.
Katkhouda N, Mouiel J. A new technique of surgical treatment of chronic duodenal ulcer without laparotomy by videocoelioscopy. *Am J Surg.* 1991;161:361–364.
Katkhouda N, Waldrep DJ, Campos GMR, et al. An improved technique for laparoscopic highly selective vagotomy using harmonic shears. *Surg Endosc.* 1998;12:1051–1054.
Taylor TV, Gunn AA, Macleod DAD, et al. Anterior lesser curve seromyotomy with posterior truncal vagotomy in the treatment of chronic duodenal ulcer. *Lancet.* 1982;320:846–848.

10 Patch for Perforated Ulcer

David W. Mercer and Matthew R. Goede

 ## INDICATIONS/CONTRAINDICATIONS

Patients with perforated peptic ulcers usually present with acute onset of abdominal pain. Patients frequently report that the pain started "as if someone flipped a switch." However, elderly patients frequently present with a less robust onset of pain. Occasionally, patients will complain of left shoulder pain from diaphragmatic irritation and some will complain of nausea and vomiting. While some patients report a history of recent gastritis, frequent steroid or nonsteroidal anti-inflammatory drug use, or use of cocaine, perforation may be the first clinical sign that patients have underlying peptic ulcer disease. On radiographic imaging, pneumoperitoneum is present in greater that 80% of patients.

Nonoperative management of perforated ulcers has been described since the 1940s; however, its use and patient selection remains a major debate. Patients who present with pneumoperitoneum who have a water-soluble contrast gastroduodenogram showing no extravasation, no signs of septic shock, and abdominal examination findings confined to the upper abdomen may be considered for nonoperative treatment. Nonoperative treatment routinely includes nasogastric decompression, antibiotics to cover enteric pathogens, antibiotics to cover *Helicobacter pylori* if present, and proton pump inhibitors. However, approximately 30% of patients treated nonoperatively do not improve and require surgical intervention. Patients treated nonoperatively also have about a 30% longer inpatient length of stay. Nonoperative management also has an extremely high failure rate (around 70%) in the elderly, patients with comorbidities, patients with hemodynamic instability, perforations greater than 48 hours old, and in patients with impaired wound healing. This creates a dilemma because the patients that you would prefer to treat nonoperatively are the ones most likely to fail nonoperative therapy. Therefore, operative treatment is the preferred modality except in an extremely selective subset of patients.

The classic indication for use of a patch for perforated ulcer is in the unstable patient with shock, the presence of extensive peritonitis or abdominal abscess formation, or patients with severe comorbidities. While patch repair of perforated ulcer was described as a damage control technique, with the development of effective medical therapy for ulcer disease and the corresponding decrease in patients requiring surgical therapy for ulcer disease, more surgeons are utilizing patch repair in the acute setting. In addition, the average age of patients presenting with perforated duodenal ulcers is increasing, with the average age now between 65 and 75 years. With this older age at presentation, it is more likely that these patients will have comorbidities that lead the surgeon to opt for a less involved procedure in the acute phase.

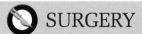 PREOPERATIVE PLANNING

While a large majority of patients do not present in hemodynamic shock, appropriate preoperative resuscitation is still needed. Placement of a nasogastric tube to decompress the stomach and limit peritoneal contamination should be performed. Antibiotics to cover enteric pathogens should be administered, along with appropriate goal-directed crystalloid resuscitation. If possible, a determination of the presence of *H. pylori* through a serum antibody test should be done to aid in operative planning. Urea breath tests should not be done in patients with suspected perforation. In addition, the operative plan should be decided based on the patient's presentation. Patients who present with hemodynamic instability, signs of end-organ failure, or shock should be classified as unstable.

- Gastric ulcer
  - Unstable patients should be treated with patch repair and biopsy of ulcer or ulcer resection depending on the location of gastric ulcer.
  - Patients with known *H. pylori* may be treated with patch repair and *H. pylori* eradication and biopsy.
  - In medication-induced ulcers, in which the medication regimen can be altered, patients may be treated with patch repair and biopsy.
  - Stable patients who are known to be *H. pylori*-negative, patients with a long history of peptic ulcer disease, or patients with essential medication needs (chronic steroid use) should undergo a definitive antiulcer procedure.
- Duodenal ulcer
  - Unstable patients should be treated with patch repair.
  - Initial presentation of duodenal ulcer disease, especially if *H. pylori* is present, can be treated with patch repair, proton pump inhibitors, and *H. pylori* eradication.
  - Stable patients with ulcer disease refractory to proton pump inhibitors and *H. pylori* eradication should be treated with a definitive antiulcer procedure.

In patients who are profoundly septic, are hypotensive, or on vasopressors, one must carefully consider if a patient can tolerate pneumoperitoneum before proceeding with a laparoscopic repair. Also in patients with extensive previous abdominal surgery, significant duodenal scarring, or concomitant bleeding ulcer, the use of laparoscopy may be limited. Given the intra-abdominal inflammatory process caused by the perforation, the technique for obtaining initial intra-abdominal access may need to be modified.

SURGERY

Open Technique

- Patient is placed supine.
- Sequential compression devices and urinary catheter are placed.
- Abdomen is entered through an upper midline incision to allow for exploration of entire abdomen if gastric or duodenal perforation is not the cause of peritonitis.
- Following repair of the perforation, a thorough irrigation of the abdomen with attention paid at the right and left subphrenic spaces and pelvis should be done.

The laparoscopic approach is becoming more widely used in these patients. Laparoscopy offers several advantages, most notably the magnification provided by the laparoscope, less postoperative pain, fewer postoperative pneumonias, and fewer wound complications. Also laparoscopy affords the ability to examine the entire abdomen without extending or relocating incisions, which is especially helpful when the exact location of the perforation has not been identified preoperatively. It also aids in performing a thorough inspection and irrigation of the entire abdomen under direct visualization.

Patch Techniques

Frequently any omental reinforcement of an ulcer perforation is referred to as a Graham patch. The original nonpedicled patch (Fig. 10.1A) described by Graham is infrequently used today in favor of pedicled omental flaps. Maintaining a vascular pedicle allows the omentum to remain alive and continue in its natural function as "watchdog" of the abdomen.

- Primary closure with omental pedicle flap (Fig. 10.1B)
  - Used in small ulcers where the tissue has minimal inflammation and can be brought together easily, without narrowing the duodenum.
  - Edges of ulcer are debrided if necessary, and the defect is closed primarily in a transverse orientation, usually in a single layer using 2-0 or 3-0 silk.
  - A vascularized pedicle of omentum is brought up to cover the repair.
    - The pedicle is secured in place with the long tails of the ulcer closure sutures or separate tacking sutures of 3-0 silk around the margins of the primary closure.
- Omental pedicle flap (Cellan–Jones repair) (Fig. 10.1C and Fig. 10.2)
  - Excise friable edges.
    - Send the gastric specimen for pathologic examination.
  - Classically place four to six 3-0 sutures through the viscera wall, transversing the ulcer.
  - Anchor an omental pedicle with a single suture beyond the ulcer.
  - Tie the previously placed sutures down like an "archway" over the length of the pedicle thereby securing the omentum firmly within the edges of the perforation.
  - The lack of primary closure decreases the risk of narrowing the duodenum in the case of a large perforation.

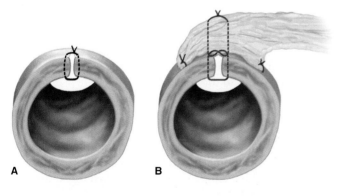

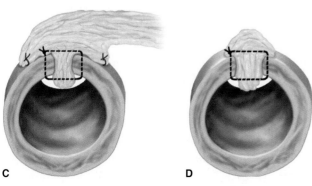

Figure 10.1 A–D: Different techniques to apply omental patch to close perforated ulcer.

A

B

C

D

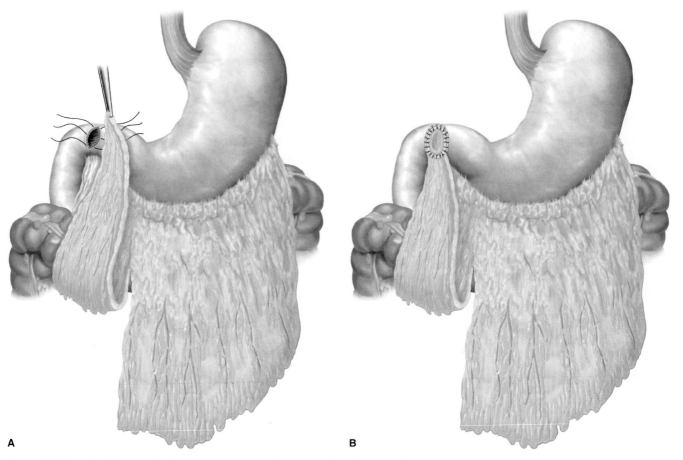

A   **B**

Figure 10.2 **A** and **B**: Different techniques to secure omental patch using long tails or tacking sutures.

- Free omental plug (Graham patch) (Fig. 10.1D)
  - The lack of primary closure decreases the risk of narrowing the duodenum in the case of a large perforation.
  - Place approximately three sutures parallel to the long axis of the duodenum across the ulcer.
  - Place a piece of free omentum within the ulcer defect and tie the sutures over the top of the free graft to secure the omentum to the ulcer defect.
    - Relies on the free piece of omentum to serve as a scaffold on which the body can secrete fibrin.
- Serosal patch
  - Used in large perforations, frequently following traumatic duodenal injuries
  - A loop of jejunum is brought up to cover the perforation and is sewn circumferentially to the edges of the ulcer once they have been debrided in a fashion similar to a small bowel anastomosis; however, the bowel is not opened.

Operative Pearls

- Unless excised, gastric ulcers should always undergo biopsy prior to closure or patch repair. These biopsies are essential given the risk of gastric cancer leading to perforation or the presence of *H. pylori* infection involved with perforation.
- The sutures used to secure the omental patch should not be overly tightened, as doing such would compromise the vascular supply to the patch.
- The repair can be tested either by filling the upper abdomen with saline and then instilling air through the nasogastric tube or by the placement of methylene blue dye down through the nasogastric tube.

■ Placement of a nasojejunal tube should be considered prior to repair of large ulcers to allow the possibility of enteral feeding beyond perforation.

  ■ In elderly or debilitated patients or in patients with a high concern of possible continued leak, placement of a jejunostomy tube for distal enteral feedings should be considered if the patient is tolerating anesthesia.

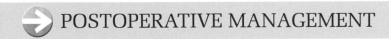 POSTOPERATIVE MANAGEMENT

Inpatient

■ While the duration of nasogastric tube decompression remains controversial, many surgeons promote at least a brief period of gastric decompression to allow time for the patch to fully adhere to the visceral wall.

■ Drains are rarely left anymore; however, if placed, drains should be closely monitored for the presence of bile. The peritonitis associated with a perforated peptic ulcer frequently leads to a significant amount of fibrin deposition, which makes drains nonfunctional after just a day or two.

■ Tachycardia may be the earliest sign of developing sepsis or a continued leak from the repair.

■ Patients should be started on intravenous proton pump inhibitors postoperatively and converted over to oral once tolerating a diet.

Outpatient

■ *H. pylori* infection is present in 80% of gastric ulcer perforations and 90% of duodenal perforations. All patients should undergo evaluation for and treatment of *H. pylori* infection if present following recovery from their perforation and discharge from the hospital.

  ■ If follow-up endoscopy is planned to evaluate for ulcer healing (required in gastric ulcers to rule out malignancy), endoscopic biopsies of the gastric antrum can be performed to evaluate for the presence/eradication of *H. pylori*.

  ■ Urea breath tests and stool antigen tests can also be done to detect *H. pylori* infection and determine whether it has been eradicated.

■ If *H. pylori* is detected, appropriate triple therapy including proton pump inhibitor and antibiotics should be administered and eradication again confirmed.

  ■ If eradication is not achieved, repeat treatment with quadruple therapy should be considered.

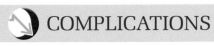 COMPLICATIONS

Continued leak has been reported in 5% to 10% of patients treated with omental patch repair. Patients with suspicion of a continued leak should be evaluated by a water-soluble contrast study. If the leak is small or contained, one could entertain treating the collection with percutaneous techniques; however, the possibility exists of developing a persistent fistula, which, depending on the patient's condition, could be a desirable outcome over reoperation.

If the persistent leak is from a gastric ulcer, a wedge resection may be possible. However, if one is going to reoperate on a patient, a definitive antiulcer procedure should be attempted unless the patient remains septic or the degree of inflammation or contamination is prohibitive.

If the persistent leak is from a duodenal ulcer, again a definitive ulcer operation needs to be strongly considered. In a septic patient, triple tube therapy including a gastrostomy for proximal drainage, a jejunostomy with the tube fed retrograde to drain the duodenum near the perforation, and a distal jejunostomy for enteral feeding should be placed. A duodenostomy should be avoided to drain the duodenum as this will limit future attempts at definitive surgical treatment.

Intra-abdominal abscess formation is possible and can usually be treated with radiographically guided percutaneous techniques. In the past, abdominal irrigation through drains left at the initial operation was attempted, which did not decrease abscess formation and significantly increased demands on the healthcare providers to monitor the continuous input and output. Likewise, the routine placement of drains in the peritoneal cavity has not decreased the incidence of abscess formation.

Sepsis is frequently the complication that leads to death in these patients. Most of these patients warrant at least brief observation in an intensive care unit postoperatively, and healthcare providers must vigilantly observe for signs of sepsis even when the patient is sent to the general surgical ward. Empiric antibiotics with a broad spectrum should be continued depending on the degree of peritoneal contamination. Empiric antifungal coverage should be considered as well given the proximal nature of this visceral perforation. Patients who develop overwhelming sepsis should be started on antifungal coverage, as frequently by the time the fungus is isolated from blood or peritoneal cultures the patient has already succumbed to the sepsis.

RESULTS

- The mortality of perforated peptic ulcers is around 3% for healthy, younger patients.
- Unfortunately the mortality rate can approach 30% in elderly and debilitated patients.
- In perforated duodenal ulcers the use of patch repair followed by effective medical acid suppression and *H. pylori* eradication has a 1-year recurrence rate of around 5%.

CONCLUSIONS

The use of patch repair for perforated ulcer is more frequent now than in past years. The introduction of effective acid-suppressing medications, a better understanding of the role of *H. pylori* and its eradication, introduction of minimally invasive techniques, and the decreasing experience with acid-reducing procedures have led many surgeons to depend on patch repair as their technique of choice in the acute setting.

Recommended References and Readings

Boey J, Wong J, Ong GB. Prospective study of operative risk factors in perforated duodenal ulcers. *Ann Surg.* 1982;195:265.

Cellan-Jones CJ. A rapid method of treatment in perforated duodenal ulcer. *Br Med J.* 1929;1(3571):1076–1077.

Crofts TJ, Park KG, Steele RJ, et al. A randomized trial of nonoperative treatment for perforated peptic ulcer. *N Engl J Med.* 1989; 320:970–973.

Donovan AJ, Berne TV, Donovan JA. Perforated duodenal ulcer: An alternative therapeutic plan. *Arch Surg.* 1998;133:1166–1171.

Feliciano DV. Do perforated ulcers need an acid-decreasing surgical procedure now that omeprazole is available? *Surg Clin North Am.* 1992;72:369.

Graham RR. The surgeon's responsibility in the treatment of duodenal ulcer. *Can Med Assoc J.* 1936;35(3):263–268.

Kauffman GL. Duodenal ulcer disease: Treatment by surgery, antibiotics or both. *Adv Surg.* 2000;34:121.

Lau H. Laparoscopic repair of perforated peptic ulcer: A meta-analysis. *Surg Endosc.* 2004;18:1013.

Ng EK, Lam YH, Sung JJ, et al. Eradication of *Helicobacter pylori* prevents recurrence of ulcer after simple closure of duodenal ulcer perforation: Randomized controlled trial. *Ann Surg.* 2000; 231:153–158.

Siu WT, Leong HT, Law BK, et al. Laparoscopic repair for perforated peptic ulcer: a randomized controlled trial. *Ann Surg.* 2002; 235: 313–319.

Taylor H. Perforated peptic ulcer; treated without operation. *Lancet.* 1946;2(6422):441–444.

11 Laparoscopic Patch of Perforated Duodenal Ulcer

Sunil Sharma and Bestoun H. Ahmed

 ## INDICATIONS/CONTRAINDICATIONS

The success of medical management of peptic ulcer disease has reduced the overall need for surgical intervention. But, the incidence of perforation, which is a serious and potentially fatal complication, remains the same (5% to 10%). The surgical intervention of simple closure of the perforation with or without omentoplasty is accepted in most of these patients. Modern antiulcer therapy (i.e., H_2 receptor antagonists or proton pump inhibitors [PPI] with anti-*Helicobacter pylori* agents) has decreased the high recurrence rate from 40% to 3–4%.

Laparoscopic patch of perforated duodenal ulcer has become an alternative method to the open procedure since its initial report in 1989 by Mouret. It offers advantages of better visualization of the peritoneal cavity, thorough lavage and lack of upper abdominal incision with its related complications, especially in high-risk patients. The need for definitive surgical procedures is diminishing. However, it depends on the chronicity and intractability of the disease.

Laparoscopic closure is a favorable method in most patients. It is especially indicated in

- those with age less than 70 years,
- symptoms persisting less than 24 hours,
- absence of shock on admission,
- American Society of Anesthesiologists grade less than III, and
- perforation smaller than 10 mm in diameter (Fig. 11.1).

There are no absolute contraindications for the laparoscopic approach. It is preferable to avoid this approach in patients with Boey's score of 2 or 3. Patients with such a score range are associated with high morbidity and mortality. Boey score (0 to 3) is the count of Boey risk factors: shock on admission, American Society of Anesthesiologists grade III to V, and prolonged perforation. A Boey score of 0 means low surgical risk; otherwise, it is considered a high surgical risk.

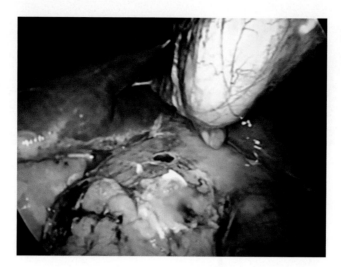

Figure 11.1 Perforated duodenal ulcer. (Image courtesy of D. Oleynikov, University of Nebraska Medical Center.)

 PREOPERATIVE PLANNING

- Diagnosis is achieved by the history of sudden onset of abdominal pain with abdominal findings indicating peritonitis. Free air under the diaphragm is expected in 85% of patients. Usually, no further diagnostic measures are indicated.
- Following diagnosis, the preoperative resuscitation is achieved by intravenous fluids (crystalloids), nasogastric intubation, and urinary catheterization.
- Therapeutic intravenous antibiotics should be started preoperatively and continued postoperatively. Once the patient tolerates oral intake, antibiotics will be switched to an oral formula which treats *H. pylori* organisms.
- H$_2$ blockers or PPI should also be started preoperatively and continued throughout the postoperative period.
- These patients must be scheduled for urgent laparoscopic exploration.
- Diagnostic laparoscopy is indicated in all patients except the minority who present with a high Boey's score. For this small group of patients, starting with exploratory laparotomy is the safest approach.

 SURGERY

Positioning

- The patient should be in supine position with sequential compression devices and safety belts on the lower extremities. Both arms should be tucked to allow freedom of movement for the surgeon and assistants.
- Some surgeons prefer to stand between the patient's legs while others perform the procedure from the patient's left side.
- Standing on the patient's right side makes suturing an easier task. But, change of position may be needed to achieve an efficient peritoneal lavage (Fig. 11.2).

SURGICAL TECHNIQUE

- Under general anesthesia, the patient is placed in a 15- to 20-degree reverse Trendelenburg position. The operating surgeon stands on the patient's left. This initial position allows better diagnostic exploration and more efficient peritoneal lavage. An

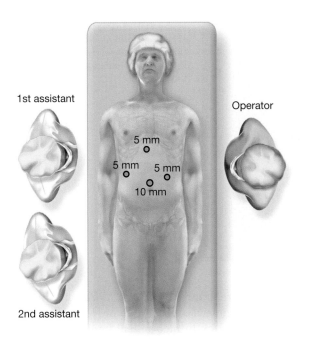

Figure 11.2 An example of port site placement.

assistant stands on the right side. Later the surgeon may switch the position to the right side for easier suturing.

- All port sites should be infiltrated both subdermally and preperitoneally with 0.5% bupivacaine prior to incision or creation of the trocar path.

- Through a 2-mm-long left hypochondrial stab incision just inferior to the costal margin at the midclavicular line, the carbon dioxide pneumoperitoneum (up to 15 mm Hg) is established with a Veress needle.

- After establishing the pneumoperitoneum, through a 10-mm-long supraumbilical curvilinear incision a 10-mm trocar is placed and an angled laparoscope with 30° or 45° is introduced and the entire abdominal cavity is thoroughly investigated. If the laparoscopic findings correspond with the preliminary diagnosis of perforated ulcer, additional trocars are placed under laparoscopic view.

- A 5-mm port is placed one hand-breadth below the left costal margin at the midclavicular line. This port is used as the right-handed working port and can be used to introduce the ski-needle and suture or could be exchanged for a 12-mm port if a regular curved needle or an Endostitch (Covidien, Norwalk, CT, USA) is used. Another 5-mm port is placed in the right hypochondrium at the midclavicular line one hand-breadth from the liver edge on the abdominal wall below the costal margin. This port is the left-handed working port.

- If the liver is covering the perforation site, a 5-mm trocar is placed in the midepigastric region and used for liver and gallbladder retraction (Fig. 11.3).

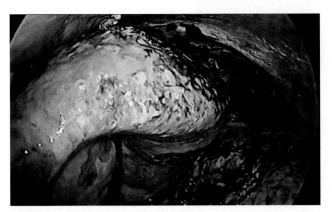

Figure 11.3 The liver is covered by bile-stained fibrinous membrane.

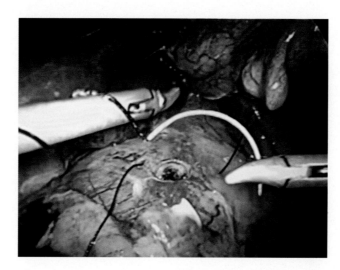

Figure 11.4 Laparoscopic primary closure of perforated duodenal ulcer. (Image courtesy of D. Oleynikov, University of Nebraska Medical Center.)

- After the ulcer size is carefully measured with reference to the 5-mm-diameter working laparoscopic instrument, the perforation is closed with double or triple Vicryl or silk sutures (Fig. 11.4). The perforation is closed by intracorporeal knotting with an omental patch (omentopexy) directly applied to the perforation site (Modified Graham's technique). This approach avoids tension on the inflamed ulcer margin and cutting through the tissue (Figs. 11.5 and 11.6).
- It is critical to avoid anchoring the posterior duodenal wall when these sutures are applied. The best approach is to pull the needle through the perforation and reinserting it through the perforation to complete the next half of the stitch.
- Giant duodenal ulcer perforations (greater than 2 cm in diameter) are better to be dealt with by open exploration and definitive acid reduction operation. Great care should be practiced to avoid duodenal narrowing when closing larger perforations.
- Intracorporeal knotting is the preferred method. Extracorporeal suturing technique could be used for small ulcers with little inflammation. This should be done with care to avoid cutting through the friable ulcer margin.
- The air–fluid leak test is optional as this may lead to overdistension of the bowel.
- Thorough peritoneal lavage is another key intervention of the operation. This is performed using 3 to 5 L of warm normal saline with the patient in various positions. Special attention is given to potential spaces for collection. These are bilateral subdiaphragmatic, subhepatic, lateral paracolic gutters, and pelvic cavities.
- Drainage of the peritoneal cavity is not necessary.
- All ports larger than 5 mm are closed with the help of a transabdominal suture passer device using 0-Vicryl suture material to close the fascia.

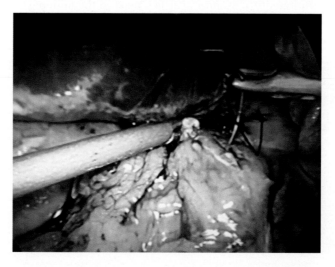

Figure 11.5 Placing tacking sutures for patch repair of perforated duodenal ulcer. (Image courtesy of D. Oleynikov, University of Nebraska Medical Center.)

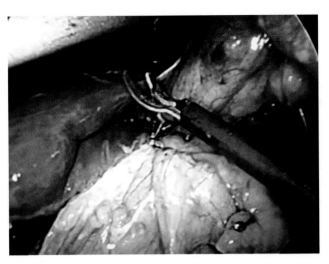

Figure 11.6 Completed pedicled omental patch of perforated duodenal ulcer. (Image courtesy of D. Oleynikov, University of Nebraska Medical Center.)

Alternative Techniques

Alternative methods have been described to close the perforation if suture repair is challenging. Examples of these methods are as follows:

- Closure of the perforation by a gelatin sponge glued into the perforation
- The perforation is closed by fibrin glue.
- The automatic stapler has been used for perforation site closure.
- The simple "one-stitch" repair with omental patch.
- Use of running suture to avoid intracorporeal or extracorporeal knotting,
- Combined laparoscopic–endoscopic repair.

Definitive Ulcer Surgery

- The policy of simple closure alone without definitive procedures is sufficient, provided it is followed by anti-*H. pylori* antibiotics and PPI management.
- This is especially true for patients who are poor surgical risks with severe peritonitis.
- Performing an elective definitive procedure is now restricted to
  - those patients with a long history of dyspepsia (more than 3 months) with rapid recurrence of symptoms following discontinuation of H_2 blockers or PPI;
  - those with true recurrence
  - those with other complications of ulcer (e.g., stricture);
  - Giant duodenal ulcer.
- Definitive procedures such as posterior truncal vagotomy and anterior highly selective vagotomy or anterior seromyotomy can be performed laparoscopically.

➔ POSTOPERATIVE MANAGEMENT

- All patients receive intravenous fluids, nasogastric tube decompression, and parenteral analgesics.
- The nasogastric tube should be removed after 24 to 48 hours according to its output.
- Upper GI study to confirm absence of leak is optional and depends on the magnitude of inflammation and delay in presentation.
- Oral intake is started in general after 48 hours, beginning with clear liquids and advanced accordingly. This depends on the degree of peritonitis and hence the duration of bowel recovery.

- Perioperative administration of intravenous antibiotics to cover bowel organisms is essential as well as intravenous PPI or H_2 blockers.
- Once oral intake is established, the triple therapy regimen is initiated which consists of clarithromycin and amoxicillin for 14 days, in addition to a PPI for 4 weeks.
- This is followed by esophagogastroduodenoscopy after 2 months to check the healing status of the ulcer and existence of persistent *H. pylori* organisms.

RESULTS

- The incidence of perforated duodenal ulcer has not been reduced comparably despite the overall decline in the incidence of complicated peptic ulcer disease. That may be due to the widespread use of nonsteroidal anti-inflammatory drugs in the last three decades.
- Laparoscopic closure of the perforation offers important advantages:
  - Decreasing postoperative pain
  - Less abdominal wall complications
  - Improved quality of visualization and peritoneal lavage.
- Some argue against the laparoscopic choice as being a time-consuming procedure, in addition to the equipment costs; however, the operative time decreases with experience.
- No significant difference has been found in the time of postoperative recovery and hospital stay in comparison to the open method (laparotomy), which is probably due to the degree of peritonitis and intestinal ileus. But, it leads to earlier return to the previous lifestyle.

COMPLICATIONS

- The pooled estimate of the effect in the meta-analyses of multiple randomized controlled trials showed that the incidence of complications was no higher after laparoscopic (17.2%) than open repair (17.8%), $p = 0.50$.
- Comparing the laparoscopic group to the open approach, the incidence of complications are as follows:
  - Suture-site leakage after using laparoscopic omental patch repair is statistically comparable to the traditional laparotomy repair.
  - The incidences of thoracic complications (pneumonia and pleural complications), prolonged postoperative ileus, and intra-abdominal abscess formation were no different.
  - The wound complications rate: the pooled estimate favored laparoscopic over open repair.
  - Meta-analysis showed a higher reoperation rate after laparoscopic repair, but the difference was not significant ($p = 0\cdot10$).
  - The pooled estimate of the mortality rate favored laparoscopic repair and the difference was statistically significant ($p < 0\cdot001$). However, meta-analysis of randomized controlled trials did not demonstrate any significant reduction in mortality following laparoscopic repair ($p = 0\cdot63$).

CONCLUSIONS

- In case of suspected perforated duodenal ulcer, laparoscopy should be advocated as a diagnostic and a potential therapeutic tool.
- Laparoscopic omental patch repair with intracorporeal knotting is the preferred approach.
- Triple anti-*H. pylori* and PPI therapy is required in the postoperative period.
- Closure of perforated duodenal ulcer allows early return to normal lifestyle and has a lower incidence of abdominal wall complications.

Recommended References and Readings

Al Aali AY, Bestoun HA. Laparoscopic repair of perforated duodenal ulcer. *MEJEM*. 2002;2(1):15–19.

Alvarado-Aparicio H, Moreno-Portillo M. Multimedia article: management of duodenal ulcer perforation with combined laparoscopic and endoscopic methods. *Surg Endosc*. 2004;18:1394.

Bergamaschi R, Mårvik R, Johnsen G, et al. Open vs laparoscopic repair of perforated peptic ulcer. *Surg Endosc*. 1999;13:679–682.

Bertleff M, Lange J. Laparoscopic correction of perforated peptic ulcer: first choice? A review of literature. *Surg Endosc*. 2010; 24(6):1231–1239.

Kirshtein B, Bayme M, Lantsberg L, et al. Laparoscopic treatment of gastroduodenal perforations: comparison with conventional surgery. *Surg Endosc*. 2005;19:1487–1490.

Lam O, Lam M, Hui E, et al. Laparoscopic repair of perforated duodenal ulcers: the "three-stitch" Graham patch technique. *Surg Endosc*. 2005;19(12):1627–1630.

Lau H. Laparoscopic repair of perforated peptic ulcer. *Surg Endosc*. 2004;18:1013–1021.

Lunevicius R, Morkevicius M. Comparison of laparoscopic vs open repair for perforated duodenal ulcers. *Surg Endosc*. 2005;19:1565–1571.

Lunevicius R, Morkevicius M. Systematic review comparing laparoscopic and open repair for perforated peptic ulcer. *Br J Surg*. 2005;92:1195–1207.

Mahvi DM, Krantz SB. Stomach. Chapter: 49. In: Townsend, ed. *Sabiston Textbook of Surgery*. 19th ed. Philadelphia, PA: Elsevier Saunders; 2012.

Millat B, Fingerhut A, Borie F, et al. Surgical treatment of complicated duodenal ulcers: controlled trials. *World J. Surg*. 2000;24: 299–306.

Mouret P, Francois Y, Vagnal J, et al. Laparoscopic treatment of perforated peptic ulcer. *Br J Surg*. 1990;77:1006.

Sebastian M, Chandran VP, El Ashaal YI, Sim AJ. *Helicobacter pylori* infection in perforated peptic ulcer disease. *Br J Surg*. 1995;82:360–362.

Siu W, Leong H, Law B. Laparoscopic repair for perforated peptic ulcer. A randomized controlled trial. *Ann Surg*. 2002;235(3):313–319.

SO JB, Kum CK, Fernandes ML, et al. Comparison between laparoscopic and conventional omental patch repair for perforated duodenal ulcer. *Surg Endosc*. 1996;10:1060–1063.

Song K, Kim K, Park C, et al. Laparoscopic repair of perforated duodenal ulcers: the simple "one-stitch" suture with omental patch technique. *Surg Endosc*. 2008;22:1632–1635.

12 Ligation Bleeding Ulcer, Vagotomy, Pyloroplasty

Eric S. Hungness

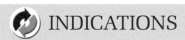 INDICATIONS

Despite the significant decrease in the surgical treatment of complicated peptic ulcer over the past two decades, duodenal ulcer remains one of the most common sources of upper gastrointestinal (UGI) bleeding. The incidence of bleeding from duodenal ulcers that is severe enough to necessitate emergency endoscopic or operative intervention also has not decreased over the past decade.

Patients may present with hematemesis or melena in varying degree of hypovolemic shock. If the patient is unstable, he or she should be taken to an intensive care unit and resuscitated immediately. Resuscitation of an unstable patient is begun by establishing a secure airway and ensuring adequate ventilation. Oxygen should be given, with a low threshold for endotracheal intubation. Isotonic crystalloid is infused after reliable intravenous (two large bore, short peripheral catheters) catheters are placed. For patients in class 3 or 4 shock or those with poor peripheral access, a single lumen 8 French central line should be considered. A urinary catheter should be inserted with close monitoring of urine output. A complete blood count, blood chemistries (including tests of liver function and renal function), and measurement of the prothrombin time and the partial thromboplastin time should be drawn, and a specimen should be sent to the blood bank for typing and crossmatching.

Attempts to establish the cause of bleeding should only be attempted after the initial measures to protect the airway and stabilize the patient have been completed. The next step is nasogastric (NG) aspiration. A bloody aspirate is an indication for esophagogastroduodenoscopy, as is a clear, nonbilious aspirate if a bleeding site distal to the pylorus has not been excluded. The source of the bleeding is unlikely to be the stomach or duodenum with a nonbloody, bile-stained aspirate. Nonetheless, if subsequent evaluation of the lower GI tract for the source of the bleeding is unrewarding, a duodenal ulcer that had stopped bleeding prior to NG tube passage should still be considered. Esophagogastroduodenoscopy should then be performed to confirm the presence of a duodenal ulcer. Most bleeding duodenal ulcers may be controlled endoscopically, although the degree of success to be expected in individual cases varies according to the expertise of the endoscopist.

In general, a 6-unit blood transfusion or bleeding that is not able to be controlled endoscopically mandates surgical intervention. Likewise, ongoing hemorrhage in a hemodynamically unstable patient (especially an elderly one) calls for immediate surgical therapy. The following endoscopic findings for patients whose bleeding is controlled endoscopically should also be strongly considered for surgical therapy: (1) a visible vessel, (2) active bleeding, (3) adherent clot, and (4) giant ulcers.

If the bleeding is controlled endoscopically, intravenous proton pump inhibitor therapy should be given either in a bolus twice daily or by continuous infusion. Antibiotics directed against *Helicobacter pylori* (e.g., a 14-day course of metronidazole, 500 mg p.o., t.i.d.; omeprazole, 20 mg p.o., b.i.d.; and clarithromycin, 500 mg p.o., b.i.d.) should be administered if the organism is present, as treatment has been shown to reduce rebleeding rates. If bleeding recurs, a second attempt at endoscopic control should be made. Repeat endoscopic treatment reduces the need for surgery without increasing the risk of death and is associated with fewer complications than surgery.

For patients who do require urgent operative intervention from a bleeding duodenal ulcer, duodenotomy, suture control of hemorrhage, and subsequent pyloroplasty and truncal vagotomy allows for best balance between expeditious and effective treatment. Some have advocated selective vagotomy or highly selective vagotomy to reduce postvagotomy syndromes; however, selective vagotomy affords little advantage over truncal vagotomy. Moreover, highly selective vagotomy is a procedure that most surgeons are unfamiliar with and requires significant expertise to effectively reduce the chance of rebleeding. The proximal (truncal) vagus nerve anatomy is more consistent resulting in the fact that truncal vagotomy is more easily reproduced and expeditious when performed by the majority of surgeons.

 PREOPERATIVE PLANNING

There is limited preoperative planning as these cases are usually performed in an urgent or emergent basis. All patients who present with UGI bleeding should routinely have

- type and cross for 6 units,
- two sites of reliable intravenous access,
- correction of coagulopathy.

 SURGERY

Positioning

Patients should be placed in a supine position and prepped and draped in standard fashion for general anesthesia so that the anesthesia team has easy access to the IV lines. A reliable arterial line should be placed for continuous blood pressure monitoring and arterial blood gas analysis. These patients are prone to relative hypothermia due to the large volume of crystalloid and blood products infused, thus an upper or lower Bair hugger should be placed and fluid warmers used as necessary. Mechanical compression devices are applied for thromboprophylaxis, and patients should receive appropriate preoperative IV antibiotics. A Bookwalter or Omni retractor is usually necessary for these cases, so having one arm tucked may be useful. A functional NG tube and urinary catheter should have been placed preoperatively.

Exposure

An upper midline celiotomy is made from the xiphoid to just above the umbilicus. This usually provides adequate exposure for both parts of the operation. It is often necessary to extend the incision proximally to the left of the xiphoid to gain adequate exposure to the hiatus. A Bookwalter or Atlas retractor is usually required, particularly for the vagotomy portion of the operation to elevate the rib cage. It may also be necessary to take down the triangular ligament and mobilize the left lobe of the liver to optimize hiatal exposure. Care must be taken with adequate padding to retract the left lobe medially and avoid liver laceration.

Duodenotomy and Ligation of Bleeding Vessel

After the abdomen is carefully inspected and any adhesiolysis completed, retractors are placed to optimize exposure of the distal stomach and duodenum. Appropriate positioning of the NG tube is confirmed. After the pylorus is located, two 3-0 traction sutures are placed cephalad and caudal approximately 1 cm apart on the pylorus muscle, and a 6-cm enterotomy is made to expose the posterior bleeding ulcer (Fig. 12.1). Typically, the well-described "vein of Mayo" can help identify the pylorus. Manual finger pressure can temporarily control active bleeding to allow the anesthesia team to restore the intravascular volume in patients with hypovolemic shock. The bleeding vessel is usually from the gastroduodenal artery that runs cephalad to caudad or a branch of the gastroduodenal artery that may have a more medial course toward the pancreas. Therefore, a superior, inferior, and "U" stitch should be placed to ensure adequate vascular control (Fig. 12.2). Care must be made not to take excessively deep bites as to avoid injury to the common bile duct. Once the bleeding is stopped, attention is placed on closing the duodenotomy with a Heineke–Mikulicz pyloroplasty.

Heineke–Mikulicz Pyloroplasty

The pyloroplasty is started by placing the initial traction sutures on tension to create the cephalad and caudad corners of the transverse closure (Fig. 12.3). The full thickness

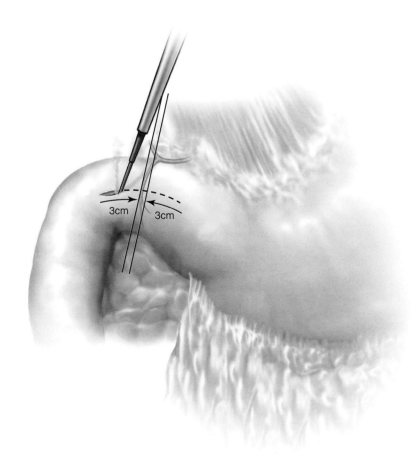

Figure 12.1 Traction sutures are placed using the "vein of Mayo" to help identify the pylorus. A 6-cm longitudinal is positioned midway at the pylorus to adequately expose the posterior duodenal bulb and identify the bleeding duodenal ulcer.

3cm   3cm

Figure 12.2 Tension on the traction sutures allows visualization of the posterior duodenal wall and the bleeding gastroduodenal artery. Adequate suture ligation requires three sutures: superior, inferior, and the "U-stitch" to control the lateral pancreatic branch.

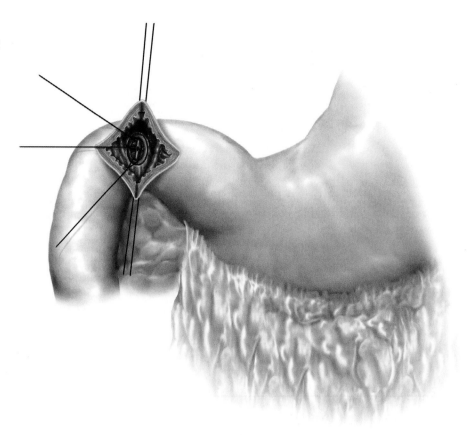

Figure 12.3 A Heineke–Mikulicz pyloroplasty is performed using the traction sutures as the superior and the inferior corners of the transverse closure.

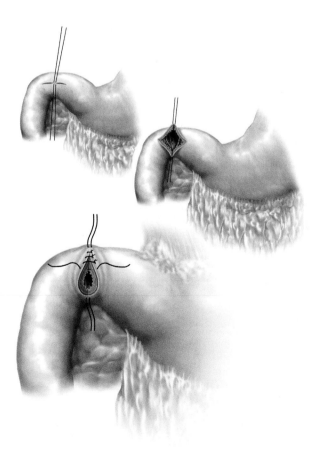

closure with 3-0 silk sutures can be either single- or two-layered. With a single-layered closure, the corners usually appear "dog-eared," tempting surgeons to add a second layer. Care must be taken to avoid narrowing the lumen if the corners are turned in or a second layer of Lembert sutures are placed. If there appears to be excessive tension on the closure, the duodenum should be mobilized by freeing the lateral attachments with a full Kocher maneuver. A tongue of omentum can be mobilized to buttress the repair.

Truncal Vagotomy

The choice of vagotomy is highly dependent on the surgeon's experience and the patient's characteristics; however, truncal vagotomy is the procedure of choice for patients requiring surgical treatment for bleeding duodenal ulcer. The operating surgeon should stand on the patient's right side. This procedure is started by gaining adequate exposure to the upper abdomen and esophageal hiatus. A liver retractor for the Bookwalter is used to elevate the left lobe of the liver. Another option is to free the triangular ligament and fold the left hepatic lobe medially. The stomach is retracted inferiorly with Babcock clamps. The pars flaccida is opened and proximally divided toward the phrenoesophageal ligament which is likewise divided transversely at the esophageal hiatus (Fig. 12.4). The anterior mediastinum is entered with gentle manual blunt dissection using the thumb and index finger to develop the mediastinal dissection (Fig. 12.5). The esophagus is circumferentially dissected using the NG tube as a guide, and the anterior and posterior vagus branches are identified. The placement of a Penrose drain around the esophagus is sometimes useful for inferior retraction of the esophagus. The anterior vagus branch is usually directly anterior at the hiatus and gently courses to the patient's left as it ascends in the mediastinum. The posterior branch is usually toward the right posterior side and is the more difficult of the two branches to identify. If there is any question as to the location of this branch, additional posterior mediastinal dissection is needed to identify it. After identification, both nerve branches are sharply dissected away from the esophagus, and a 2-cm specimen is resected from both (Figs. 12.6 and 12.7). Intraoperative frozen section can be performed to verify nerve tissue if any doubt exists, otherwise permanent specimens suffice. Additional anterior and posterior branches are divided by skeletonizing the esophagus for at least 2 cm

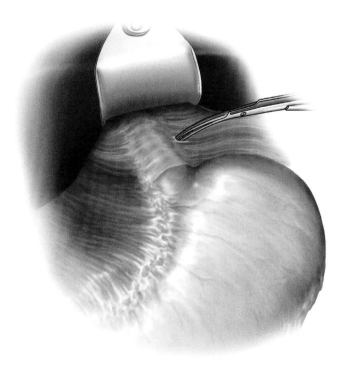

Figure 12.4 Truncal vagotomy is begun by opening the phrenoesophageal membrane transversely.

Figure 12.5 Gentle manual dissection with the thumb and index finger is used to create the retroesophageal window using the nasogastric tube as a guide to free the esophagus circumferentially.

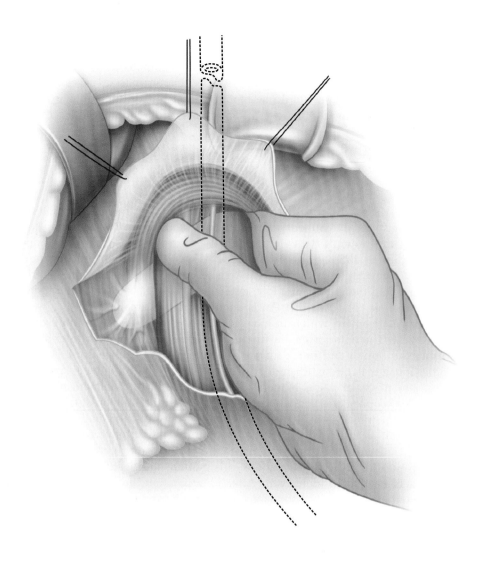

circumferentially, ensuring that the posterior nerve of Grassi is taken. A final check of hemostasis in the mediastinum is made before the esophageal hiatus is approximated with interrupted permanent suture (Fig. 12.8). Placement of closed suction drains is not required. The midline fascia and skin are closed in standard fashion.

POSTOPERATIVE MANAGEMENT

Patients should be admitted to and monitored in a surgical intensive care unit. A NG tube should be left in the midbody of the stomach for 2 to 3 days for stomach decompression. Prolonged NG tube placement should be avoided as early refeeding is associated with improved ulcer healing time. The patient should be kept on intravenous proton pump inhibitors and treated appropriately for *H. pylori* infection if found. A contrast study may be obtained prior to NG removal.

COMPLICATIONS

Rebleeding can occur in up to 10% of patients and is usually a technical failure due to inadequate suture placement at the original surgery if it recurs early on. Late rebleeding is usually associated with inadequate vagotomy or failure to eradicate *H. pylori* infection.

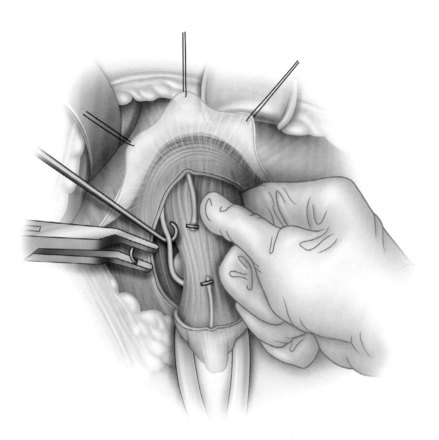

Figure 12.6 After the anterior vagus nerves is identified, a 2-cm segment is resected.

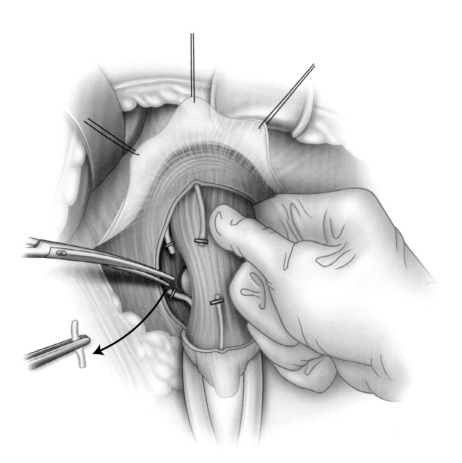

Figure 12.7 After the 2-cm segment of posterior vagus nerves is identified, the distal esophagus is then skeletonized to ensure a complete vagotomy.

Figure 12.8 The posterior crura are approximated with interrupted permanent 2-0 sutures allowing easy passage of an instrument alongside the esophagus.

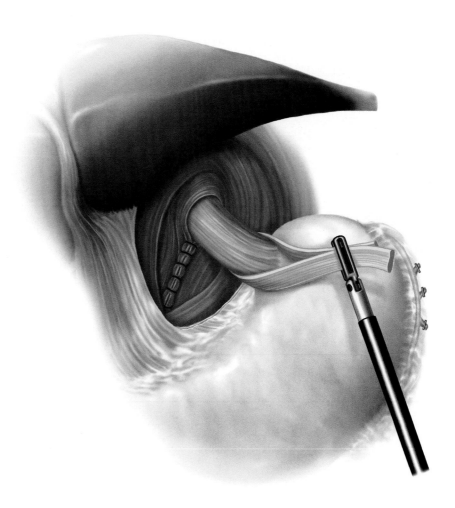

Postvagotomy diarrhea can occur in up to 30% of patients following truncal vagotomy and may be related to the passage of unconjugated bile salts into the colon. Cholestyramine (which binds bile salts) can be used in patients to help control symptoms, but most cases are self-limited.

Dumping syndrome can occur in about 15% of patients after vagotomy and pyloroplasty and can manifest in a variety of symptoms such as bloating, cramping, diarrhea, and emesis. The etiology of this is thought to be due to the rapid emptying of hyperosmotic liquid into the small intestine and should be managed by dietary measures. Dumping symptoms are also frequently self-limited and improve with time.

✸ CONCLUSIONS

Pyloroplasty and truncal vagotomy is required in the armamentarium of every general surgeon. It is straightforward, easily reproduced, and effective in the treatment of patients with bleeding duodenal ulcer.

Recommended References and Readings

Barkun AN, Cockeram AW, Plourde V, et al. Review article: acid suppression in non-variceal acute upper gastrointestinal bleeding. *Aliment Pharmacol Ther.* 1999;13:1565.

Chan VM, Reznick RK, O'Rourke K, et al. Meta-analysis of highly selective vagotomy versus truncal vagotomy and pyloroplasty in the surgical treatment of uncomplicated duodenal ulcer. *Can J Surg.* 1994;37:457.

Cooper GS, Chak A, Way LE, et al. Early endoscopy in upper gastrointestinal hemorrhage: associations with recurrent bleeding, surgery, and length of hospital stay. *Gastrointest Endosc.* 1999;49:145.

Gilliam AD, Speake WJ, Lobo DN, et al. Current practice of emergency vagotomy and *Helicobacter pylori* eradication for complicated peptic ulcer in the United Kingdom. *Br J Surg.* 2003; 90:88.

Gisbert JP, Khorrami S, Carballo F, et al. *H. pylori* eradication therapy vs. antisecretory non-eradication therapy (with or without long-term maintenance antisecretory therapy) for the prevention of recurrent bleeding from peptic ulcer. *Cochrane Database Syst Rev.* 2004:CD004062.

Lau JY, Sung JJ, Lam YH, et al. Endoscopic retreatment compared with surgery in patients with recurrent bleeding after initial endoscopic control of bleeding ulcers. *N Engl J Med.* 1999; 340:751.

Ohmann C, Imhof M, Roher HD. Trends in peptic ulcer bleeding and surgical treatment. *World J Surg.* 2000;24:282.

Reuben BC, Stoddard G, Glasgow R, et al. Trends and predictors for vagotomy when performing oversew of acute bleeding duodenal ulcer in the United States. *J Gastrointest Surg.* 2007;11:22.

Rockall TA, Logan RF, Devlin HB, et al. Incidence of and mortality from acute upper gastrointestinal haemorrhage in the United Kingdom. Steering Committee and members of the National Audit of Acute Upper Gastrointestinal Haemorrhage. *BMJ.* 1995; 311:222.

Savides TJ, Jensen DM. Therapeutic endoscopy for nonvariceal upper gastrointestinal bleeding. *Gastroenterol Clin North Am.* 2000;29:465.

13 Ligation of Bleeding Ulcer, Antrectomy, Vagotomy, and Gastrojejunostomy

Bruce Schirmer

 INDICATIONS/CONTRAINDICATIONS

Bleeding duodenal ulcer is a surgical emergency that has decreased in frequency over the past several decades due to the overall decrease in the incidence of peptic ulcer disease. However, the condition still arises and is a life-threatening one for the individual who develops it. Surgery remains an important treatment option for the patient with a bleeding duodenal ulcer. Its role has been decreased from primary line therapy in most situations to secondary treatment when the patient is stable enough to undergo less invasive therapy, in particular flexible endoscopic attempts to relieve the bleeding.

Indications

Specific indications for the performance of antrectomy, vagotomy, gastrojejunostomy, and oversewing of a bleeding duodenal ulcer are as follows:

1. Initial treatment of a patient with a bleeding duodenal ulcer causing hemodynamic changes unresponsive to intravenous fluid and blood product transfusion.
2. Treatment of a patient with bleeding duodenal ulcer who has failed attempts at endoscopic therapy to control the bleeding ulcer and for whom interventional angiographic therapy to control the bleeding is either unavailable, has failed, or is felt to be contraindicated.
3. Treatment of a patient with bleeding duodenal ulcer for whom no endoscopic or radiographic therapeutic options to arrest the bleeding are available.

In addition to the above three indications for the operation, the following parameters are also considered important by many surgeons to be present to warrant this operation:

1. The patient should have had a history of previous peptic disease to warrant resectional therapy.
2. The previous peptic disease should not have been so severe as to render the pyloric and postpyloric area severely scarred.

3. The patient's condition in the operating room must be one of hemodynamic stability once the bleeding ulcer has been oversewn.

Contraindications

Specific contraindications for the performance of antrectomy, vagotomy, gastrojejunostomy, and oversewing of a bleeding duodenal ulcer are as below. This list may not be totally comprehensive but should encompass the major contraindications.

1. Hemodynamic instability in the operating room necessitating the performance of the most rapid operation feasible (vagotomy, pyloroplasty, and oversewing of the ulcer).
2. Severe scarring of the pyloric and proximal duodenum, such that the resection staple line for the distal margin of the antrectomy would be at jeopardy for breakdown.
3. No previous history of peptic disease or potential other etiologies (e.g., aspirin or nonsteroidal anti-inflammatory drug ingestion) that may have contributed to the ulcer diathesis.
4. Previous antireflux surgery, placement of lap-adjustable band for weight loss, or other operation with extensive dissection around the gastroesophageal junction which would contraindicate easy performance of a truncal vagotomy.

PREOPERATIVE PLANNING

The overwhelming issue regarding preoperative planning for the operation is the attention to achieving hemodynamic stability in the patient and the means to monitor such stability and to provide vigorous transfusion volume should it be necessary. For any major gastrointestinal bleed, the following resuscitative and patient care measures should be instituted as the first priority of care:

1. Transfer the patient to an ICU setting where continuous monitoring of vital signs is performed
2. Central line placement for both rapid fluid resuscitation and for monitoring volume status
3. Foley catheter to measure organ perfusion and hence resuscitation success
4. Availability of appropriate blood products should the bleeding worsen or continue unabated. These could include, as most appropriate, whole blood, fresh frozen plasma, packed red blood cells, and if significant transfusion requirements occur, platelets and cryoprecipitate
5. Reversal of any potential anticoagulant medication
6. Large bore intravenous access for transfusion requirements

Confirming the diagnosis of bleeding duodenal ulcer is normally done using flexible upper endoscopy. Usually endoscopic measures to control the bleeding are performed at the time of the procedure. Lack of efficacy of such measures is considered an appropriate indication to proceed with surgical intervention. Performing an extensive operation such as antrectomy, vagotomy, gastrojejunostomy, and oversewing of a bleeding duodenal ulcer is normally not performed without a clear diagnosis of bleeding duodenal ulcer. It is feasible that such a diagnosis can be inferred by the clinical picture but not confirmed endoscopically. In such situations, endoscopic success could have been limited by excessive blood in the lumen of the duodenum or due to other technical reasons. On occasion, diagnosis by angiography with inability to perform angiographic measures to stop the bleeding or failure of such measures could also serve as an appropriate confirmation of the diagnosis of bleeding duodenal ulcer and the need to perform surgical therapy.

Prior to surgery, a thorough history of the patient's previous problems with gastrointestinal issues, including any history of previous ulcer disease or long-standing symptoms consistent with ulcer disease, is appropriate. Given such a history, the use of an antrectomy with vagotomy, rather than just vagotomy and drainage procedure, for the treatment of complications of duodenal ulcer is more justified.

Surgical Procedure

The operation is, due to its nature as an emergency procedure for life-threatening bleeding, normally conducted as an open operation through an upper midline incision. Its performance as a laparoscopic operation could be feasible, but the two major factors that would make laparoscopy more difficult are the maintenance of hemodynamic stability in the setting of creating a pneumoperitoneum and the difficulty in suctioning the actively bleeding area in order to place the sutures properly to oversew the ulcer without losing the pneumoperitoneum and the operative field of vision.

Oversewing the Ulcer

Once an upper midline incision is made and the abdominal organs are made accessible, the first priority and hence also first step of the operation is to perform the oversewing of the ulcer. The steps of this portion of the operation are as follows:

- The duodenum is exposed. A Kocher maneuver may assist in bringing the duodenum up into the field and should be used.
- The pylorus is identified.
- An anterior duodenal incision is made starting 1 cm beyond the pylorus, and extending 2 cm into the duodenum (Fig. 13.1).
- The bleeding site should be within visualization using this access. On occasion, further extension of the duodenal end of the incision may be needed.
- The bleeding ulcer is normally on the posterior surface of the duodenum, in the location of the gastroduodenal artery. The course of the artery is usually through the distal first part of the duodenum or most proximal second portion.
- The ulcer bleeding vessel is now directly oversewn with three simple silk sutures. Other materials may be used, but the suture weight must be heavy enough to allow it to be tied to gather the ligated tissue together without breaking. A 2-0 weight suture is recommended.

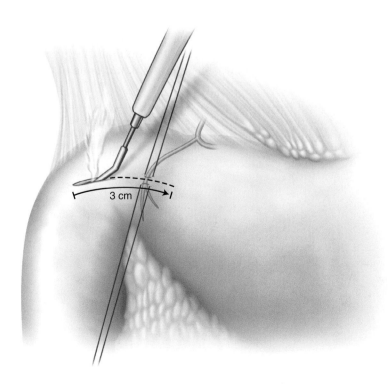

Figure 13.1 Performing an incision 1 cm distal to the pylorus and extending it 2 cm distally in the duodenum to expose the site of the bleeding ulcer.

3 cm

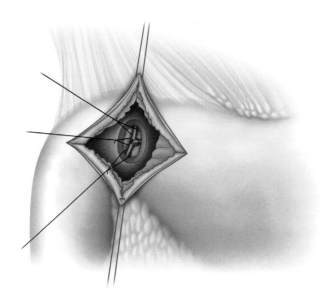

Figure 13.2 Placement of sutures for oversewing of a bleeding duodenal ulcer. Three sutures are required. One is placed proximally and one distally through the axis of the bleeding vessel. The third is placed at a 90-degree orientation medially to the gastroduodenal artery in order to ligate the frequently present medial pancreatic branch of the artery.

- The sutures are placed as illustrated in Figure 13.2. One is at right angle to the course of the artery proximal to it, a second in that same orientation distal to it, and the third at a 90-degree orientation on the medial or proximal side of the bleeding to occlude the frequently present transverse pancreatic branch of the gastroduodenal artery.
- Once the bleeding is controlled, the duodenotomy is closed with a running layer of absorbable suture.

Performing the Antrectomy

The antrectomy is now performed once it is confirmed that the most proximal duodenum is not excessively scarred and therefore is amenable to surgical closure. The steps of the antrectomy are as follows:

- The plane underneath the surface of the most proximal duodenum is dissected to allow passage of a stapler through it. Small vessels in this area may need division with an ultrasonic scalpel.
- The GIA-type stapler is fired across the most proximal duodenum at this location. The staple line should be beyond the pylorus. It should also be proximal to the closure of the duodenotomy whenever feasible (Fig. 13.3). Inclusion of the suture closure

Figure 13.3 A GIA-type stapler is fired across the proximal duodenum just beyond the pylorus.

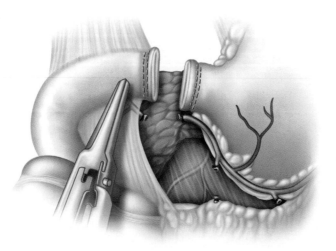

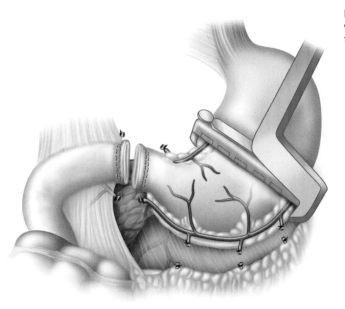

Figure 13.4 Dividing the stomach with a TA-type stapler to perform the antrectomy.

of the duodenotomy will weaken that suture line, and if this occurs, the suture line must be reinforced to prevent disruption.

- The site of proximal division of the stomach is determined. This is normally at the incisura on the lesser curvature of the stomach and in a point directly radially opposite to it on the greater curvature of the stomach. These sites are marked by local division of vessels adjacent to the lesser and greater curvatures of the stomach with the ultrasonic scalpel.

- The vessels of the right gastroepiploic artery running adjacent to the greater curvature of the stomach along the antrum are divided using either suture ligation technique or with the ultrasonic scalpel. Special care is taken to ligate the main trunk of the right gastroepiploic artery.

- The vessels along the lesser curvature of the stomach, beginning at the pyloric division, are also ligated in a similar fashion. Here the right gastric artery must be securely identified and ligated.

- The stapler is used to divide the stomach at the previously determined sites of division (Fig. 13.4). Care must be taken to be sure no nasogastric or other tubes are in the lumen of the stomach. The blue, gold, or green load of the TA-type stapler is used, depending on the thickness of the gastric tissue.

- Both the gastric staple line and the duodenal staple line are inspected for integrity and hemostasis. Simple sutures are used if any areas of concern are noted.

Performing Vagotomy

A truncal vagotomy is indicated in this setting. Optimal elimination of the cholinergic stimulation of gastric secretion is sought; hence complete or truncal vagotomy is performed. The steps of the vagotomy are as follows:

- The phrenoesophageal ligament is divided anteriorly to expose the anterior surface of the esophagus. Dissection of the peritoneum is extended to the left to the angle of His and to the right to just past the right crus of the diaphragm.

- The anterior vagus nerve is located buried within the musculature of the anterior distal esophagus (Fig. 13.5).

- A 1 cm or longer segment of the anterior nerve is resected, with small hemoclips placed on the proximal and distal resected ends of the nerve. These clips serve to achieve hemostasis but also serve as a radiographic marker to demonstrate the performance of a truncal vagotomy.

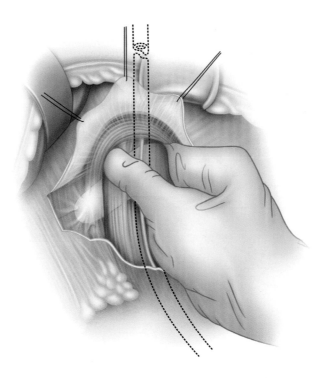

Figure 13.5 Locating the anterior vagus nerve which is buried in the anterior esophageal muscle wall.

- The posterior vagus is clearly identified. It often lies posterior to the esophagus, along the surface of the crura (Fig. 13.6). **Failure to clearly identify the posterior vagus nerve is a common technical error of this procedure.** If the nerve is not clearly palpable along the posterior surface of the esophagus, the surgeon must extend the plane of blunt dissection with a finger up along the patient's right side of the esophagus until the nerve is clearly palpated. Then it can be traced distally to assure proper identification of the posterior nerve at the hiatus.
- The posterior nerve is similarly resected and clipped as was the anterior nerve.

Performing Gastrojejunostomy

Gastrojejunostomy is performed as the preferred drainage method of the stomach after antrectomy. The creation of a single anastomosis is preferred. Resection of just the antrum

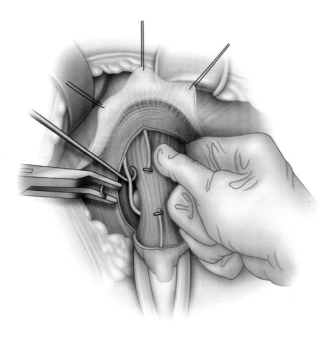

Figure 13.6 Locating the posterior vagus nerve, which is often not closely attached to the posterior esophageal wall, but instead courses more posteriorly, lying atop the area of intersection of the diaphragmatic crura.

will normally allow adequate gastric volume and peristalsis to prevent reflux of jejunal secretions into the esophagus. The key steps in this portion of the operation are as follows:

- Identification of the ligament of Treitz to identify the most proximal jejunum. The jejunum just distal to this is then brought through an opening in the transverse colon mesentery just to the patient's left of the middle colic vessels. The gastrocolic ligament is opened widely to allow good access to the posterior surface of the stomach.
- The jejunal loop is secured to the posterior surface of the distal stomach, just above the resection line, with several tacking sutures of 3-0 silk. Isoperistaltic alignment of the jejunum is ideal. In aligning the jejunum, however, the most important aspect is to avoid a kink and hence obstruction of the course of the bowel as it traverses up to and back from the anastomosis with the stomach.
- Use of a double-staple technique decreases the chance of kinking of the distal or outflow portion of the anastomosis. The midportion of the segment of jejunum that is brought up to the surface of the stomach is used for the creation of the anastomosis. This point must be at least 4 cm proximal to the distal end of the resected stomach to allow for double stapling. A gastrostomy and a corresponding enterotomy at that location are created (Fig. 13.7).
- The linear stapler, usually a 45-mm blue load, is fired first in one direction (Fig. 13.8) and then in the opposite direction through the same opening (Fig. 13.9).
- The defect from the stapling is now closed with a single layer of absorbable suture.
- Tacking sutures are placed 1 cm beyond the end of the anastomosis both proximally and distally (Fig. 13.10). These sutures are important to prevent outflow or inflow obstruction to the gastrojejunostomy. They are more important than making a very long gastrojejunostomy, since no matter what the length of the anastomosis, its emptying is eventually determined by the caliber of the lumen of the efferent limb of jejunum. If this is kinked, as may often occur without the tacking suture, then outlet obstruction occurs. **Failure to prevent outflow obstruction of the gastrojejunostomy is the most common technical error of this operation.** If the outflow obstruction is severe enough, the pressure from the obstruction will distend the duodenal limb and result in blowout of the stapled end of the duodenal stump.

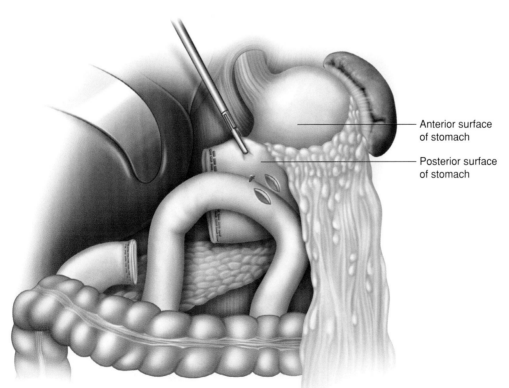

Figure 13.7 Making a gastrostomy and an enterotomy to begin stapling the gastrojejunostomy. Note the jejunum is aligned along the posterior surface of the distal stomach to facilitate emptying.

Anterior surface of stomach

Posterior surface of stomach

Figure 13.8 Firing the GIA-type stapler in one direction to begin the gastrojejunostomy.

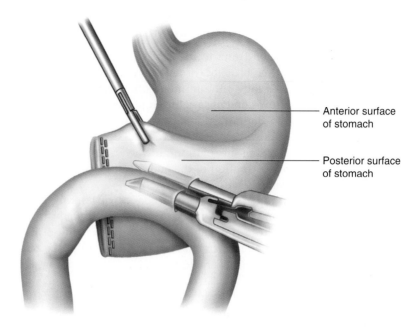

Anterior surface of stomach

Posterior surface of stomach

 The afferent and efferent limbs of the jejunum are tacked to the transverse colon mesentery to prevent another loop of intestine from migrating upward into the lesser sac. They may also be tacked to each other at this location for additional security.

→ POSTOPERATIVE MANAGEMENT

The postoperative care of the patient with a bleeding duodenal ulcer, who has undergone antrectomy and vagotomy as a curative operation, must be focused on the continued resuscitation of the intravascular space, with adequate intravenous fluid administration.

Figure 13.9 Firing the GIA-type stapler in the other direction to perform a double-stapled gastrojejunostomy anastomosis. This technique will decrease the incidence of postoperative outflow obstruction of the gastrojejunostomy.

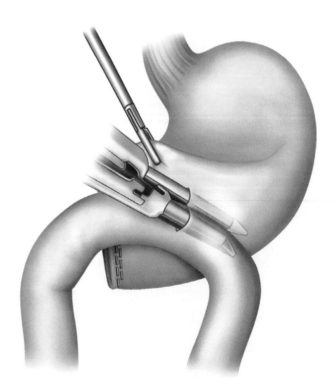

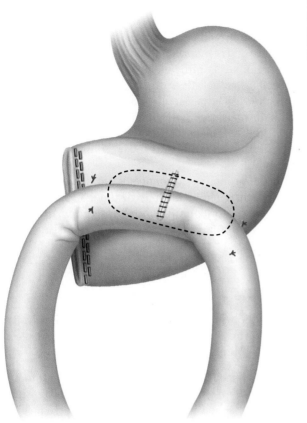

Figure 13.10 Placing tacking sutures 1 cm from the ends of the anastomosis both proximally and distally such that the jejunum is not kinked either in its inflow or outflow from the area of the gastrojejunostomy.

Hemodynamic stability, good perfusion of organs, and no signs of organ dysfunction from the stress and potential shock of the bleeding episode are the goals of therapy at this point. Careful monitoring of organ function, preferably in an ICU setting for 24 to 48 hours, is indicated. If a significant period of hypotension occurred during the bleeding, then the surgeon must be alert for signs of renal, pulmonary, neurologic, cardiac, or other organ injury secondary to the period of hypotension. Replenishment of the hemoglobin-carrying capacity of the blood to an adequate level is also indicated. This level can vary based on age and underlying medical conditions. Signs of organ dysfunction require continued treatment in the ICU setting with therapy focused on restoration of full organ function. These goals and the major other postoperative care issues and treatment are as follows:

- Monitoring for no further signs of bleeding or other hemodynamic instability
- Restoration of full vital organ function
- Restoration of adequate hemoglobin capacity
- Monitoring for adequate gastric emptying (signs of nausea, vomiting, distention are the signal that this may be an issue)
- A nasogastric tube is not indicated unless the patient does develop postoperative gastric ileus or partial outlet obstruction. Placement is based on clinical and potentially also radiographic criteria.
- If poor gastric emptying occurs, decompression with a nasogastric tube is indicated if it is severe. Otherwise, transient use of intravenous fluids and nutrition until gastric emptying is improved may be all that are necessary.
- A postoperative gastrografin swallow is variably used by surgeons to assess for gastric emptying as well as for security of all staple lines and anastomoses prior to initiating oral intake.
- Mild gastric dysfunction after vagotomy is usually the rule. The patient should be counseled that poor food tolerance may be present initially, but this will improve. On occasion pharmacologic therapy such as erythromycin may be used.

- Treatment of the underlying ulcer diathesis has been largely accomplished by the operation, but the patient should be tested for *Helicobacter pylori* presence in the resected stomach specimen. In many cases, surgeons will empirically give the patient a course of triple therapy for treatment of *H. pylori.* Subsequent hydrogen breath testing to confirm eradication of the organism is indicated.
- The patient must be counseled about postoperative dumping and diarrhea, not uncommon after vagotomy and antrectomy. These usually occur in tandem, though may be manifested individually. Dietary measures will alleviate most symptoms of dumping and diarrhea. Avoidance of highly concentrated carbohydrates and fats is the hallmark of such diet modification. Slower eating and lower volumes of food at a sitting improve these problems as well.
- Past experience has shown that, with the proper performance of antrectomy, truncal vagotomy, and gastrojejunostomy, the recurrence of ulcer is in the 1% range. Most surgeons do not recommend prolonged proton pump inhibitor therapy for these patients. However, recurrence of peptic symptoms may warrant their reinstitution.

COMPLICATIONS

Some of the most severe complications which may be seen after this operation have already been alluded to in the above text. These complications may be thought of as constituting four general areas. They are as follows:

- Overall typical complications that one may see following any abdominal laparotomy.
- Sequelae and complications from the period of gastrointestinal hemorrhage, particularly episodes of hypotension and organ ischemia that may have occurred. This group of complications is the most life-threatening.
- Complications specific to the operation. These would further be broken down into short-term or long-term complications.
- Potential complications that may arise if the ulcer disease were to recur or persist.

Overall complications that one would anticipate after a laparotomy include atelectasis, wound infection, venous thromboembolism, and postoperative ileus. Cardiovascular events would be less anticipated but not rare. Attention to postoperative pulmonary toilet, early ambulation, and adequate pain control without excessive sedation all are paramount to combating the complication of postoperative atelectasis. Appropriate prophylactic antibiotics administered parenterally before the performance of the incision are known to have the greatest impact on decreasing postoperative wound infection. Broad-spectrum antibiotics effective against both gram-positive and some gram-negative bacteria are used (cefazolin is the usual choice). However, careful tissue handling, hemostasis, irrigation, and minimization of wound contamination are all also important in minimizing wound infection rates.

Complications which occur after an episode of hemorrhagic shock may include organ dysfunction from any and all organs sensitive to the effects of the period of hypotension. The most frequently affected are the renal and pulmonary systems, with acute tubular necrosis/acute renal failure and acute respiratory distress syndrome resulting from this injury. Cardiac ischemia may result, leading to some degree of myocardial infarction if severe enough. Neurologic sequelae may arise, especially if pre-existing cerebrovascular disease is present. Cholestasis and acute hepatic injury is common but is usually more reversible than others due to liver capacity. Pre-existing liver disease, however, could result in acute decompensation of liver function. Treatment for all these conditions rests in now what is generally much better understood by intensive care specialists: measures to restore perfusion, maintain organ viability, minimize infectious complications, and support organ function until recovery occurs.

Complications specific to the operation include short-term and long-term complications. For these complications, it is also relevant to discuss the most common measures known to successfully prevent them. The short-term commonly expected complications include the following:

■ Persistent or recurrent bleeding from the ulcer: This would be a technical failure of the oversewing and would potentially require reoperation to place additional sutures to achieve hemostasis. Careful attention to suture placement and correct technique are the best measures to avoid this complication.

■ Bleeding from a staple line or anastomosis: This is best avoided by observing all staple lines at the time of surgery for hemostasis. If wider staple loads (such as green cartridges) are used to divide the stomach, consideration for oversewing the staple line should be given, since such staple sizes are more prone to postoperative bleeding.

■ Gastric outlet obstruction: This is a common technical error caused by improper attention to the outflow tract of the gastrojejunostomy. It must be secured in a position such that the bowel will not kink and collapse the lumen of the opening. Placement of the anastomosis on the posterior surface of the stomach facilitates emptying. There should be a smooth curvature of the intestine both going up to and exiting away from the posterior surface of the stomach and the gastrojejunostomy.

■ Breakdown of the duodenal stump: This is perhaps the most feared complication of this operation and one which is associated with significant morbidity and mortality. There are two major causes. The first is that the closure is technically inadequate. The second is that distal obstruction creates enough pressure for the staple line to rupture. Treatment is adequate drainage and intravenous antibiotics, which may or may not involve reoperation.

Complications from recurrence of the ulcer disease include recurrent abdominal pain, possible recurrent bleeding, and gastric outlet obstruction from marginal ulceration. Confirmation that a complete vagotomy was performed is one step in treatment; reoperation is needed if it was incomplete. Medical therapy is otherwise usually adequate to overcome recurrence of ulcer diathesis when it occurs. Rarely a neoplastic (gastrinoma) cause may be responsible.

RESULTS

This operation is done primarily for patients with urgent or emergent bleeding problems. They often have associated hypotension and are critically ill in most situations. Therefore, the outcomes of this procedure must be judged by the clinical setting under which it is performed and the patient population for which it is performed. Most results published in the literature date back to the days when surgery for ulcer disease was more common, the prevalence of ulcers was more common, and medical treatment of ulcer disease was not as effective. The operation described in this chapter is now very selectively used by surgeons for the treatment of patients with bleeding duodenal ulcer.

The literature, and practical experience, has shown that patients who are poor candidates to begin with for surgery have multiple medical problems or who have become *in extremis* from a prolonged period of shock and hypotension from gastrointestinal bleeding are likely to have a very high mortality rate from surgical therapy. Furthermore, for patients who are at high risk for surgery, a resectional operation such as antrectomy would be relatively contraindicated in favor of a less involved operation such as simple oversewing of the ulcer with pyloroplasty and possibly truncal vagotomy.

Most reports of surgical therapy in the literature combine a variety of operations and a variety of degree of severity of illness in patients in their reports.

Historically speaking, the generally quoted mortality rate overall for patients with hemorrhage from duodenal ulcer disease is in the 12% range. First-line therapy for such bleeding patients is normally endoscopic therapy, which has an expected success rate of 85% to 95% of stopping the bleeding. This figure is influenced by local expertise.

The success of endoscopic therapy for rebleeding, or failed first-time therapy, is lower at about 58% to 72%.

The literature has shown that overall surgical therapy and repeat endoscopy after an initial failed endoscopic treatment have roughly equivalent success rates and mortality rates. The decision to perform surgery at the time of a failed initial endoscopic therapy is the judgment of the surgeon and again is based on local expertise, patient condition, and other qualifying factors. Antrectomy and vagotomy with gastrojejunostomy could be used in this setting, but it would generally be applied to more fit patients with less transfusion requirements and greater hemodynamic stability. Factors that predict failure of endoscopic therapy include

- initial hypotension
- an ulcer size greater than 2 cm in diameter.
- vessel size of 1 mm in diameter or larger

Initial endoscopic findings of a large duodenal ulcer with a visible bleeding vessel of 1 mm or greater would likely lead to surgery if any sign of rebleeding did occur or if the initial endoscopic therapy was unsuccessful.

If endoscopic therapy fails, then the surgeon faces the option of performing salvage surgery or, more recently, referring the patient for a transcatheter arterial embolization (TAE) therapy. A recent comparison of results of TAE versus surgical therapy was published by Venclausakas et al.. This report showed that the mortality for such patients was comparable at 21% for the TAE group of patients and 22% for the surgical patients. The rebleeding rate was higher, but not statistically so, for the TAE group, which is not unexpected. Though overall mortality for the group was comparable, the authors noted the TAE group had a higher age and Apache II score, meaning they were overall poorer risk candidates. For patients with an Apache II score of 16.5 or greater, the TAE mortality was 23% versus the surgical mortality of 50%.

Another review by Eriksson et al. showed that in such a situation the mortality for TAE was less than for surgery, at 3% vs. 14%. In that surgical group, 35 of 51 operations involved resection, whereas only 14% involved simple oversewing of the ulcer. Use of the latter approach may have decreased the surgical mortality. Also, the average age of the patients who died after surgery was 80, suggesting operative therapy in this elderly a patient population may not have been the best choice versus TAE.

Certainly the surgeon should be the ultimate decision maker in the choice of therapy for bleeding duodenal ulcer. Lower risk patients are probably better treated earlier with surgical therapy. A history of peptic ulcer disease, previous bleeding, and hemodynamic stability are the optimal settings under which to perform antrectomy, vagotomy, oversewing of the ulcer, and gastrojejunostomy. However, reports of a pure series of such patients alone are difficult to find in the literature, and those that exist are very dated and do not reflect improvements in modern surgical perioperative care, critical care, patient resuscitation, and improved antibiotic and medical therapy. Given the traditional overall mortality of surgical therapy for bleeding ulcer as being approximately 12%, selected patients today should be expected to have improved outcomes over that figure.

The difficult patient for the surgeon becomes the patient who has failed endoscopic therapy and then the decision of whether to perform salvage surgical therapy or TAE must be determined. The role of TAE is largely influenced by the local expertise of that group of radiologists in a given institution. However, the overall literature results show that

- TAE is technically successful in over 90% of cases
- control of hemorrhage is between 50% to 90% in case series in TAE
- rebleeding after TAE is reported to occur between 8% and 40% of cases
- higher mortality is associated with rebleeding in TAE
- overall mortality for patients with bleeding duodenal ulcer treated by TAE has been reported as being between 0% and 25%
- mortality is less if TAE is successfully performed early in the course of the bleeding, as would be expected

A recent review of the experience at a large teaching hospital reviewing the incidence of peptic ulcer disease showed that in the decade from 1995 to 2004, the incidence of surgery for gastric or duodenal ulcers decreased from 6.7% to 3.8% of cases, with the gastric ulcer group representing the major decrease. The incidence of surgery for duodenal ulcer was constant at about 7.5% of cases. During the decade, the incidence of using an acid-reduction operation such as is described in this chapter for the operative treatment of bleeding duodenal ulcer fell from 50.6% to 31.6% over that time frame, showing that recent trends are to just perform an operation focused on stopping the bleeding and not reducing acid secretory capacity. The overall results of surgical therapy for patients with gastric or duodenal ulcers was a mortality of 6.0%, morbidity of 23.9%, and an average length of hospital stay of 15.9 days.

The shift away from performing an acid-reducing operation was in part borne out by studies that examined the effectiveness of using medical therapy to eradicate *H. pylori* as part of the therapy to treat duodenal ulcer disease and to prevent recurrent duodenal ulcer disease. Duodenal ulcer disease is felt to occur as a result of a hypersecretory state of acid production, stimulated in large part by antral D-cell dysfunction secondary to *H. pylori*-induced antral gastritis, which in turn limits somatostatin release and exacerbates acid production. Such acid production in the face of *H. pylori* colonization of the duodenal mucosa leads to ulceration. A study by Ng and associates showed that appropriate treatment of *H. pylori* with four drug medical therapy at the time of closure of perforated duodenal ulcer resulted in a 5% ulcer recurrence rate over the next year versus 38% recurrence for patients who did not receive such therapy against *H. pylori*. The ability to thus treat potential ulcer recurrences in the future for patients with previously unknown peptic ulcer disease have led in large part to the shift in surgical thinking regarding treatment for patients with duodenal ulcer, with a clear trend away from acid-reducing operations to simple closure of perforation or oversewing of bleeding ulcer. Patients who are candidates for acid-reducing operations would be those for whom risk factors still exist or cannot be diminished:

- chronic refractory nonsteroidal anti-inflammatory drug ingestion
- smoking
- noncompliance with medical therapy for *H. pylori* or acid secretion

Salvage surgery is often one of the main indications for performing surgery for bleeding duodenal or gastric ulcer in recent years. In this situation, where patients are often quite critically ill, mortality from surgery or any therapy can be very high. Walsh et al. described a series of 50 patients who had failed endoscopic therapy (an average of over two procedures each), many of whom developed their GI bleeding after hospital admission while in an intensive care setting. The Apache scores of 79 and the 64% incidence of organ failure as well as the average transfusion amount of 24 units of blood puts these patients in a very high risk for death from any treatment. In this group, 12 patients underwent salvage surgery for bleeding duodenal ulcer, with a resection performed in seven and a simple oversewing of the ulcer in five. The mortality for such surgery was 50%.

✥ CONCLUSIONS

The performance of antrectomy, vagotomy, gastrojejunostomy, and oversewing of a bleeding duodenal ulcer is now a relatively rarely performed operation due to improved medical therapy against the causative agent of most duodenal ulcers, *Helicobacter pylori*. Nevertheless, when it is indicated, surgeons must be familiar with the procedure and adequately skilled to perform it to produce good outcomes. The patients who are potential candidates for such an operation may be threatened by significant duodenal hemorrhage. Therapeutic endoscopy is the first-line treatment for bleeding duodenal ulcer in most settings. Failure of such therapy may then be an indication for the performance of surgical therapy. Performing an antrectomy, vagotomy, gastrojejunostomy, and oversewing of a bleeding duodenal ulcer is indicated largely for those patients who have other risk factors for duodenal ulcer disease other than simple presence of *H. pylori,* or who have a previous history of such ulcers, and who are hemodynamically stable enough and good surgical candidates to undergo a major resective operation. For most patients with bleeding duodenal ulcer and no other risk factors, simple oversewing of the ulcer along with adequate medical therapy for *H. pylori* has proven to be appropriately effective for most patients. When any surgery is used for salvage after failure of multiple endoscopic therapies and/or transarterial catheter embolization therapy, the mortality of such operations is high. Use of antrectomy, vagotomy, gastrojejunostomy, and oversewing of a bleeding duodenal ulcer in such settings probably should be rarely done in favor of a more simple operation to oversew the bleeding ulcer.

When antrectomy, vagotomy, gastrojejunostomy, and oversewing of a bleeding duodenal ulcer is performed, careful attention to technical considerations outlined in the chapter above will produce optimal results and prevent unnecessary complications.

Recommended References and Readings

Eriksson LG, Ljungdohl M, Sundbom M, et al. Transcatheter arterial embolisation versus surgery in the treatment of upper gastrointestinal bleeding after therapeutic endoscopic failure. *J Vasc Intervent Radiol.* 2008;19:1413–1418.

Lau JYW, Sung JT, Lam YH, et al. Endoscopic treatment compared with surgery in patients with recurrent bleeding after initial endoscopic control of duodenal ulcers. *NEJM.* 1999;340:751–756.

Ng EK, Lam YH, Sung JJ, et al. Eradication of *Helicobacter pylori* prevents recurrence of ulcer after simple closure of duodenal ulcer perforation: Randomized controlled trial. *Ann Surg.* 2000; 231:153–158.

Smith BR, Stabile BE. Emerging trends in peptic ulcer disease and damage control surgery in the *H. pylori* era. *Am Surgeon.* 2005; 7:797–801.

Venclauskas L, Bratlie SO, Zachrisson K, et al. Is transcatheter arterial embolization a safer alternative than surgery when endoscopic therapy fails in bleeding duodenal ulcer? *Scand J Gastroenterol.* 2010;45:299–304.

Walsh RM, Anain P, Geisinger M, et al. Role of angiography and embolization for massive gastrointestinal hemorrhage. *J Gastrointest Surg.* 1999;3:61–65.

14 Operation for Giant Duodenal Ulcer

Michael S. Nussbaum and Keyur Chavda

Introduction

Giant duodenal ulcer (GDU) is a variant of peptic ulcer disease and is defined as a duodenal ulcer crater that is benign and at least 2 cm in diameter. This subset of duodenal ulcers have historically resulted in greater morbidity than usual duodenal ulcers since, by definition, they involve the full thickness of the duodenal wall and occupy a significant portion of the duodenal bulb. Brdiczka first called attention to this entity in 1931 and emphasized the difficulty in diagnosing them with barium roentgenogram. Although once thought to be a rare variant, with the advent of flexible endoscopy and awareness of this entity numerous case reports and case series have been published in the literature. GDUs comprise approximately 1% to 2% of all duodenal ulcers and 5% of peptic ulcers requiring surgical intervention. In the initial reports, few patients were successfully treated with medical therapy. Surgery was favored as the treatment of choice for this disease, and high mortality rates were reported despite surgical intervention. Improvements in surgical techniques have revolutionized the operative treatment and outcome of this condition. However, today, with the widespread use of endoscopy, the introduction of histamine-2 receptor antagonists and later proton pump inhibitors (PPIs), medical treatment has replaced operation as the first line of treatment for the patient with GDU. Because of the large, penetrating nature of these ulcers, when not recognized and treated promptly, complications such as hemorrhage and perforation remain common, and GDUs are still associated with high rates of morbidity and mortality. Thus, surgical evaluation of a patient with GDU should remain an integral part of patient care in all cases. There are important differences when comparing GDUs to classic peptic ulcers, and they must be approached differently than their more common counterpart.

Standard-sized ulcer disease affects males greater than females at a rate of approximately 2 to 1, whereas it is 3 to 1 for GDU. The etiology of standard-sized and GDUs has been associated with two major contributing causes: recent usage of nonsteroidal anti-inflammatory drugs (NSAIDs) and *Helicobacter pylori* infection. However, the percentage of GDUs caused by *H. pylori* is less when compared to standard-sized ulcers, and NSAID use plays a more prominent role.

The most common presenting symptom is abdominal pain. Most patients describe the pain as involving the epigastric region, and some experience involvement of the right hypochondrium and/or radiation into the back, particularly when the ulcer penetrates into the pancreas. The pain is more intense and persistent than the pain found with usual ulcer patients. The pain is generally not relieved with food or antacids and weight loss is a frequent comorbidity.

Diagnosis

The most common emergency presentation of GDU is hemorrhage, which may manifest as melena, hematochezia, hematemesis, or any combination of the above, associated with anemia. The size of the ulcer and the surrounding inflammation may cause gastric outlet obstruction with nausea, vomiting, and weight loss. An inflammatory mass in the upper abdomen with associated weight loss, cachexia, malnutrition, and chronic abdominal pain can frequently mislead the clinician to suspect malignancy as the most likely diagnosis. Other important historical features include a past history of ulcer disease and the recent use of NSAIDs.

The size of the ulcer often causes replacement of the duodenal bulb, and as a result GDUs may be missed or misinterpreted as a deformed bulb, diverticulum, or pseudo-diverticulum during a barium upper GI series. The advent and widespread use of endoscopy has markedly improved the ability to detect GDUs with greater accuracy. It is not uncommon to encounter a GDU during an endoscopy without the expectation of finding one, and it is important to measure the ulcer so as not to misdiagnose it as a simple peptic ulcer. The ulcers usually are quite deep and involve over 50% of the mucosal circumference of the duodenal bulb. It is essential to exclude a neoplastic source as the cause of ulcer formation with biopsy in the setting of GDUs, particularly when there is nodularity at the edge. A recent review of 52 cases of duodenal ulcers larger than 2 cm found a malignancy rate of approximately 19% (primary duodenal carcinoma in 15%, lymphoma and tuberculosis in 2% each).

Management

Medical Treatment

Prior to the introduction of histamine-2 receptor antagonists in the late 1970s, GDUs were managed primarily surgically. Before 1982, there were very few published reports of long-term successful medical management of GDUs. With the advent of new acid suppression medication, the discovery of *H. pylori* and its role in ulcer formation with the importance of eradication therapy, successful medical management of most GDUs is now possible. The most recent studies have demonstrated that PPI therapy is a safe and effective first-line treatment in stable patients and should decrease the eventual need for operative intervention. Thus, attempts at medical treatment of GDUs should consist of PPIs. Discontinuation of NSAIDs and antimicrobial treatment of *H. pylori* infection in conjunction with PPI therapy are important treatment adjuncts in the presence of these risk factors.

Surgical Treatment

Indications

Despite the marked improvement in outcome with medical therapy, GDUs are still associated with high rates of morbidity, mortality, and complications. All patients diagnosed with GDU should be evaluated promptly by a surgeon. Operation is indicated in patients with acute complications of GDU such as hemorrhage and perforation.

Intractability, recurrent disease, incomplete healing despite proper medical therapy, and gastric outlet obstruction may require surgical intervention. GDU with adherent clot or a visible vessel on index esophagogastroduodenoscopy (EGD) is a marker of an ulcer that is more likely to require early surgical intervention. Uncontrolled hemorrhage and perforation are the most common emergent indications for operation. Unresolving obstruction, intractable or recurrent bleeding, and fistula formation are some of the elective indications for operation. The chronic inflammatory changes associated with these conditions often make the operations in these patients technically quite challenging.

Preoperative Assessment

A detailed clinical history and physical examination is required before elective surgery. Radiological study with contrast (upper gastrointestinal series) is useful in the evaluation of the duodenum and is useful in defining the anatomy of the upper digestive tract. EGD is useful in establishing the diagnosis of GDU and identifying features that may preclude successful medical treatment. EGD is also useful for monitoring the healing of the ulcer after medical therapy in cases of intractability or recurrent disease. Other conditions which may mimic GDU are pseudodiverticulum of the bulb or true diverticulum of the postbulbar area and a neoplasm such as carcinoma or lymphoma of the duodenal bulb. These conditions when suspected must be ruled out prior to surgery. If there is a suspicion of neoplasm, EGD is required for examination and biopsy to rule out malignancy.

The nutritional and immune status of the patient should be assessed prior to operation. Patients with chronic ulcer disease and gastric outlet obstruction are more prone to malnutrition with a higher incidence of perioperative complications. Severely malnourished patients may benefit from a course of preoperative enteral or parenteral nutrition. Patients with significant medical comorbidities will require thorough evaluation and optimization of their medical conditions prior to elective operation.

Operation

A definitive acid-reducing operation is the procedure of choice for patients with GDU requiring surgical intervention. Truncal vagotomy and antrectomy with removal of the involved duodenum is the procedure of choice whenever possible. When the inflammation and edema of the duodenum is not a factor, a Billroth I reconstruction can occasionally be performed (see Chapter 1 for truncal vagotomy, antrectomy, and Billroth I). Frequently, however, due to the nature of GDU, the involved duodenum is so inflamed and indurated that duodenal dissection and anastomosis would be hazardous. Thus, a Billroth II gastrojejunostomy is the most frequent method of reconstruction utilized in these patients (see Chapter 3 for truncal vagotomy, antrectomy, and Billroth II).

Because of the large size of the ulcer bed and its proximity to such vital structures as the pancreas, common bile duct, and their blood supply, it may be best to leave the ulcer bed in situ, resecting the duodenum around the ulcer bed and closing the duodenal stump. Duodenal stump leak is a major source of morbidity and mortality after resection of duodenum in these patients. Numerous methods and modifications of the standard duodenal stump closure have been described in an effort to prevent leakage in this setting. The use of a duodenostomy tube is a safe, rapid, and effective means of managing the difficult duodenal stump so often encountered in this setting. Tube duodenostomy involves insertion of a tube through the second portion of the duodenum to encourage formation of a controlled duodenocutaneous fistula. Similarly, a retrograde tube can be threaded through the wall of the jejunum downstream at the site of the placement of antegrade feeding jejunostomy (*drain-me feed-me tubes*) to provide decompression of this portion of the afferent limb.

The Nissen closure of the duodenal stump can be used to reinforce a difficult stump. After the duodenum is transected, the open lumen is sutured to the capsule of the pancreas (Fig. 14.1A). Another technique is the Bancroft procedure and its various modifications which entail performing an antrectomy but leaving the distal 3 to 4 cm of antrum proximal to the pylorus and performing a mucosectomy in which the mucosal layer of the antral stump and the pylorus are dissected away from the submucosa and

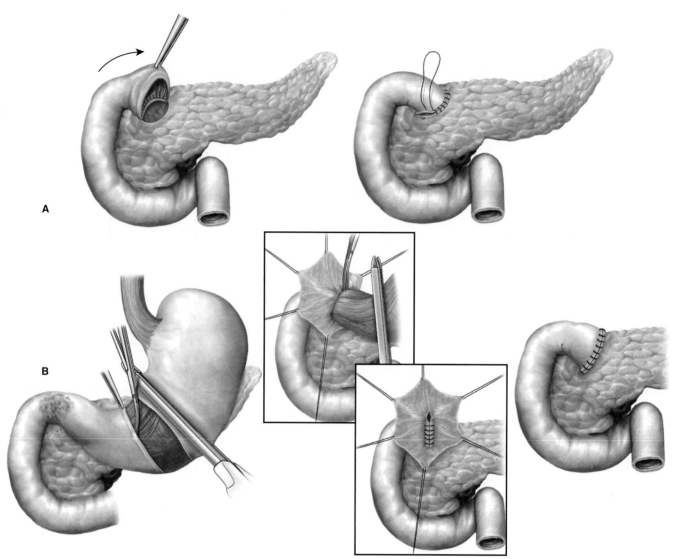

Figure 14.1 (A) Nissen closure. This method, often employed when the duodenum is scarred to the pancreatic capsule, is performed by first transecting the duodenum. The duodenal stump is then sutured to the pancreatic capsule or duodenal wall left in place on the pancreatic capsule. **(B)** Bancroft closure. In this method of duodenal stump closure, the stomach is transected 3 to 4 cm proximal to the pylorus, where tissue is less fibrotic. The antral mucosa in the duodenal stump is then dissected away from the submucosa beyond the pylorus and into the duodenum. This is secured with a purse-string suture, and the seromuscular layer is closed over the stump.

removed. A purse-string suture is then used to close the pylorus from inside; then the submucosa and the muscularis layers of the prepyloric stomach are used to reinforce the closure of the duodenal stump (Fig. 14.1B). An important principle is preservation of the distal antral blood supply because necrosis of the stump is a risk with this procedure. Either of these closure techniques can be combined with duodenostomy tube decompression.

When emergency surgery is required for continuing hemorrhage from a duodenal ulcer, it is common practice to oversew the bleeding ulcer and at the same time perform a vagotomy and pyloroplasty. But in the case of a GDU, where the blood may be coming directly from the gastroduodenal or pancreaticoduodenal artery, this approach is insufficient and carries a high risk of recurrent bleeding. Truncal vagotomy and either pyloroplasty or gastrojejunostomy should be avoided. The ulcer must be separated from the duodenum and the blood supply to the ulcer must be appropriately ligated.

Laparoscopic approaches for gastroduodenal disease are well established. The minimally invasive approach allows for the possible benefits of less pain, less wound complications, and shorter hospital stay (see Chapter 2 for laparoscopic vagotomy,

Part I: Procedures for Ulcer Disease

antrectomy, and Billroth I and Chapter 4 for laparoscopic vagotomy, antrectomy, and Billroth II). However, because of chronic inflammation around the ulcer area and surrounding organs, the laparoscopic approach is sometime difficult when treating GDU. The surgeon should be prepared to convert to an open approach if duodenal inflammation makes it difficult to perform a safe and expeditious resection.

CONCLUSIONS

Historically, the two key features of GDU disease were the difficulties in prompt diagnosis and the failures of medical management. The advent and widespread use of endoscopy has made prompt diagnosis of GDU more accurate and easy to obtain. Once a diagnosis has been made, initiation of therapy can begin. Uncontrolled hemorrhage, perforation, and unstable patients should undergo prompt operative management with vagotomy and antrectomy. Stable patients may be safely treated initially with medication. However, close observation and repeat endoscopic evaluation is essential in the successful medical management of these patients. Furthermore, a malignant etiology may be more common than previously suspected, and liberal use of endoscopic biopsies are warranted in the setting of GDU, particularly those with nodular-appearing edges. Due to evolving endoscopic and medical therapies, the management of GDUs has changed. What was once a disease that was difficult to diagnose and managed solely with surgical intervention has become one easily diagnosed and potentially treated medically. It is of utmost importance that physicians recognize GDUs as being different than their standard-sized counterparts and that we continue to further our understanding of this entity.

Recommended References and Readings

Agrawal NM, Campbell DR, Safdi MA, et al. Superiority of lansoprazole vs ranitidine in healing nonsteroidal anti-inflammatory drug-associated gastric ulcers: results of a double-blind, randomized, multicenter study. NSAID-Associated Gastric Ulcer Study Group. *Arch Intern Med.* 2000;160:1455–1461.
Bader JP, Delchier JC. Clinical efficacy of pantoprazole compared with ranitidine. *Aliment Pharmacol Ther.* 1994;8(Suppl 1): 47–52.
Bancroft FW. A modification of the Devine operation of pyloric exclusion for duodenal ulcer. *Am J Surg.* 1932;16:223–230.
Bennett JM. Modified Bancroft procedure for the duodenal stump. *Arch Surg.* 1972;104:219–222.
Brdiczka JG. Das Grosse ulcus duodeni in rontgenbild. *Fortschr Geb Rontgenstr.* 1931;44:177–181.
Burch JM, Cox CL, Feliciano DV, et al. Management of the difficult duodenal stump. *Am J Surg.* 1991;162:523–524.
Collen MJ, Santoro MJ, Chen YK. Giant duodenal ulcer. Evaluation of basal acid output, nonsteroidal antiinflammatory drug use, and ulcer complications. *Dig Dis Sci.* 1994;39:1113–1116.
Fischer DR, Nussbaum MS, Pritts TA, et al. Use of omeprazole in the management of giant duodenal ulcer: Results of a prospective study. *Surgery.* 1996;126:643–649.

Gustavsson S, Kelly KA, Hench VS, et al. Giant gastric and duodenal ulcers: a population-based study with a comparison to nongiant ulcers. *World J Surg.* 1987;11:333–338.
Jaszewski R, Crane SA, Cid AA. Giant duodenal ulcers. Successful healing with medical therapy. *Dig Dis Sci.* 1983;28:486–489.
Klammer TW, Mahr MM. Giant duodenal ulcer: a dangerous variant of a common illness. *Am J Surg.* 1978;135:760–762.
Mistilis SP, Wiot JF, Nedelman SH. Giant duodenal ulcer. *Ann Intern Med.* 1963;59:155–164.
Newton EB, Versland MR, Sepe TE. Giant duodenal ulcers. *World J Gastroenterol.* 2008;14:4995–4999.
Nussbaum MS, Schusterman MA. Management of giant duodenal ulcer. *Am J Surg.* 1985;149:357–361.
Rathi P, Parikh S, Kalro RH. Giant duodenal ulcer: a new look at a variant of a common illness. *Indian J Gastroenterol.* 1996;15: 33–34.
Walan A, Bader JP, Classen M, et al. Effect of omeprazole and ranitidine on ulcer healing and relapse rates in patients with benign gastric ulcer. *N Engl J Med.* 1989;320:69–75.
Yeomans ND, Tulassay Z, Juhasz L, et al. A comparison of omeprazole with ranitidine for ulcers associated with nonsteroidal antiinflammatory drugs. Acid Suppression Trial: Ranitidine versus Omeprazole for NSAID-Associated Ulcer Treatment (ASTRONAUT) Study Group. *N Engl J Med.* 1998;338:719–726.

15 Distal Subtotal Gastrectomy and D1 Resection

K. Roggin and Mitchell C. Posner

 INDICATIONS/CONTRAINDICATIONS

Gastric adenocarcinoma is the fourth most common malignancy and the second leading cause of death worldwide annually. In the United States, it remains a relatively rare cancer (in 2010, approximately 22,000 new cases were diagnosed). Gastric carcinoma is associated with chronic exposures to environmental carcinogens (*Helicobacter pylori,* nitrosamines, tobacco exposure), inflammatory conditions of the stomach (atrophic gastritis), pernicious anemia, blood type A, and less commonly, genetic mutations in the E-cadherin gene, *CDH-1* (hereditary diffuse gastric cancer). The relatively poor overall survival reported in most Western series is likely influenced by the high percentage of patients who are diagnosed with locally advanced or metastatic disease. Symptoms remain nonspecific early in the course of the disease, but advanced tumors can cause GI hemorrhage, gastric outlet obstruction, and profound weight loss. Curative treatment requires an appropriate gastrectomy with adequate regional lymphadenectomy. Peri- or postoperative treatment with chemotherapy and/or radiation has been shown to reduce recurrence and improve survival. Tumor location, clinical stage of disease, and patient performance status influence the decision to perform a subtotal versus total gastrectomy. Lymphatic metastases should be treated with an appropriate lymphadenectomy for optimal locoregional control of disease. Early-stage cancers may be cured by complete endoscopic mucosal resection (e.g., T1a cancers) or surgical gastrectomy; chemotherapy and/or radiation are effective adjuvant treatments that have been associated with improved disease-free and overall survival in stage II and III disease. Optimal management should be individualized with the input of a multidisciplinary tumor board. Two treatment paradigms are accepted as standards of care:

- Perioperative chemotherapy using EOX (Epirubicin–Oxaliplatin–Capecitabine) or equivalent chemotherapy for three cycles (nine weeks) before and after radical gastrectomy (MAGIC trial regimen).
- Subtotal or total gastrectomy followed by chemotherapy and external beam radiation (McDonald regimen, SWOG 0116).

PREOPERATIVE PLANNING

NCCN guidelines (www.nccn.org) suggest a comprehensive staging workup for patients with resectable gastric cancer.

- Comprehensive history and physical examination
- Complete upper endoscopy defining the location of the tumor within the stomach, extent of intragastric spread, and relationship of the cancer to the gastroesophageal junction.
    - All biopsies should be reviewed by a dedicated GI pathologist to determine the histologic subtype (intestinal, Lauren's diffuse type, signet ring cell adenocarcinoma, adenosquamous carcinoma) and degree of differentiation.
- Endoscopic ultrasonography should be considered in select patients who are candidates for neoadjuvant chemotherapy protocols. This modality is accurate at assessing the depth (T stage) of invasion, presence of metastatic regional lymphadenopathy, and distant metastatic disease to the liver or peritoneal cavity (liver metastases, peritoneal implants, and/or ascites).
- Contrast-enhanced, triphasic (pre-, arterial-weighted, and portovenous phases) multirow detector computed tomography of the chest, abdomen, and pelvis.
- Positron-emission tomography (PET scans) remains an experimental diagnostic staging modality in gastric adenocarcinomas, as only two-thirds of these mucin-producing or signet ring adenocarcinomas have the ability to concentrate the radiotracer fluorodeoxyglucose. PET–CT fusion scanning has been reported to improve the diagnostic accuracy compared with either CT or PET scans alone.
- Staging laparoscopy ± peritoneal washings (cytology) should be considered in patients with ≥T3 or node-positive cancers; as many as 20 to 30% of patients with negative radiographic and endoscopic imaging will have occult M1 or stage IV disease on laparoscopy.
    - Peritoneal cytology appears to be an independent predictor associated with death from gastric adenocarcinoma.

SURGERY

Complete surgical resection of gastric cancers is the only treatment modality associated with long-term survival. The tumor stage, location, and performance status of the patient influence the optimal type of resection (subtotal vs. total gastrectomy). Two randomized prospective trials have shown that the estimated overall survival after distal subtotal gastrectomy is equivalent to total gastrectomy for distal gastric cancers. Total gastrectomy is associated with higher postoperative complication rates, more frequent concomitant splenectomy, and longer inpatient length of stay. In addition, it is often associated with significant long-term protein-calorie malnutrition and functional impairment. Proximal gastrectomy has not been rigorously compared with total gastrectomy, but it offers a reasonable alternative to total gastrectomy for cancers of the cardia and gastroesophageal junction (GEJ). In general, this procedure has a higher frequency of recalcitrant postoperative biliary reflux. Radical gastrectomy requires a comprehensive understanding of the arterial supply of the stomach and duodenum (Fig. 15.1), lymphatic drainage basins, and physiologic consequences of decreasing the volume of the gastric reservoir. The optimal extent of regional lymphadenectomy remains controversial. Two landmark-randomized controlled trials failed to show a short-term survival benefit with D2 lymphadenectomy. Results from both a recent trial by Wu et al. and a 15-year re-analysis of the Dutch gastric cancer trial suggest a small absolute survival benefit for patients who were treated with extended lymphadenectomy (>D1).

Operative principles include the following:

- Complete laparoscopic and open assessment of occult, sub-radiographic metastases to the liver, peritoneal cavity, adrenal glands, and distant lymphatic basins.

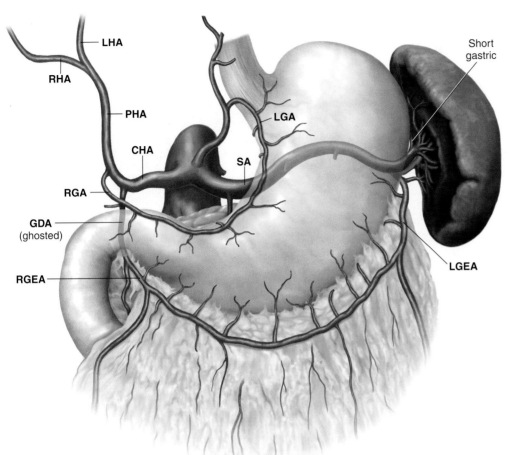

Figure 15.1 Arterial supply to stomach and duodenum. LGA, left gastric artery; SA, splenic artery; CHA, common hepatic artery; PHA, proper hepatic artery; LHA, left hepatic artery; RHA, right hepatic artery; RGA, right gastric artery; GDA, gastroduodenal artery; RGEA, right gastroepiploic artery; IGEA, gastroepiploic artery.

Part II: Procedures for Neoplastic Disease

- Complete resection of the primary tumor with at least 5-cm proximal and distal margins.
- Appropriate regional lymphadenectomy as indicated by the location of the primary tumor (proximal, middle, and distal stomach) and stage of disease. In the absence of clinical lymphadenopathy in the D2 drainage basins (celiac axis distribution), a complete D1 lymphadenectomy may be sufficient treatment. Resecting at least 15 lymph nodes appears to ensure adequate staging accuracy.
    - D1 lymphadenectomy involves removal of the perigastric lymph nodes along the lesser curvature (stations 1, 3, and 5) and greater curvature (stations 2, 4, and 6) (Fig. 15.2).
    - D2 lymphadenectomy extends the lymphatic sampling to all of the lymph nodes around the celiac axis and its named vessels (stations 7–11).
- Gross and histologic intraoperative margin assessment.
- Reconstruction of GI tract continuity with appropriate conduit to maximize function and reduce the incidence of postgastrectomy syndromes.

Operative Positioning and Setup

Patients are positioned on the operating room table in the supine position with appropriate padding. Sequential compression devices and a single dose of 5,000 units of subcutaneous heparin are administered prior to induction of anesthesia to reduce the incidence of perioperative thromboembolic events. An oro- or nasogastric tube and Foley catheter are placed into their respective locations after the patient has been sedated and successfully intubated. Complete pharmacologic neuromuscular blockade is essential to maximize operative exposure and minimize incision length. Broad-spectrum antibiotics covering gastric flora (e.g., second-generation cephalosporins) are given intravenously

Figure 15.2 D1 lymphadenectomy stations.

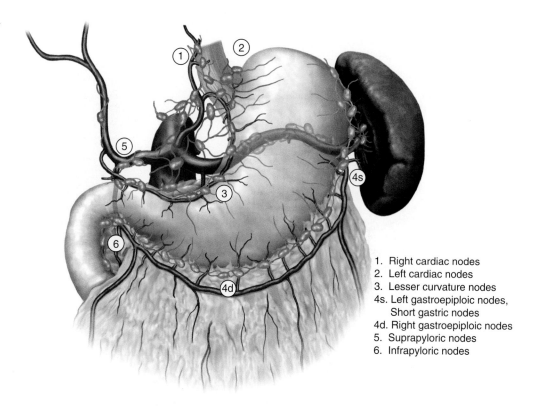

1. Right cardiac nodes
2. Left cardiac nodes
3. Lesser curvature nodes
4s. Left gastroepiploic nodes,
    Short gastric nodes
4d. Right gastroepiploic nodes
5. Suprapyloric nodes
6. Infrapyloric nodes

within 1 hour prior to the incision; antibiotics are routinely re-dosed within one-half life (generally 4 to 6 hours) if needed. The patient's left arm is usually padded and tucked to facilitate the placement of the retractor arm. The skin is prepared with a chlorhexidine solution and allowed several minutes to completely dry before draping the patient. An antibiotic-impregnated impermeable barrier is placed on the abdominal skin.

Operative Technique

Diagnostic Laparoscopy

All patients with gastric cancer operation require complete operative staging prior to resection. A formal diagnostic laparoscopy is performed to rule out radiologically occult metastatic disease. Generally, two trocars are used: a 12-mm supraumbilical incision for the Hasson port and a 5-mm port in the subcostal position along the left midclavicular line. The peritoneal cavity should be systematically explored to identify intrahepatic metastases, peritoneal carcinomatosis, drop metastases (i.e., Krukenberg tumors), or local extension into surrounding viscera (e.g., linitis plastica). If peritoneal washings are required, the laparoscopy is usually performed as a staged procedure. In general, the results of the peritoneal washings take 24 to 48 hours to be completed. Approximately 50 to 100 mL of normal saline is instilled into the left upper quadrant, right upper quadrant, and pelvis; 30 mL of fluid from each location is collected and sent in separate containers for cytology evaluation.

Exploratory Laparotomy

The peritoneal cavity is thoroughly explored through an upper midline (preferred) or bilateral subcostal incision to confirm the absence of metastatic disease. We prefer an Omni or Thompson retractor to separate the wound edges for optimal exposure. The falciform ligament should be divided and the liver thoroughly evaluated by palpation and if needed, hand-held ultrasonography. The entire small bowel and abdominal viscera are examined.

Distal Subtotal Gastrectomy Resection of the Stomach

- The nasogastric tube is advanced into the duodenal bulb and used as a "handle" to elevate the gastric body. The transverse colon is retracted in a caudal direction to facilitate mobilization of the greater omentum off the transverse colon with the electrosurgery device. The micronodular, granular appearance of the greater omentum is reflected in a cranial direction and the homogenous, light yellow fat of the transverse mesocolon is retracted caudally and preserved. The dissection in the avascular plane is extended posteriorly down to the inferior border of the pancreas. If possible, you should remove the visceral peritoneum off the anterior surface of the body and tail of the pancreas. The soft tissue dissection continues to the celiac axis. If a D2 lymphadenectomy is performed, the lymphatic stations (7–11) around the celiac-named vessels will be harvested.

- The duodenal bulb is mobilized off the retroperitoneum and hepatic flexure colonic mesentery. It is critical to identify and preserve the suprapancreatic portion of the extrahepatic bile duct. The gastroduodenal artery is identified and preserved.

- The omental mobilization continues laterally to the hepatic and splenic flexures of the colon. The lateral borders of the omentum are divided using a tissue transection device (i.e., Ligasure or Enseal). On the right side, special care is taken to avoid injuring the duodenal sweep and head of pancreas. On the left side, the omental resection is facilitated by dividing the white line of Toldt to ensure that the splenic flexure of the colon is fully mobilized and not inadvertently injured. The omentum is divided along the splenic hilum with great care taken to avoid capsular traction injuries to the spleen or splenic artery/vein.

- The short gastric vessels are divided up to the level of the gastric fundus using the tissue transection device.

- The right gastroepiploic artery and vein are divided at the level of the superior mesenteric vein between 2-0 silk ties; the proximal end is usually reinforced with a 4-0 prolene suture ligature.

- All lymphatic tissue along the gastroepiploic vessels is reflected toward the planned gastric specimen.

- The supra- and infraduodenal lymph nodes are included in the D1 dissection.

- The duodenal bulb is circumferentially skeletonized by dividing all small feeding vessels between 3-0 silk ties.

- The duodenum is divided with a linear mechanical stapling device with either a 2.5-mm or 3.5-mm load. Hemostasis is achieved along the staple line with the electrosurgery device. Although not necessary, the staple line can be inverted with interrupted 3-0 silk or 3-0 Maxon sutures.

- The lesser (gastrohepatic) omentum is divided sharply from medial to lateral after ruling out the presence of a replaced left hepatic artery. The right gastric artery is divided close to its origin off the common/proper hepatic artery; the proximal end is usually reinforced with a 4-0 prolene suture ligature.

- The lymphatic tissue along the lesser curvature of the stomach is reflected toward the planned specimen. The left gastric artery and vein are divided at its origin (usually along the superior border of the pancreas) between Kelly clamps, ligated with 2-0 silk ties, and the proximal end is reinforced with a 4-0 prolene suture ligature. The left gastric artery is identified because it tends to have a short (posterior to anterior) course before curving laterally along the proximal lesser curvature of the stomach.

- At this point, the proximal body of the stomach should be completely skeletonized and prepared for transection.

- It can be helpful to perform an intraoperative upper endoscopy to confirm the precise proximal extent of the tumor prior to resection. We usually have our assistant mark this location on the serosa of the stomach with an identifiable silk stitch. The stomach is decompressed and the nasogastric tube, endoscope, and esophageal temperature probe are completely removed.

- The stomach is transected at least 5 cm proximal to the superior extent of the tumor. The stomach can be divided with a 90-mm TA™ stapler (Covidien Surgical, Mansfield,

MA), sequential fires of the Endo GIA™ Ultra Universal reticulating stapler (Covidien) with Tri-Staple™ technology (purple medium/thick loads with 3.0-mm, 3.5-mm, 4.0-mm staples). If the TA stapler is used, the distal transected end of the stomach should be occluded with a long atraumatic bowel clamp to avoid spillage. Hemostasis is achieved along the staple line with the electrosurgery device. Additional topical hemostasis along the staple line can be controlled with interrupted 3-0 silk horizontal mattress sutures under the staple line. The gastric staple line is often inverted with 3-0 silk sutures in Lembert fashion. We keep the corner sutures attached to small Kelly clamps for traction during the construction of the anastomosis.

■ The specimen should be transferred to a back table for orientation. We generally mark the proximal margin with an easily identifiable suture. The specimen is hand-delivered to pathology to have all the margins inked and the specimen completely opened. If there is at least a 5-cm gross margin proximal and distal to the mass and no evidence of linitis plastica, frozen sections are not routinely performed. If there is concern about either margin, it is reasonable to request a frozen section of the proximal or distal margin. It should be noted that most pathologists cannot assess the entire circumferential margin and usually sample random portions of the margin closest to the tumor.

Distal Subtotal Gastrectomy Reconstruction
■ The peritoneal cavity is copiously irrigated with normal saline.
■ Reconstruction of the GI tract (Fig. 15.3) can either be accomplished with a
  ■ Billroth I gastroduodenostomy
  ■ Billroth II gastrojejunostomy ± enteroenterostomy (Omega loop)
  ■ Roux-en-Y gastrojejunostomy

Figure 15.3 Reconstruction of the gastric remnant.

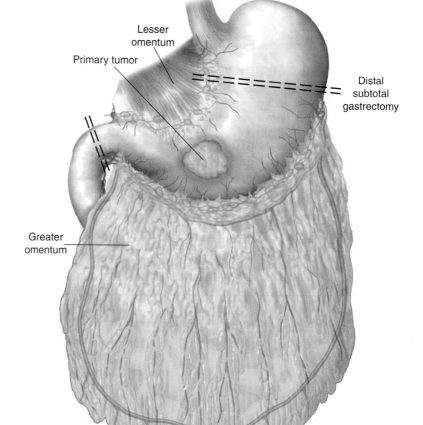

Lesser omentum

Primary tumor

Distal subtotal gastrectomy

Greater omentum

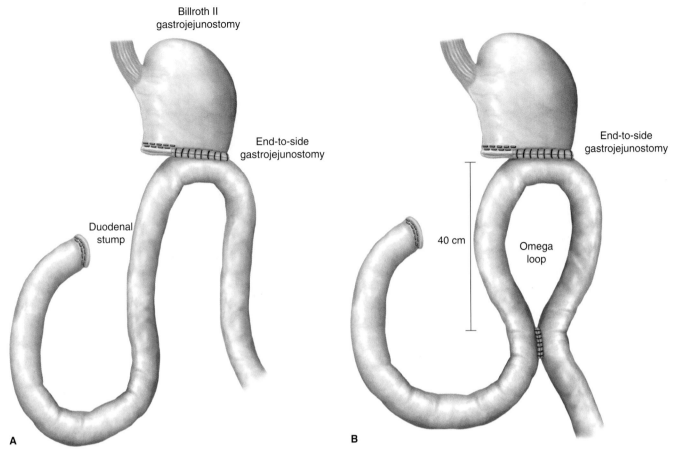

Billroth II
gastrojejunostomy

End-to-side
gastrojejunostomy

Duodenal
stump

End-to-side
gastrojejunostomy

40 cm

Omega
loop

A

B

Figure 15.4 Billroth II gastrojejunostomy (**A**) and with an enteroenterostomy to prevent alkaline reflux (**B**).

Part II: Procedures for Neoplastic Disease

■ The choice of reconstruction depends on the likelihood of recurrence, body habitus, flexibility of the small bowel mesentery, estimated recurrence-free survival, and life expectancy of the patients. In general, we prefer to use the Roux-en-Y gastrojejunostomy.

■ A Billroth II gastrojejunostomy (Fig. 15.4A), ± an Omega loop (40 cm enteroenterostomy to prevent alkaline reflux, Fig. 15.4B) can be completed using a hand-sewn technique or with mechanical stapling devices. We use either interrupted 3-0 silk or continuous Maxon (monofilament polyglyconate synthetic absorbable sutures, Covidien) sutures for both anastomoses. The mucosal reapproximation is performed in Connell fashion. The gastrojejunostomy is typically performed along the posterior wall of the stomach (1 to 2 cm from the staple line) to facilitate drainage of the gastric remnant. A stapled anastomosis is constructed by aligning the sides of the stomach and jejunum with 3-0 silk sutures at least 1 cm away from the gastric staple line. A small gastrotomy and antimesenteric jejunotomy are created to accommodate an endo- or open Endo-GIA™ stapler (3.5-mm or 3.8-mm/blue loads). A generous common channel is created and special care is taken to inspect and control bleeding from the staple line. The common enterotomy is aligned transversely with Allis clamps and closed with a 45-mm or 60-mm TA™ stapler (4.8-mm/green load); alternatively, this can be closed in two layers with sutures.

■ Roux-en-Y gastrojejunostomy (Fig. 15.5) is the best method of reducing the long-term complications that have been associated with Billroth II reconstructions (i.e., marginal ulceration, alkaline reflux gastritis, afferent loop syndrome, etc.). This may be more technically challenging in short/obese patients with a foreshortened or tethered small bowel mesentery. The jejunum is divided approximately 40 cm from the ligament of Treitz with an Endo-GIA™ stapler (3.5-mm/blue load). A window is created in the transverse mesocolon to the left of the middle colic vessels. The roux limb should be delivered without tension and with proper mesenteric orientation. The hand-sewn gastrojejunostomy is created along the posterior wall of the stomach

Figure 15.5 Roux-en-Y gastrojejunostomy.

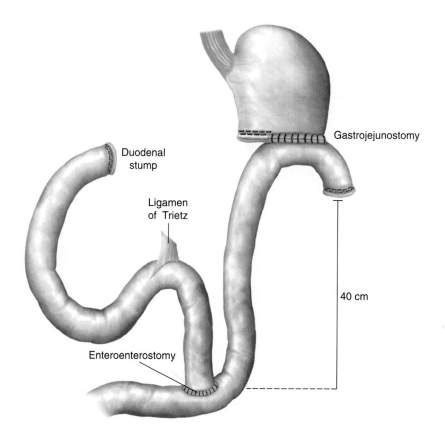

using either 3-0 silk or Maxon sutures in two layers; in general, we try to construct the anastomosis along the lateral aspect of the gastric remnant to avoid the "angle of sorrow" along the lesser curvature near the GEJ. The mesocolic defect is closed with 3-0 polysorb sutures in interrupted fashion; special care should be taken to avoid narrowing the aperture leading to obstruction of the gastric limb. A side-to-side enteroenterostomy is created in a similar fashion so that the total length of the roux limb (distance from the gastrojejunostomy to enteroenterostomy) is at least 35 to 40 cm in length. This is performed to prevent biliary reflux into the gastric remnant. This technique can be performed using either hand-sewn or stapled anastomoses.

■ Billroth I gastroduodenostomy has excellent long-term functional results by preserving the passage of food through the native duodenum. This appears to preserve the proper physiologic balance of GI endocrine secretion (pancreatic exocrine enzyme secretion, bile flow) and may contribute to the inhibition of gastric acid secretion through the production of somatostatin and other hormones. The reconstruction is typically performed in an end-to-end fashion and can be performed using an EEA™-type mechanical stapling device. This technique should be avoided in cancers that are likely to recur locally (i.e., diffuse type, linitis plastica, or node-positive primary tumors.)

■ The anastomosis is visually inspected for integrity. A repeat endoscopy can be performed to visualize the anastomosis for hemorrhage. The distal bowel is occluded with an angled atraumatic bowel clamp prior to insufflation. The patient is placed into a steep Trendelenburg position and the upper abdomen is filled with warm normal saline. An air leak test is performed with maximum distention of the stomach. If no leak is identified, the scope is withdrawn after the stomach has been completely deflated.

Conclusion of Surgical Procedure

■ The peritoneal cavity is copiously irrigated with normal saline lavage and antibiotic irrigation (e.g., bacitracin).

- Meticulous hemostasis is achieved, especially along the retroperitoneal dissection planes and on all named arterial transection sites.
- Nasogastric tubes are generally not replaced.
- Feeding jejunostomy tubes are not routinely placed unless the patient is frail or severely malnourished.
- After the preliminary sponge, needle, and instrument counts are verified, the anterior abdominal wall fascia is closed in a single layer using an absorbable monofilament suture (i.e., #0 or #1 looped Maxon).
- Meticulous hemostasis is obtained in the subcutaneous tissues with the electrosurgery device. The subcutaneous tissues are irrigated with bacitracin solution.
- The skin is closed with staples and the wound is covered with a water-repellant dressing.

→ POSTOPERATIVE MANAGEMENT

- Most patients can be safely managed in a multispecialty bed unit. We only admit to the intensive care unit if the patient has significant medical comorbidities, excessive intraoperative blood loss/case length, or if there were respiratory difficulties during the case.
- Gum and hard candy are encouraged as an economical method of stimulating bowel activity.
- In general, we do not restrict oral intake until the patient passes flatus or has a bowel movement. Instead, we individualize the decision to advance oral intake based on the clinical status of the patient. Aspiration pneumonia is a serious adverse event and should be vigilantly prevented by minimizing narcotics, keeping the head of bed elevated at 30 degrees, and examining the patient frequently for distention that could indicate ileus or obstruction.
- Pain is controlled via patient-controlled analgesic devices (e.g., PCA). We encourage patients to limit narcotics to prevent acute delirium and ileus. Ketorolac can be used for a limited duration (generally 4 to 6 doses) to relieve the musculoskeletal pain associated with the incision and facilitate dose reductions in narcotic analgesics. Since these agents potentiate anticoagulants, we do not concomitantly administer blood thinners during the time that ketorolac is being used. This medication should be used with caution or at a reduced dosage in elderly patients to prevent acute renal failure.
- DVT prophylaxis begins in the OR (subcutaneous heparin and sequential compression devices) and continues postoperatively. Our practice has been to give prophylactic enoxaparin for 28 days postoperatively to reduce the risk of life-threatening thromboembolic events.
- Routine upper GI contrast studies are not routinely performed unless clinical symptoms suggest an anastomotic leak.

COMPLICATIONS

Complications following distal subtotal gastrectomy include hemorrhage, surgical site infection (superficial or organ space), deep venous thrombosis, aspiration/nosocomial pneumonia, and cardiac events. Rare complications specific to the procedure include

- Anastomotic leak
- Afferent loop syndrome
- Duodenal stump leak
- Delayed gastric emptying
- Alkaline reflux gastritis
- Peptic ulcer disease
- Marginal ulceration

Long-term complications include adhesive small bowel obstruction, ventral hernia, internal small bowel hernia (Peterson's hernia with Roux-en-Y gastrojejunostomy), and anastomotic stricture.

RESULTS

The 5-year overall survival rate of all patients with gastric cancer is approximately 15 to 20%. If the disease is confined to the stomach, complete resection is associated with long-term survival rates >50%. Independent predictors of survival after complete R0 resection include age, sex, primary site, histologic subtype (e.g., diffuse, mixed, intestinal), number of positive lymph nodes, and depth of primary tumor invasion.

CONCLUSIONS

The optimal oncologic treatment of distal and midgastric cancer is radical subtotal gastrectomy and regional lymphadenectomy. Extended lymphadenectomy (>D1 nodal resection) improves the accuracy of pathologic staging, increases postoperative morbidity, and may improve survival in a subset of patients with clinically positive nodal metastasis. Perioperative chemotherapy for locally advanced tumors has been shown to increase the rates of resectability and improve long-term survival.

Acknowledgments

The authors thank Roberta Carden for proofreading and editing this manuscript.

Recommended References and Readings

Bentrem D, Wilton A, Mazumdar M, et al. The value of peritoneal cytology as a preoperative predictor in patients with gastric carcinoma undergoing a curative resection. *Ann Surg Oncol.* 2005;12:1–7.

Bonenkamp JJ, Hermans J, Sasako M, et al. Extended lymph node dissection for gastric cancer. *N Engl J Med.* 1999;340:908–914.

Bozzetti F, Marubini E, Bonfanti G, et al. Subtotal versus total gastrectomy for gastric cancer. Five-year survival rates in a multicenter randomized Italian trial. *Ann Surg.* 1999;230:170–178.

Brennan M. Current status of surgery for gastric cancer: A review. *Gastric Cancer.* 2005;8:64–70.

Cunningham D, Allum WH, Stenning SP, et al. Perioperative chemotherapy versus surgery along for resectable gastroesophageal cancer. *N Engl J Med.* 2006;355:11–20.

Cuschieri A, Weeden S, Fielding J, et al. Patient survival after D1 and D2 resections for gastric cancer: Long-term results of the MRC randomized surgical trial. *Br J Cancer.* 1999;79:1522–1530.

Edge SB, Byrd DR, Compton CC, eds. *AJCC Cancer Staging Manual.* 7th ed. Chicago, IL: Springer; 2010:117–126.

Gouzi FL, Huguier M, Fagniez PL, et al. Total versus subtotal gastrectomy for adenocarcinoma of the gastric antrum. *Ann Surg.* 1989;209:162–166.

Kattan MW, Karpeh MS, Maxumdar M, et al. Postoperative nomogram for disease-specific survival after an R0 resection for gastric carcinoma. *J Clin Oncol.* 2003;21:3647–3650.

MacDonald JS, Smalley SR, Benedetii J, et al. Chemoradiotherapy after surgery compared with surgery alone for adenocarcinoma of the stomach or gastroesophageal junction. *New Engl J Med.* 2001;345:725–730.

Sarela AI, Lefkowitz R, Brennan MF, et al. Selection of patients with gastric adenocarcinoma for laparoscopic staging. *Am J Surg.* 2006;191:134–138.

Songun I, Putter H, Kranenbarg EM, et al. Surgical treatment of gastric cancer: 15-year follow-up of the randomized nationwide Dutch D1D2 trial. *Lancet Oncol.* 2010;11:439–449.

Vogel SB. Gastric Cancer. In: Bland KI, Karakousis CP, Copeland EM, eds. *Atlas of Surgical Oncology.* Philadelphia, PA: W.B. Saunders; 1195:419–430.

Wu C, Hsiung CA, Lo S, et al. Nodal dissection for patients with gastric cancer: A randomized controlled trial. *Lancet Oncol.* 2006;7:309–315.

16 Laparoscopic Subtotal Gastrectomy and D1 Resection

Namir Katkhouda, Helen J. Sohn, John C. Lipham, and Joerg Zehetner

 INDICATIONS/CONTRAINDICATIONS

Resectable gastric cancers involving the body and antrum are the main indication for subtotal gastrectomy with Roux-en-y gastrojejunostomy and regional lymphadenectomy (D1-resection: includes the perigastric lymph nodes stations 1–6 and the nodes along the left gastric artery station 7). A minimum of 5 cm proximal margin is required. Laparoscopic approach can be used when there are no contraindications for laparoscopy, such as multiple prior upper gastrointestinal operations, liver cirrhosis, poor cardiac status proven on stress test, pregnancy, or inability for the patient to give consent for laparoscopy.

Uncommon Indications

- Benign tumors of the stomach such as gastrointestinal stromal tumor located in the proximal stomach that is too large for a wedge resection. No lymphadenectomy is required.
- Complications of ulcer diseases such as bleeding and obstruction.
- Gastroparesis with uncontrollable vomiting. Near total gastrectomy can be performed after all medical and other therapies have been exhausted. No lymphadenectomy is required.
- Conversion of distal gastrectomy with gastroduodenostomy or loop gastrojejunostomy.

Contraindications for subtotal gastrectomy are cancers of the proximal stomach or diffuse gastric cancer both of which will necessitate a total gastrectomy for an R0 resection with disease-free microscopic margins. Metastatic cancers are treated by chemotherapy unless bleeding, obstruction, or perforation is present. Bleeding or perforated gastric cancers should be treated with a resection and obstructed cancers can be treated by either a resection or a bypass. Invasion of adjacent organs such as colon, liver, or spleen is not a contraindication to resection.

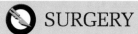 PREOPERATIVE PLANNING

- Upper endoscopy is performed to assess the location and the extent of the disease.
- Endoscopic ultrasound is performed to assess the lymph nodes in the celiac axis and obtain a fine needle biopsy for staging and planning treatment.
- CT scan of the chest, abdomen, and pelvis is important to assess the presence of metastasis in distant lymph nodes, peritoneum as studding and ascites, or distant organs.
- PET scan is used to further assess for metastatic diseases. There may be limited usefulness if the primary tumor does not show increased uptake of the tracer.
- Standard cardiopulmonary workup should be done to assess operability of the patient.

SURGERY

Laparoscopic surgery should be performed using the same principle as open surgery.

Positioning

Patient is supine in low lithotomy position to allow the surgeon to stand between the legs. Both arms should be tucked to allow placement of retractor posts onto the bed at the nipple level. Patient is placed in steep reverse Trendelenburg position to expose the upper abdominal structures with gravity. This is the ideal position for all upper gastrointestinal operations, and the surgeon faces the screen above the head of the patient. The first assistant is to the right and the camera assistant to the left of the patient. This enables the surgeon to have a straight view of the relevant screen. A Mayo stand for the surgeon's instruments is usually placed to the surgeon's right and the scrub technician stands to the left. It is important in this position for advanced upper abdominal procedures to avoid deep venous thrombosis by using bilateral lower extremity sequential compression devices and comfortably padding the knees, ankles, and legs.

Port Placement

Before starting the operation it is important to insert a nasogastric tube to decompress the stomach, thus avoiding any injury to the stomach upon insertion of the Veress needle.

The first 12-mm trocar is introduced after the creation of the pneumoperitoneum with the Veress needle using an optical port in the midline superior of the umbilicus (Fig. 16.1). The reason for midline rather than left paramedian for this port is to extend this incision later in the procedure for specimen removal and introduction of the circular stapler if used. This small incision can also be used for jejunojejunostomy and optional feeding jejunostomy tube placement. This port is used for the camera.

A second 12-mm trocar is placed in the left subcostal position in the midclavicular line as a primary working port.

Three additional 5 mm or 10 mm trocars are used:

- One in the subxyphoid position used to make a subcutaneous tract for the introduction of the Nathanson Hook Liver Retractor (Automated Medical Products Corporation, Sewaren, NJ). This retractor is secured to the right bed post using an Iron Intern (Automated Medical Products Corporation, Sewaren, NJ).
- Two retracting ports are placed in the right and left subcostal margins.

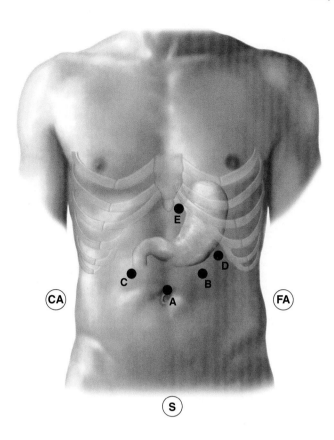

Figure 16.1 Port position for laparoscopic gastrectomy. A, umbilicus; B, surgeon's right hand (scissors); C, surgeon's left hand (grasper), D, assistant's grasper; and E, subxiphoid port. S, surgeon; FA, first assistant; and CA, camera assistant.

Technique

We will describe two common techniques:

Greater Curvature First Technique

Before the actual dissection starts, it is important to check on the various landmarks: the curvatures of the stomach, the gastrocolic ligament and the gastroepiploic arcade, the inferior aspect of the antrum, the duodenum, the pyloric muscle, the lesser sac, and the right gastric artery. The limit of the antrum and the proposed site of the gastrojejunostomy is marked using electrocautery. The assistant begins the procedure by retracting the greater curvature of the stomach using the lateral port. The surgeon uses a grasper and the ultrasonic shears to create windows in the gastrocolic ligament (Fig. 16.2). It is advisable to start outside the gastroepiploic arcade and divide the arcade at the end of the dissection. The first step to follow is the mobilization of the greater curvature followed by the second step of dissection of the antrum and inferior aspect of the duodenum. At this point the right gastroepiploic artery is divided between clips rather than applying electrocautery or using the ultrasonic shears alone.

Using a right-angled dissector, exactly as it is used for dissection of the esophagus, a retroduodenal passage is created starting at the inferior aspect of the duodenum. Dissection then proceeds to the superior aspect of the duodenum, and the right gastric artery is ligated between clips and divided. Again, the right-angled 10-mm dissector is introduced into the subxyphoid port to complete the dissection behind the duodenum, as this port is immediately in line with the dissection (Fig. 16.3). When the retroduodenal space has been created, an umbilical tape is passed around the duodenum, and the window is enlarged to introduce a 60-mm linear cutter through the same subxyphoid port in the same direction to perform the transection. Blue loads are typically used, but green loads can be used if the duodenum is thickened. After dissection the stomach can be pulled upward and the lesser curvature is skeletonized. The posterior attachments of the stomach to the pancreas are divided to allow full mobilization of the stomach. Proximal resection is also performed using an endoscopic linear stapler to the previous dissection limits of the lesser and the greater curvature.

Figure 16.2 Initiation of the gastrectomy. An asterisk marks the beginning of the dissection (division of the gastroepiploic arcade).

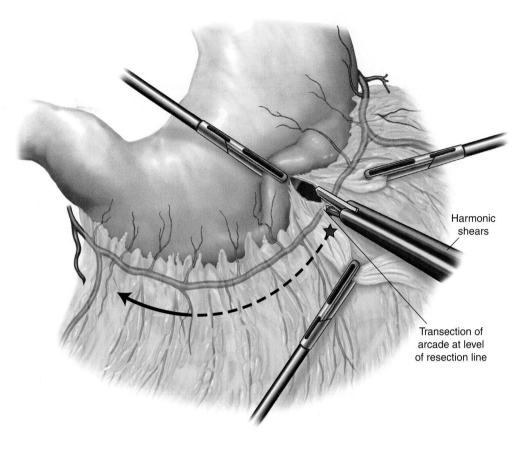

Harmonic shears

Transection of arcade at level of resection line

Figure 16.3 Creation of a retroduodenal passage using the subxyphoid port.

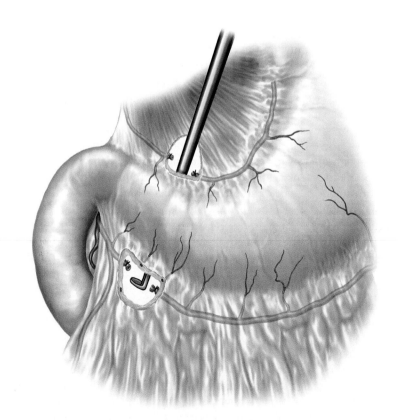

Alternative Lesser Curvature First Technique

The gastrohepatic ligament is divided to enter the lesser sac. The proximal extent of the dissection is the lesser curvature incisura where the left gastric vessels enter the stomach. The distal extent of the dissection is the pylorus, ligating and dividing the right gastric vessels.

The omentum is lifted up and its attachment to transverse colon and mesocolon is divided to enter the lesser sac inferiorly. Dissection is carried proximally to the fundus of the stomach ligating approximately the distal half of the short gastric vessels along the greater curvature including all lymph nodes. The right gastroepiploic vessels should be identified and ligated using a linear cutter stapler with vascular loads, and any posterior adhesions from stomach to pancreas should be divided.

Distal resection is done using a linear cutter stapler at the duodenal bulb just distal to the pylorus. If the tumor abuts the pylorus, the first portion of the duodenum should be taken to the point where it is safe and the margins should be checked with frozen sections. The duodenal stump is not routinely oversewn. The proximal resection is also performed using a linear cutter stapler to the previous dissection limits of the lesser and the greater curvature. Every attempt should be made for an R0 resection.

D1-Lymphadenectomy

The resection includes the removal of the specimen en bloc with the omentum and the regional perigastric lymph nodes stations 1–6, which are around the lesser and greater curvature, as well as the removal of the nodes along the left gastric artery (station 7). It does not include lymph node removal along the common hepatic artery, celiac axis, splenic artery, and proper hepatic artery.

Specimen Retrieval

The camera port site is enlarged to approximately 5 cm, a wound protector is placed, and the gastrectomy specimen is removed and inspected grossly. The size of the incision can be varied depending on the size of the tumor. Frozen sections can be done as needed of the proximal, distal, or radial margins. The proximal jejunum is eviscerated and is divided using the linear cutter stapler between 10 and 20 cm from the ligament of Treitz where the mesentery will reach the remnant stomach without tension in the antecolic position. Then a stapled side to side jejunojejunostomy is created between the biliary limb and the distal jejunum leaving approximately 50 cm of the alimentary limb in order to prevent bile reflux. If feeding jejunostomy tube is indicated, it is placed in the alimentary limb in an appropriate position to avoid tension in the yet to be made proximal gastrojejunostomy anastomosis.

Anastomosis

Gastrojejunostomy can be made by hand-sewn sutures or circular EEA staplers, both done intracorporeally. In order to achieve pneumoperitoneum again, a gel port can be attached to an appropriately sized wound protector. It is difficult to prevent all leakage of pneumoperitoneum, but enough space can be achieved for adequate anastomosis.

Hand-sewn Anastomosis
- End to side gastrojejunostomy in single layer using absorbable sutures such as 3-0 Polydioxanone (Ethicon, Somerville, NJ) after lining them up in the two corners.
- Anastomosis should be 6 cm in length.
- An alternative technique is to reconstruct the gastrojejunostomy with a 70-cm Roux-en-Y limb, in the same technique as a hand-sewn laparoscopic gastric bypass technique.

Stapled Anastomosis
- A circular stapler can be used for anastomosis. EEA with a 25-mm OrVil (Covidien, Norwalk, CT) , which is the largest size made, is used. The tube end of the OrVil is introduced transorally prior to enlarging the incision. This is done to minimize the pneumoperitoneum time after the manipulation of the incision when leak is common.

The OrVil should be well lubricated and the anesthesiologist is asked to pass it transorally until the tip can be seen inside the remnant stomach. A small gastrotomy is made to allow passage of the tube which is pulled and guided gently out of a working port while the anesthesiologist guides the well lubricated anvil into the mouth. The tube is pulled until the post of the anvil is out of the gastrotomy and the suture is seen. The suture is cut, which straightens the previously flat anvil. Then the anvil is left in this position until the time of the anastomosis. The EEA stapler is introduced through the gel port. The staple line of the proximal end of the alimentary limb is excised and the EEA stapler is placed inside. Then it is advanced approximately 5 cm, and the spike is opened at the anti-mesenteric border. The anvil and the stapler are mated carefully to avoid any twisting of the jejunum, and the stapler is fired creating the anastomosis. The EEA with the anvil is removed with gentle twisting motion, and the opening at the end of the hockey stick is closed using a linear cutter stapler.

■ A linear stapler can be used for anastomosis. The anastomosis can be performed on the anterior or posterior aspect of the stomach (Fig. 16.4). After performing an enterotomy on the jejunal limb and the remnant stomach, it is advisable to use several firings of a

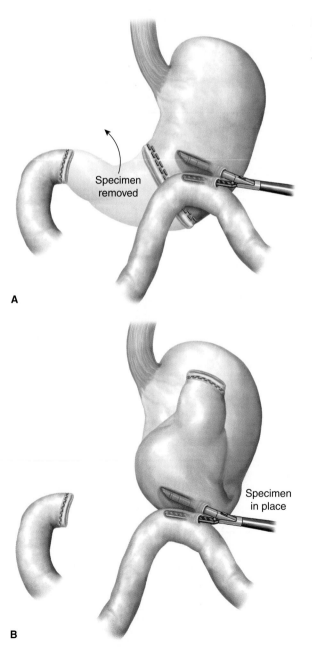

Figure 16.4 Intra-abdominal Billroth II reconstruction: (**A**) resection of the specimen first; (**B**) Billroth II reconstruction first, specimen in place.

Specimen removed

A

Specimen in place

B

30-mm linear cutter rather than a single firing of a 60-mm linear cutter which is bulky and more difficult to handle in this instance. Green staples are preferable if the stomach is thickened. After stapling, the enterotomies are closed using intracorporeal suturing techniques with a running 3-0 Prolene suture. This is preferable to the application of linear cutters that could narrow the anastomosis. It is also advisable to leave the nasogastric tube in the jejunal loop to calibrate the loop and avoid any bites in the posterior wall while suturing the gastrotomies and enterotomies.

OTHER TECHNICAL NOTES

One Jackson Pratt drain is placed in a dependant position to run adjacent to the gastrojejunostomy anastomosis and the duodenal stump. Omentectomy and regional lymphadenectomy are omitted if resection is done for benign disease. Adjacent organs are resected as needed en bloc if either gross inspection or frozen section reveals extension. At the end of the procedure there are two important final steps: First, a leak test should be performed with methylene blue and/or air insufflation of the stomach; second, the patient should be placed in Trendelenburg position to remove all fluid with suction, as some enteral fluid may remain otherwise and promote abscess formation in the postoperative period.

 POSTOPERATIVE MANAGEMENT

Routine postoperative prophylaxis against deep vein thrombosis and atelectasis includes early ambulation and incentive spirometry.

Routine use of nasogastric tube is controversial, but we place it routinely with the tip across the anastomosis, and it is connected to low continuous wall suction until the output is minimal, which usually takes 1 to 2 days.

Contrast studies to assess for leak are not routinely used in subtotal gastrectomies unless it is clinically indicated. Jejunostomy tube, if placed, needs routine flushing in order to prevent clogging, and tube feeding is started on day 2 and used in the immediate postoperative period as nutritional supplementation until patients are able to take in adequate nutritional requirements orally. It can be removed after 4 weeks if it is not needed but should be left in longer if the patient is receiving adjuvant therapy, so it can be used if the patient experiences nausea from the medications. If the feeding tube gets clogged or is removed accidentally, it can be replaced with a wire and fluoroscopic guidance by interventional radiology.

The Jackson Pratt drain is removed when output is low after the patient is started on a diet.

The patient should be followed by the oncologist for any adjuvant therapy, surveillance, and vitamin B12 supplementation.

 COMPLICATIONS

Patients generally recover quickly from the procedure with low complication rates. Anastomotic leak rate is very low at 1 to 2% but can be higher in irradiated or malnourished patients. Patients with a jejunostomy tube can rely on tube feeding for all of their nutritional requirements while the leak heals. Duodenal stump leak or other leak from jejunojejunostomy or feeding jejunostomy site is extremely uncommon but should be suspected if the patient has peritonitis or has enteric output from the drains. Undrained leaks can be treated by percutaneous drain placement in stable patients or operative drainage in sick patients.

Wound infections of the mini-midline wound occur more frequently in patients who are immunocompromised and in grossly contaminated cases. Wound protector usage has not been associated with complete elimination of infections. The overall postoperative morbidity rate is around 10% and mortality rate approaches 0 to 1%.

RESULTS

In experienced hands, the laparoscopic approach shows similar results to the open approach with similar number of lymph nodes harvested and overall survival.

CONCLUSIONS

Laparoscopic subtotal gastrectomy with regional lymphadenectomy should be the procedure of choice in patients with resectable gastric cancer. Novel minimally invasive approaches such as natural orifice translumenal endoscopic surgery, single-incision laparoscopy, sentinel node biopsy, and robotic operations have been reported but the benefits are yet to be determined.

Recommended References and Readings

Etoh T, Shiraishi N, Kitano S. Laparoscopic gastrectomy for cancer. *Dig Dis.* 2005;23(2):113–118.

Huscher CG, Mingoli A, Sgarzini G, et al. Laparoscopic versus open subtotal gastrectomy for distal gastric cancer: Five-year results of a randomized prospective trial. *Ann Surg.* 2005;241(2):232–237.

Jeong O, Park YK. Intracorporeal circular stapling esophagojejunostomy using the transorally inserted anvil (OrVil) after laparoscopic total gastrectomy. *Surg Endosc.* 2009;23(11):2624–2630.

Kitano S, Iso Y, Moriyama M, et al. Laparoscopy-assisted Billroth I gastrectomy. *Surg Laparosc Endosc.* 1994;4(2):146–148.

Kitano S, Shiraishi N, Fujii K, et al. A randomized controlled trial comparing open vs. laparoscopy-assisted distal gastrectomy for the treatment of early gastric cancer: An interim report. *Surgery.* 2002;131:S306–S311.

Kitano S, Shiraishi N, Uyama I, et al. A multicenter study on oncologic outcome of laparoscopic gastrectomy for early cancer in Japan. *Ann Surg.* 2007;245(1):68–72.

Martínez-Ramos D, Miralles-Tena JM, Cuesta MA, et al. Laparoscopy versus open surgery for advanced and resectable gastric cancer: A meta-analysis. *Rev Esp Enferm Dig.* 2011;103(3):133–141.

Strong VE, Devaud N, Karpeh M. The role of laparoscopy for gastric surgery in the West. *Gastric Cancer.* 2009;12(3):127–131.

Tonouchi H, Mohri Y, Kobayashi M, et al. Laparoscopy-assisted distal gastrectomy with laparoscopic sentinel lymph node biopsy after endoscopic mucosal resection for early gastric cancer. *Surg Endosc.* 2007;21(8):1289–1293.

17 Subtotal Gastrectomy and D2 Resection

Carmine Volpe and Bestoun H. Ahmed

 ## INDICATIONS/CONTRAINDICATIONS

The worldwide geographical distribution of gastric carcinoma is variable. It is more common in Japan and other far eastern countries. It is the second worldwide leading cause of cancer death. In the west the incidence of distal gastric cancers has been decreasing for decades; however, cancer of esophagogastric junction and cardia is increasing. Histologically, gastric cancer can be divided into two types, intestinal type and diffuse type, according to Lauren classification. The intestinal type is more common in high-incidence countries like Japan, more likely found in the distal stomach and associated with *Helicobacter pylori.* The diffuse type is more common in young patients, in hereditary gastric cancer, in proximal locations, and is associated with a worse prognosis. Distal subtotal gastrectomy (50% to 75%) is the recommended surgical treatment for distal cancer of the stomach with fewer complications, shorter hospital stays, better quality of life, and no difference in overall survival compared to total gastrectomy.

The east and west remain sharply divided regarding the extent of lymph node dissection (D1, D2) for gastric adenocarcinoma. The general rules of the Japanese Research Society for Gastric Cancer divide the anatomic perigastric lymph nodes into 16 groups (Table 17.1). The anatomic location of the perigastric and extragastric lymph nodes are shown in Figure 17.1. The nodal groups are further subdivided into three regions (N1, N2, and N3), and their designations vary depending on whether the gastric cancer is located in the proximal, middle, or distal third of the stomach. The N1 and N2 lymph node groups of the distal third of the stomach are illustrated in Table 17.2. Removing only the N1 lymph nodes constitutes a D1 gastric resection while the more extended D2 resection requires the removal of both N1 and N2 lymph node groups. The current pathologic N stage is defined by the number of metastatic lymph nodes and not their anatomic location relative to the primary tumor. The American Joint Committee on Cancer recommends that retrieval of at least 15 lymph nodes is necessary to accurately stage a gastric cancer.

TABLE 17.1	Perigastric and Regional Lymph Node Groupings
Location	**Group no.**
Right cardiac	1
Left cardiac	2
Lesser curvature	3
Greater curvature	4
Suprapyloric	5
Infrapyloric	6
Left gastric artery	7
Common hepatic artery	8
Celiac artery	9
Splenic hilum	10
Splenic artery	11
Hepatoduodenal ligament	12
Retropancreatic	13
Base of SMA	14
Middle colic artery	15
Para-aortic	16

From Japanese Research Society for Gastric Cancer: The general rules for gastric cancer study in surgery and pathology. *Jpn J Surg* 1981;111:127.

TABLE 17.2	Lymph Node Groups Resected for Distal Gastric Cancers According to Extent of Resection
D1 Gastrectomy	**D2 Gastrectomy**
No. 3—lesser curve	No. 1—right cardiac
No. 4—greater curve	No. 3—lesser curve
No. 5—suprapylorus	No. 4—greater curve
No. 6—infrapylorus	No. 5—suprapylorus
	No. 6—infrapylorus
	No. 7—left gastric
	No. 8—hepatic artery
	No. 9—celiac artery

From Japanese Research Society for Gastric Cancer: The general rules for gastric cancer study in surgery and pathology. *Jpn J Surg* 1981;111:127.

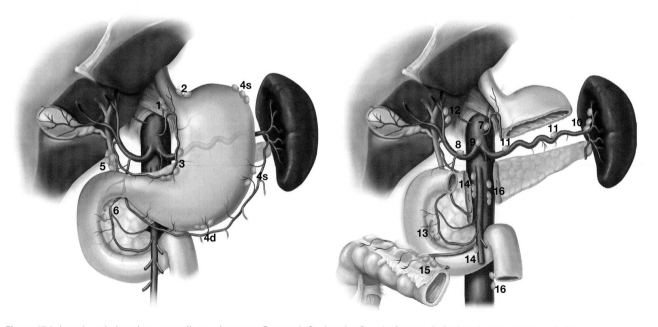

Figure 17.1 Lymph node locations according to Japanese Research Society for Gastric Cancer. **A:** D1 lymph node stations. **B:** D2 lymph node stations.

Indications for Distal Subtotal D2 Gastrectomy

- Patients should be medically fit.
- Adenocarcinoma of the distal third of the stomach
- Gastric tumor that does not cross the line extending from the bare area on the greater curvature (between portion of the stomach supplied by the gastroepiploic artery and the area supplied by the short gastric) to a point on the lesser curvature 5 cm below the cardioesophageal junction.
- Intestinal-type gastric cancer according to the Lauren classification
- T3/T4 tumors after neoadjuvant therapy

Contraindications

- N3 lymph node involvement
- Diffuse type histology
- Cancers within 5 cm of the gastroesophageal junction
- M1 disease

 # PREOPERATIVE PLANNING

The goals of preoperative planning and assessment are to obtain a tissue biopsy for diagnosis, stage the extent of disease, and to address the patient's nutritional status and significant medical comorbidities prior to surgery. Tumor-related complications such as, gastric outlet obstruction, and bleeding may require hospital admission for resuscitation and replacement therapy prior to surgery.

Preoperative assessment includes the following:

- Fiberoptic esophagogastroduodenoscopy for diagnostic biopsy and to determine the location of the primary tumor in relation to the EG junction and pylorus
- To optimize tumor staging endoscopic ultrasonography has been utilized to assess tumor invasion into the gastric wall (T stage), invasion into adjacent organs such as, spleen, pancreas, and left lobe of the liver, and fine needle aspiration of perigastric lymphadenopathy.
- CT scan of the abdomen and pelvis to determine tumor resectability and tumor involvement of peritoneum, lymph nodes, and liver (M1).
- Diagnostic laparoscopy is recommended for patients with advanced tumors T3/T4 who are not obstructed or bleeding, patients considered at high risk for M1 disease and patients deemed candidates for neoadjuvant therapy.
- Nutritional support and nasogastric decompression for patients with gastric outlet obstruction
- Preoperative blood transfusions for patients with hemocrit <25%, hemoglobin <8 g
- Start a beta blocker 1 week prior to surgery for patients over 65-years old or those who have a significant cardiac history.
- Preoperative prophylactic heparin should be given after placement of epidural catheter.

 # SURGERY

The aim of surgical therapy is to resect the gastric tumor with negative margins (4 cm proximal, 2 cm distal) and to retrieve at least 15 lymph nodes for pathologic examination. The surgical specimen should include 50% to 75% of the stomach en bloc with the greater and lesser omentum, lesser sac bursa, lymph nodes from the lesser, and greater curvature of the stomach (N1), from above and below the pylorus (N1), right cardia, celiac axis, and its branches (N2). Since splenectomy or pancreatectomy does not offer a survival advantage the recommended procedure is a D2 lymph node dissection with adjacent organ preserving distal subtotal gastrectomy.

Positioning

The patient should be placed in the supine position with the arms abducted. Reverse Trendelenburg positioning will facilitate exposure. After general anesthesia is obtained via endotracheal intubation a nasogastric tube should be placed in the stomach for decompression. Place sequential compression devices on the lower extremities.

Technique

A variety of standard abdominal incisions are available that provide adequate exposure for gastric resections; we prefer a bilateral subcostal incision (Chevron) because this affords wide exposure of the upper abdomen and excellent retraction of the costal margin.

Diagnostic laparoscopy is indicated prior to incision if advanced disease is suspected.

Upon entering the abdomen, careful exploration should be performed looking for gross metastatic disease. The location and mobility of the primary tumor and the need for bloc resection of adjacent organs and structures are evaluated. A small aliquot of the abdominal fluid is aspirated and sent for cytologic evaluation. A mechanical retractor is placed in the incision to elevate the costal margin and retract the liver.

- The procedure begins with omentobursectomy, the greater omentum is detached from the transverse colon along with the anterior leaf of the transverse mesocolon (Fig. 17.2).
- With cephalad retraction of the greater omentum an avascular plane is entered just above the transverse colon. Bleeding at this point indicates that dissection is too deep into the transverse mesocolon proper (Fig. 17.3).
- Dissection proceeds over the anterior aspect of the pancreas. The pancreatic capsule is opened and the anterior layer of the capsule which is part of the lesser sac is mobilized toward the specimen up to the common hepatic artery.

Figure 17.2 Lesser bursectomy, dissecting en bloc the anterior sheet of the transverse mesocolon and anterior capsule of the pancreas along with its associated lymphatics.

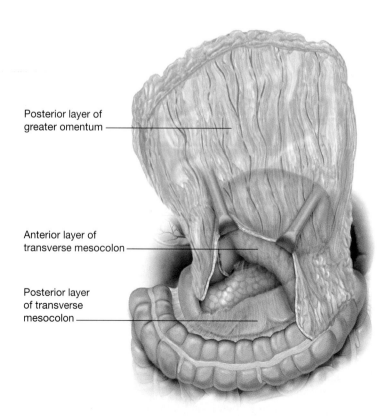

Posterior layer of greater omentum

Anterior layer of transverse mesocolon

Posterior layer of transverse mesocolon

A

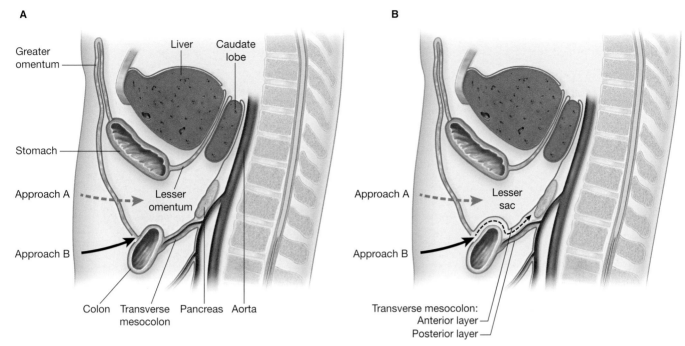

B

Figure 17.3 Proper plane of dissection for complete lesser bursectomy. **A:** Approach "A" demonstrates plane of entry that is too shallow, which would leave behind the posterior aspect of the lesser sac. Approach "B" is the proper plane of entry, which is deep to the anterior leaf of the transverse mesocolon. **B:** Once the proper plane is entered as shown by approach "B" the posterior aspect of the lesser sac is removed along with specimen allowing complete bursectomy.

- Continue dissecting in this plane toward the superior margin of the pancreas; the right gastroepiploic vessels are identified, clamped divided, and ligated; and the infrapyloric lymph nodes 6 are dissected toward the specimen (Fig. 17.4).
- Perform a Kocher maneuver elevating the duodenum out of the retroperitoneum and dissecting the first portion of the duodenum off the head of the pancreas.
- *Lesser omentectomy:* Incise the triangular ligament of the left lobe of the liver with electrocautery avoiding the left phrenic vein. Elevate the lateral segment of the left lobe to expose the attachment of the lesser omentum to the ductus venosus on the

Figure 17.4 Ligation of the right gastroepiploic vessels at the superior border of the pancreas near its origin off the gastroduodenal artery.

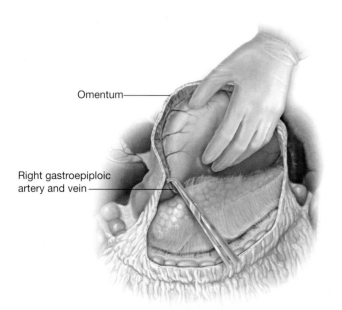

Figure 17.5 Stomach reflected superiorly displaying the celiac axis.

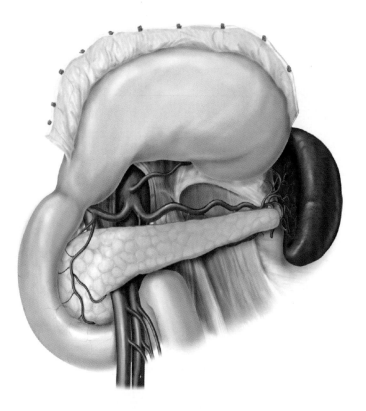

undersurface of the liver running from the left portal vein to the left hepatic vein. Detach the lesser omentum from the ductus venosum with electrocautery along its entire length over the caudate lobe from the right paracardial region down to the anterior leaf of the hepatoduodenal ligament where the right gastric artery is identi-fied. Clamp divide and ligate the right gastric artery at its origin from the common hepatic artery. This ensures complete removal of the lesser sac bursa.

■ Complete circumferential dissection of the first portion of the duodenum by ligating supraduodenal arterial branches off the gastroduodenal artery and transect the duodenum with a linear stapler (blue load) approximately 2 cm distal to the pylorus. Request frozen section to confirm a negative surgical distal margin. These maneuvers will ensure that lymph node groups 3 and 5 are included with the specimen.

■ *Celiac axis dissection:* The divided stomach is reflected superiorly and to the left (Fig. 17.5). Dissection proceeds along the superior border of the pancreas and along the common hepatic artery toward the celiac axis, including lymph nodes 8 and 9. The left gastric artery is ligated and divided at the celiac axis removing lymph nodes 7. For 75% distal subtotal gastrectomy: dissect the splenic artery near its origin from the celiac axis toward the splenic hilum sweeping lymph nodes 11 toward the specimen.

■ With the specimen retracted superiorly, the area of proximal gastric resection on the greater curvature is determined with the goal of achieving a 4-cm proximal margin. The greater omentum is liberated from the greater curvature at this point and one or two short gastric vessels are ligated and divided as necessary to free this area. In order to maintain the viability of the gastric remnant some of the short gastric vessels must be preserved when the left gastric artery is taken at its origin.

■ Proximal gastric resection is complete with a TA-90 or GIA linear green stapler in a manner to ensure complete removal of a rim of lesser curvature up to the cardia. Frozen section analysis is obtained to confirm a histologic negative proximal margin.

Reconstruction

Our preference is to perform a retrocolic Billroth II reconstruction with a two-layer hand-sewn Hofmeister-type anastomosis. We prefer the retrocolic location due to the shorter distance to travel and posterior location behind the stomach.

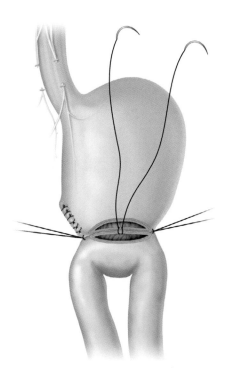

Figure 17.6 Closure of the posterior mucosal layer consists of two continuous sutures of absorbable material starting in the middle and running to each corner.

- The transverse colon is retracted upward and the transverse mesocolon inspected for the identification of an avascular area to the left of the middle colic vessels. A proximal loop of jejunum is delivered through this avascular window in the transverse mesocolon to lie opposed to the gastric remnant. The distance from the ligament of Treitz to the gastric remnant should be no more than 20 cm.
- Align the loop of jejunum up to the greater curvature of the gastric remnant.
- *Posterior serosal layer:* Place interrupted 3-0 silk seromuscular Lembert sutures about 5 mm apart between the posterior gastric wall and the antimesenteric border of the jejunum. Tag the corner sutures with a hemostat and cut the remaining silk tails. Sutures in the gastric wall should be placed about 1 cm from the gastric staple line.
- Excise approximately 3 cm of the gastric staple line from the greater curvature. Make a corresponding incision in the jejunum with electrocautery along the antimesenteric border about two-thirds the size of the gastric opening.
- *Posterior Mucosal layer:* Place two 3-0 absorbable sutures next to each other in the midpoint of the posterior layer inserted full thickness through the jejunal and gastric walls. Tie the sutures and then tie the tails together (Fig. 17.6). Run each suture from the midpoint in a continuous fashion to their corresponding corner. Sutures should be placed in a "V" configuration with a larger serosal bite compared to mucosa. The final corner suture should pass from inside to outside of the anterior gastric wall. This suture will be tied to the interrupted corner stitch from the anterior mucosal layer.
- *Anterior Mucosal Layer:* This is a full thickness layer closure with interrupted 3-0 absorbable sutures with knots tied outside the lumen. Place the corner sutures first next to the suture from the posterior mucosal layer. Tie the interrupted sutures to itself and then to the strand from the posterior mucosal layer. Sutures placed in this layer resemble an inverted "^" configuration. Prior to completing the anastomosis ask the anesthesiologist to place the nasogastric tube in the gastric remnant just above the anastomosis.
- *Anterior Serosal layer:* Place a row of interrupted 3-0 silk seromuscular Lembert sutures between the anterior gastric wall and the jejunum inverting or dunking the anterior mucosal layer.

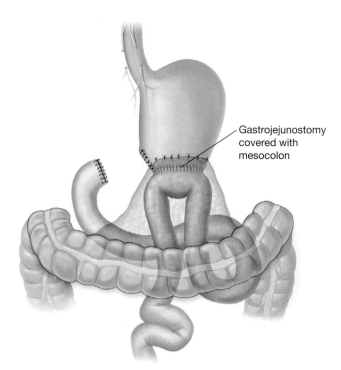

Figure 17.7 Completed Billroth II retrocolic gastrojejunostomy.

Gastrojejunostomy
covered with
mesocolon

- To prevent tension on the anastomosis and internal herniation of small bowel through the opening in the transverse mesocolon, suture the jejunal loop to the peritoneum of the transverse mesocolon with interrupted 3-0 absorbable sutures being careful to avoid the mesenteric vessels. Figure 17.7 illustrates the completed anastomosis.
- We do not drain the anastomosis or the lesser sac routinely unless there is concern of a possible pancreatic injury or leak. If necessary we use a closed suction 10 French Jackson–Pratt flat drain exteriorized through a separate incision.
- The incision is closed in two layers, the posterior sheath with a nonabsorbable suture and anterior sheath with absorbable suture.
- The skin is approximated with skin staples.
- Alternatively, gastrojejunostomy Billroth II reconstruction can be created with GIA and TA stapling devices.
- Oppose the posterior gastric wall to the antimesenteric border of the jejunum with traction sutures. The anastomotic site on the posterior gastric wall is 2 to 3 cm proximal to the gastric staple line closure.
- Create a small gastrotomy on the greater curvature side and opposing enterotomy in the jejunum on the antimesenteric surface with electrocautery.
- Insert the GIA limbs into the gastric remnant and jejunum (Fig. 17.8).
- Engage the limbs of the GIA, and before deploying the device inspect to ensure that the serosal surfaces are directly apposed with nothing between them.
- Withdraw the limbs of the GIA and inspect the anastomosis for hemostasis.
- Close the resultant gastroenterotomy with a TA stapler placing the GIA staple lines at the corners to splay open the anastomosis (Fig. 17.9).

Laparoscopic Approach
- The patient is placed on the table in the supine split leg position. A slight reverse Trendelenburg (15 to 30°) position is very helpful. The surgeon alternates position in between legs and the patient's right side, and the camera assistant is on the left side.
- Pneumoperitoneum is established via Veress needle in the left upper quadrant or Hasson technique to reach an intra-abdominal pressure of 15 mm Hg.

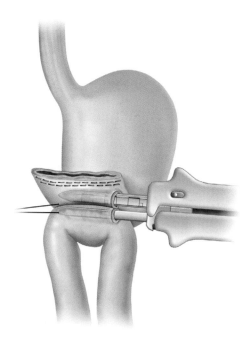

Figure 17.8 Stapled gastrojejunostomy. (Insertion of the GIA limbs into the stomach and jejunum.)

- Access to the abdominal cavity is obtained by the use of four 5-mm laparoscopic trocars and two 12-mm trocar. These ports are placed in a V-shaped arrangement around the umbilicus (Fig. 17.10).
- The gastrocolic ligament is divided using ultrasonic shears (Ultracision-Harmonic Scalpel, Ethicon Endo-Surgery Inc., Cincinnati, OH) along the border of the transverse colon, including the greater omentum in the resected specimen and allowing access to the lesser sac.
- Dissection continues toward the pylorus to include the infrapyloric nodes (group 6) and division of the right gastroepiploic artery at its origin off the gastroduodenal artery.
- Create a window in the hepatoduodenal ligament with electrocautery.
- Identify the right gastric artery; divide and ligate it near its origin off the common hepatic artery.

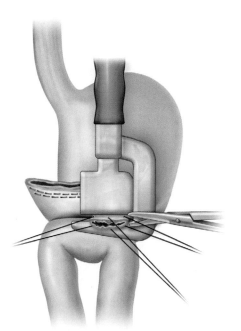

Figure 17.9 The anastomosis is completed with the application of a TA stapler.

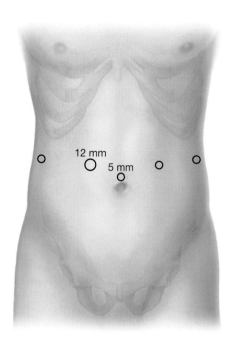

Figure 17.10 Laparoscopic port placement.

▪ Dissect the first portion of the duodenum off the head of the pancreas and divide it 2 cm distal to the pylorus with 35-mm linear endostapler.

▪ Retract the lateral segment of the left lobe of the liver and incise the lesser omentum from the undersurface of the liver up to the right paracardial region exposing the common hepatic artery and celiac axis.

▪ Continue dissection along the common hepatic artery toward the celiac axis. Identify the left gastric artery at its origin from the celiac artery and divide it. If necessary dissect the splenic artery from its origin toward the splenic hilum sweeping the lymph nodes toward the specimen (lymph node groups, 7, 8, 9, 11).

▪ Retract the stomach superiorly and determine the site of proximal resection along the greater curvature. Dissect this area free of the greater omentum and take 1 or 2 short gastric vessels if necessary.

▪ Resect the stomach with a 60-mm linear Endo-GIA stapler (green load) with the goal of achieving a 4-cm proximal margin and removing most of the lesser curvature (group 1 lymph nodes).

▪ Gastrojejunal anastomosis is performed using Billroth II antecolic technique. Bring a loop of jejunum anterior to the transverse colon up to the gastric remnant. The afferent limb should be no more than 20 cm in length beyond the ligament of Treitz.

▪ Place a posterior layer of seromuscular running absorbable suture to hold the stomach and jejunum in apposition.

▪ With electrocautery make a small gastrotomy along the greater curvature of the stomach 2 cm proximal to the gastric staple line closure.

▪ Make a corresponding enterotomy on the antimesenteric side of the jejunum.

▪ Insert the limbs of the 35-mm linear GIA stapler into the stomach and jejunum

▪ Engage the limbs of the device and fire the instrument.

▪ Close the GIA defect with an interrupted layer of absorbable sutures followed by a running outer layer of seromuscular Lembert silk suture.

▪ The specimen is retrieved through an enlarged 12-mm port-site incision via an Endocatch bag. A small wound protector should be used. The specimen retrieval could be delayed to the end of operation provided it is placed in the endobag.

▪ Close fascial wounds more than 5 mm in size with an absorbable suture followed by subcuticular skin closure.

▪ Laparoscopic D2 lymphadenectomy is feasible. Use of the robot, Da Vinci® Surgical System (Intuitive Surgical Inc., Sunnyvale, CA) is very helpful in this context secondary to achieving the most flexible and delicate intracorporeal laparoscopic movements.

In difficult cases, a 5-cm minilaparotomy is made 3 cm below the xiphisternum. This can be used to introduce a hand through a hand port. This helps in the dissection, creation of the anastomosis, and removal of the specimen.

POSTOPERATIVE MANAGEMENT

We routinely request the anesthesiologist to extubate the patient at the conclusion of the operation preferably in the operating room. If further cardiopulmonary monitoring is not indicated the patient will be transferred to the surgical floor unit. In addition to standard postoperative intravenous fluid resuscitation, pain management, and DVT prophylaxis we make every attempt to adhere to the following postoperative clinical pathway in order to expedite postoperative recovery:

- Postoperative day 1: The patient is out of bed to a chair. Prophylactic antibiotics are stopped after 24 hours
- Postoperative day 2: Remove nasogastric tube, maintain nothing by mouth, remove surgical dressing and expose the wound to air.
- Postoperative day 3: Hold the A.M. dose of subcutaneous heparin; remove the epidural catheter, followed by the Foley catheter 2 hours later. Order a liquid diet low in carbohydrates.
- Postoperative day 4: Advance to postgastrectomy diet as tolerated, switch to oral medications, hep-lock IV fluids
- Postoperative day 5: Administer diuretic as needed. Remove the JP (if placed) drain if the daily volume is less than 50cc and the drain amylase concentration is less than three times the serum amylase level.
- Postoperative day 6: Stop subcutaneous heparin if fully ambulating
- Postoperative day 7: Upon discharge warn the patient of transitory dumping symptoms which will subside in 4 to 6 weeks after surgery and recommend a diet consisting of 3 to 4 small meals per day low in carbohydrates. Avoid sweet drinks and consume liquids 30 minutes to 60 minutes after a meal.

COMPLICATIONS

Complications following radical D2 distal subtotal gastrectomy result from gastric storage dysfunction, loss of osmolar regulatory capability, and technical errors in the GI reconstruction performed to re-establish GI continuity. The impaired gastric function leads to symptoms associated with postoperative sequelae known collectively as the postgastrectomy syndromes.

- Dumping syndrome
- Afferent loop syndrome
- Efferent loop syndrome

Dumping Syndrome

Dumping symptoms develop in almost half of all patients undergoing gastric resection but is severe in less than 5% of patients. In the majority of patients the symptoms are transitory and improve spontaneously with time. Surgical intervention is required in only 1% of patients. There are two forms of the dumping syndrome: early and late, with the former being by far the more common of the two. The basic pathophysiology appears to be the same in both, the rapid discharge of hypertonic chyme from the stomach into the small intestine that induces a rapid shift of extracellular fluid into the intestinal lumen in order to restore a state of isotonicity. Early dumping usually occurs within 10 to 30 minutes after a meal characterized by a complex of gastrointestinal and vasomotor symptoms, including abdominal fullness, cramping, nausea, explosive diarrhea, palpitations, tachycardia, diaphoresis, and lightheadedness. Late dumping symptoms develop 2 to 3 hours after a meal and are typical of hypoglycemia. Symptoms are caused by the rapid gastric emptying of chyme with a high carbohydrate concentration into the small intestine leading to hyperglycemia and subsequent excessive insulin release. The insulin response overshoots its mark causing a reactive hypoglycemia and onset of neuroglycopenic symptoms. A diet of frequent small meals, separating liquids from solids, ingesting liquids after a meal, and avoiding simple carbohydrates in lieu of complex carbohydrates alleviates dumping symptoms in most patients. Lying down after a meal can pre-empt the annoying vasomotor symptomatology. If these simple measures are not effective, the long-acting synthetic somatostatin analogue, octreotide acetate, may help to control dumping symptoms in patients unresponsive to simple dietary modifications. The usual starting dose is 200 micrograms per day in divided doses administered subcutaneously before each meal. For the rare patient with severe dumping refractory to medical therapy the preferred surgical treatment is conversion of a Billroth II to a Roux-en-Y gastrojejunostomy. For patients with an initial Roux-en-Y reconstruction the best treatment for intractable dumping symptoms is construction of a 10-cm antiperistaltic (reversed) segment within the Roux-en-Y limb.

Afferent Loop Syndrome

When the afferent limb of a Billroth II is greater than 30 cm in length it is more likely to obstruct secondary to kinking, herniation, and twisting (volvulus) leading to a symptom complex known as the afferent loop syndrome. Obstruction of the afferent limb can also occur at the gastrojejunal anastomosis from ulceration, stricture formation, and recurrent tumor. Chronic intermittent obstruction of the afferent loop tends to occur more commonly than the less frequent but potentially lethal acute presentation. Chronic afferent loop syndrome may occur at any time after gastrectomy and is due to partial mechanical obstruction of the afferent limb. Typically patients develop postprandial epigastric discomfort and fullness due to rapid accumulation of biliary and pancreatic secretions in the obstructed limb after a meal. As the intraluminal pressure within the afferent limb continues to raise it overcomes the obstruction leading to the hallmark features of this syndrome of projectile bilious vomiting without food particles and dramatic relief of symptoms.

Acute afferent loop syndrome is a form of closed-loop obstruction and considered a surgical emergency. Delay in diagnosis is associated with high mortality. It usually occurs in the early postoperative period with the sudden onset of abdominal tenderness and a palpable epigastric mass. If the obstruction is severe enough the intraluminal pressure of the afferent limb may not be able to overcome the outflow resistance resulting in ischemic necrosis of the intestinal mucosa. If this condition is not recognized early perforation of the afferent limb or disruption of the duodenal stump may ensue. The Braun enteroenterostomy, an anastomosis between the afferent and the efferent limbs, is the most suitable emergency surgical treatment for the acutely ill patient with acute afferent loop syndrome (Fig. 17.11). Recommended surgical treatment for the chronic afferent loop syndrome is conversion to a Roux-en-Y gastrojejunostomy.

The afferent loop syndrome can be prevented with the reconstruction of a *retrocolic* Billroth II gastrojejunostomy with an afferent limb no longer than 20 cm.

Efferent Loop Syndrome

Efferent loop syndrome is caused by the obstruction of the efferent limb distal to the gastrojejunostomy anastomosis. It is less common than the afferent loop syndrome and can occur early in the postoperative period or years later. The clinical presentation of the efferent loop syndrome is that of a proximal small bowel obstruction.

Etiologies include postoperative adhesions, internal herniation, and jejunogastric intussusception of the efferent limb. The diagnosis is confirmed by either a gastrointestinal contrast study or a CT scan with oral contrast. Treatment of the efferent loop

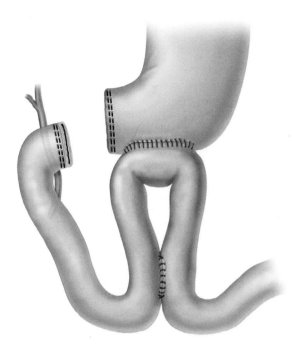

Figure 17.11 The Braun procedure, a *downstream* enteroenterostomy diverts biliopancreatic secretions distally bypassing the gastrojejunostomy is often utilized to treat the acute afferent loop syndrome.

syndrome usually requires surgical intervention. For postoperative adhesive disease lysis of adhesions is all that is necessary. For patients with obstruction due to internal herniation, reduction of the internal hernia and anchoring the efferent limb to the anterior abdominal wall or transverse mesocolon depending on whether it is reconstructed antecolic or retrocolic respectively should be performed. Jejunogastric intussusception is an uncommon cause of the efferent loop syndrome in which the efferent limb intussuscepts into the stomach. The majority of patients with jejunogastric intussusception can be managed nonoperatively; however, for those who fail conservative therapy, reduction of the intussusception and pexy of the afferent and efferent limbs to the abdominal wall or transverse mesocolon is indicated.

RESULTS

There is considerable controversy regarding the appropriate extent of lymph node dissection for patients with gastric cancer. In 1981, Kodama and associates reported the first study that showed a significant survival advantage for patients undergoing a D2 gastrectomy. Patients with node-positive gastric cancer who underwent a D2 resection had 5-year survival rate of 39% compared to 18% for patients treated with a D1 gastric resection. Since then several studies from Japan which were largely retrospective involving thousands of patients have reported 5-year overall survival rates of 50% to 60% for gastric cancer patients undergoing D2 gastrectomy clearly superior to the 15% to 20% 5-year survival rates reported from Western centers after D0 or D1 gastric resection. The discrepancy in outcome between Japan and Western countries led to the development of two large multicenter prospective trials: the Dutch Gastric Cancer Trial and the British Medical Research Council Trial, both two arm studies randomizing patients to a D1 or D2 Japanese-style gastrectomy.

- Summary of the results from the two trials:
  - Both studies showed no survival advantage with the extended lymph node dissection.
  - Higher morbidity and mortality in the D2 arm
  - Longer length of hospital stay in the D2 arm
  - The D2 resection did offer a statistically significant survival advantage for patients with stage II and stage IIIA gastric cancer in the Dutch trial.

- In the Medical Research Council (MRC) trial the majority of the morbidity and mortality in the D2 arm was attributed to the routine performance of splenectomy and pancreatectomy.
- In the MRC trial the D2 arm was associated with better survival than the D1 arm and comparable morbidity and mortality when the spleen and pancreas were preserved.
- The risk of recurrence was significantly lower among D2 patients (29% vs. 41%) in the Dutch trial.
- In both studies the overall 5-year survival rate of the D1 group increased from an expected 20% survival rate to an observed 34% (MRC) and 45% (Dutch) suggesting a strong association between survival and an adequate lymph node dissection.

✣ CONCLUSION

Although the two large European trials did not show a survival benefit, surgeons in Japan, Germany, Italy, and high-volume centers in the United States continue to support the D2 extended lymph node dissection for the treatment of gastric adenocarcinoma. Recent prospective studies suggest that D2 gastric resection markedly improves the long-term survival in patients with stage II and stage IIIA gastric cancer. Practice guidelines of the D2 gastrectomy include the following:

- En bloc resection of the greater and lesser omentum
- Involves removal of the N1 (3–6) and N2 (1, 7–9, +/–11) lymph nodes for distal third cancers
- Resection of the anterior peritoneal leaf of the transverse mesocolon, pancreatic capsule, and lesser sac bursa
- Due to the lack of a survival benefit and associated increased morbidity and mortality, routine splenectomy and distal pancreatectomy are not part of the D2 lymphadenectomy.
- The most recent edition (7th) of the *AJCC Tumor Staging Manual* requires the removal and examination of a least 15 lymph nodes for adequate staging.
- The extent of gastric resection (amount of stomach removed) depends on tumor location and not on the extent of lymph node dissection (D1 or D2).
- For patients with serosa-negative, node positive distal gastric adenocarcinoma, D2 adjacent organ preserving distal subtotal gastrectomy should be considered.

Recommended References and Readings

Bonenkamp JJ, Hermans J, Sasako M, et al. Extended lymph-node dissection for gastric cancer. Dutch Gastric Cancer Group. *N Engl J Med.* 1999;340:908–914.

Bozzetti F, Marubini E, Bonfanti G. Subtotal versus total gastrectomy for gastric cancer. *Ann Surg.* 1999;230(2):170–178.

Cushieri A, Weeden S, Fielding J, et al. Patient survival after D1 and D2 resections for gastric cancer: Long term results of the MRC randomized surgical trial. Surgical Co-operative Group. *Br J Cancer.* 1999;79:1522–1530.

Dicken BJ, Bigam DL, Cass C, et al. Gastric adenocarcinoma: Review and considerations for future directions. *Ann Surg.* 2005;241(1):27–39.

DiSiena MR, Taneja C, Wanebo HJ. Radical gastrectomy and lymphadenectomy: Historical overview, surgical trends, and lessons from the past. *Surg Onc Clin of North Am.* 2005;14(3): 511–532.

Edge SB, Byrd DR, Compton CC, et al. *AJCC Cancer staging manual.* 7th ed. New York: Springer-Verlag; 2010:119.

Glasgow RE, Mulvihill SJ. Postgastrectomy syndromes. *Probl Gen Surg.* 1997;14(3):132–152.

Haglund UH, Wallner B. Current management of gastric cancer. *J Gastrointest Surgery.* 2004;8(7):907–914.

Japanese Research Society for Gastric Cancer. The general rules for gastric cancer study in surgery and pathology. *Jpn J Surg.* 1981; 11:127–135.

Kodama Y, Sugimachi K, Soejima K, et al. Evaluation of extensive lymph node dissection for carcinoma of the stomach. *World J Surg.* 1981;5:241–248.

McCulloch P, Nita ME, Kazi H, et al. Extended versus limited lymph node dissection technique for adenocarcinoma of the stomach. *Cochrane Database Syst Rev.* 2004;18(4):CD001964.

Miller TA, Savas JF. Postgastrectomy syndromes. In: Yeo CJ, Dempsey DT, Klein AS, Pemberton JH, Peters JH, eds. *Shackelford's Surgery of the Alimentary Tract.* Philadelphia, PA, Saunders Elsevier; 2007:870–881.

Nakamura K, Ueyama T, Yao T, et al. Pathology and prognosis of gastric carcinoma. Findings in over 10,000 patients who underwent primary gastrectomy. *Cancer.* 1992;70:1030–1037.

Otsuji E, Toma A, Kobayashi S, et al. Long-term benefit of extended lymphadenectomy with gastrectomy in distally located early gastric carcinoma. *Am J Surg.* 2000;180:127–132.

18 Laparoscopic Subtotal Gastrectomy and D2 Lymphadenectomy for Gastric Carcinoma

Vivian E. Strong

 ## INDICATIONS/CONTRAINDICATIONS

The only known curative treatment for gastric adenocarcinoma involves surgical resection. With recent advances in neoadjuvant and adjuvant treatment in combination with surgery, the curative potential as measured by overall survival has improved, although overall cure rates are still low with 58% 1-year survival and 28% 5-year survival according to national U.S. statistics. This is partly due to the late stage at which most gastric adenocarcinomas are identified. Nevertheless, in recent years more early-stage gastric cancers have been identified, allowing for earlier treatment and better outcomes. Indications for gastrectomy for adenocarcinoma include patients with pathologically proven adenocarcinoma and staging work-up that demonstrates nonmetastatic disease. In addition, those patients with very early-stage (T1a) disease who met specific criteria may be considered for endoscopic mucosal resection. Indications for gastrectomy include gastric cardia tumors and gastroesophageal junction adenocarcinomas that meet criteria of Siewert type III and in some cases Siewert type II cancers. For these tumors a total gastrectomy with D2 lymphadenectomy is required.

Indications for a laparoscopic approach depend largely on surgeon skill and training with both advanced laparoscopic techniques and with appropriate oncologic principles for resection of gastric cancer. As few centers see more than a dozen such cases per year, it may be advisable to refer such patients to high-volume gastric cancer centers. Contraindications are relative to the specific patient; however, relative contraindications may include patients with multiple prior laparotomies, those with locally invasive or very large tumors, or those with a high body mass index rendering safe and timely resection more difficult. Additionally, patients with neoadjuvant treatment sometimes have intense peritumoral fibrosis that prompts an open approach. In cases that are borderline for the laparoscopic approach, starting minimally invasively in order to assess the patient is reasonable as long as the operating surgeon has a low threshold for conversion. The primary goal of resection is an oncologically safe and complete resection. Minimally invasive removal is the secondary goal, and this should be emphasized to the patient prior to resection.

PREOPERATIVE PLANNING/STAGING

All patients with gastric cancer who are being considered for operative resection need a complete staging work-up. This includes an upper endoscopy with biopsy, computed tomography of the chest, abdomen, and pelvis, and for locally advanced tumors, a positron emission tomography scan. Patients require endoscopic ultrasound as an important aspect of staging. Patients who are found to have ultrasonic penetration up to and into the muscularis propria (T1 and T2) are potential candidates for upfront surgical resection. Those patients with endoscopic ultrasound findings of penetration into the subserosal connective tissue (T3 or higher) or N+ (node positive) disease require additional staging with diagnostic laparoscopy and cytologic washings. This same-day operative procedure requires general anesthesia and staging includes inspection of the surface and undersurface of the liver, the peritoneum and remainder of the abdominal cavity (and ovaries for female patients), and in addition, peritoneal fluid cytology is obtained. If results are positive for cancer cells in biopsies of distant tumor deposits or in the collected fluid samples, these patients are staged as metastatic or stage IV gastric cancer and are not candidates for gastric resection. Patients with washings that are negative and with no other intra-abdominal deposits are staged as locally advanced and usually undergo a treatment with neoadjuvant chemotherapy prior to operation. Postoperative treatment for patients varies depending on final pathology from the operation and may include chemotherapy (MAGIC trial) or chemotherapy and radiation treatment (MacDonald trial).

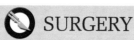 SURGERY

Laparoscopic Subtotal Gastrectomy with D2 Lymphadenectomy and Roux-en-Y Reconstruction

Patients are admitted the morning of surgery after being on clear liquids prior to surgery and being NPO after midnight the day of the operation. In select cases, where a conversion to an open approach is considered likely, an epidural catheter may be placed pre-operatively. When in the operating room, patients have sequential compression devices placed on their lower extremities and undergo general anesthesia. Unless other medical conditions exist to prompt more extensive monitoring, large bore intravenous catheters are placed in addition to a Foley catheter. The operative set-up and steps are as follows;

Instrumentation and Equipment

In addition to the typical laparoscopic set-up, special instruments include

  i. Nathanson liver retractor with Elmed or other anchoring device for the retractor
 ii. Ultrasonic scalpel or sonosurg device (Ligasure may be used as well)
iii. Universal Endo-GIA stapler with stapling loads for vessels, bowel, and stomach
 iv. 5-mm argon beam coagulator (optional)
  v. laparoscopic needle holder
 vi. split-leg bed with foot pads
vii. gastroscopy set-up with a separate tower for intraoperative tumor localization and marking.

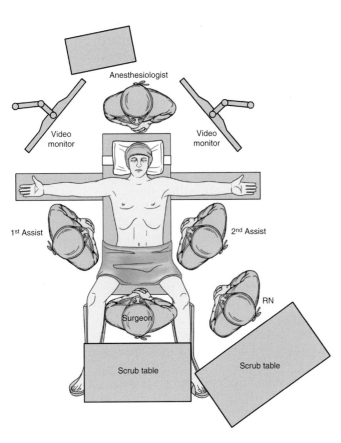

Figure 18.1 Patient positioning in the operating room.

Positioning and Trocar Placement

- Place the patient in the supine position in the split leg position with spreader bars and foot pads (Fig. 18.1).
- Place five trocars into the lower abdomen (Fig. 18.2), typically four 5-mm ports and one 12-mm port (in the right periumbilical position). Carbon dioxide insufflation is maintained at a pressure of 15 mm Hg.

Port Placement

Figure 18.2 Trocar site placement for laparoscopic total gastrectomy.

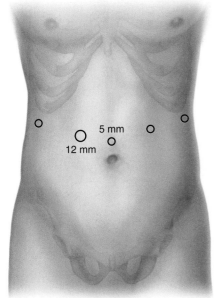

- The Nathanson liver retractor is placed to retract the left lobe of the liver via a 3-mm skin incision made in the midline at the subxiphoid position, and the retractor is then held into place with a stationary retractor. The patient is placed in steep reverse Trendelenburg position.

Operative Technique

Part I: Tumor Localization and Entry into the Lesser Sac

- Prior to beginning resection, visualize the tumor and the intended extent of resection. If the tumor cannot be visualized from outside the stomach, then begin with intra-operative endoscopy to mark the exact tumor site with a stitch.
- Lift the greater omentum in the cephalad direction to visualize the transverse colon.
- Enter the lesser sac via the top of the transverse colon. Carefully dissect under the omentum with care to preserve the transverse mesocolon, until the posterior wall of the stomach is visualized (Fig. 18.3).
- Grasp the posterior stomach wall with a large bite using the bowel grasper and retract toward the left diagonal position to view the omentum from below and proceed with the omentectomy. Care must be taken to periodically visualize and preserve the splenic flexure of the colon and the colon mesentery.
- Transect some of the short gastric vessels allowing for dissection of the splenic hilar as well as the greater curvature lymph node stations and the splenic hilar lymph nodes (Fig. 18.4).
- Mobilize the greater curvature up to the level of proximal transection.

Part 2: Greater Curvature and Pyloric Mobilization with Lymphadenectomy

Keep the patient in steep reverse Trendelenburg and change the positioning of the camera to view the posterior stomach toward the direction of the pylorus.

- Continue the omentectomy to facilitate resection along the transverse colon toward the direction of the gallbladder.
- Once the omental attachments are free, attention can be redirected toward dissection along the posterior wall of the stomach. Keep the pancreas in view and avoid injury.

Figure 18.3 Entering the lesser sac and visualization of the greater omentum.

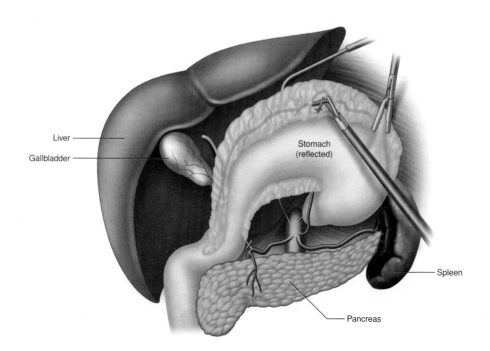

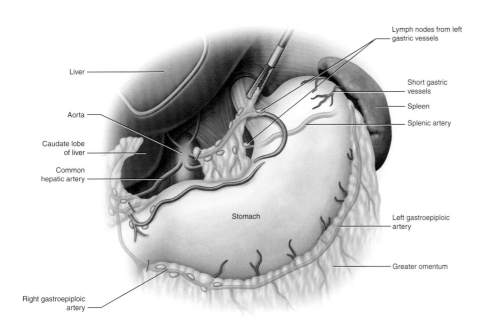

Figure 18.4 Lymphadenectomy of the right gastroepiploic vessels, right gastric artery and common hepatic lymph nodes, left gastric artery and vein, and pericardial nodes.

Liver

Aorta

Caudate lobe of liver

Common hepatic artery

Stomach

Right gastroepiploic artery

Lymph nodes from left gastric vessels

Short gastric vessels

Spleen

Splenic artery

Left gastroepiploic artery

Greater omentum

- As the dissection continues toward the pylorus posteriorly, the right gastroepiploic vessels are encountered and the lymph node bundle is carefully dissected en bloc in an upward direction to be included with the gastric resection. The base of the gastroepiploic vessels is seen here and great care must be taken to avoid injury to the pancreas. The base of the right gastroepiploic vessels is visualized and transected with a vascular stapling device or with endoclips (Fig. 18.5).
- At this point, the pylorus is visualized from a posterior position and freed carefully from any periduodenal and pancreatic tissue. Care must be taken to use hemostatic instruments here such as the sonosurg to avoid bleeding from the many periduodenal vascular branches. The pylorus is also visualized and mobilized from above, and all surrounding attachments are cleared to a point about 2 cm distal to the pylorus. However, do not devascularize duodenum that will remain or be part of the staple-line (Fig. 18.5).

Figure 18.5 Lymphadenectomy of the peripyloric nodes and duodenum.

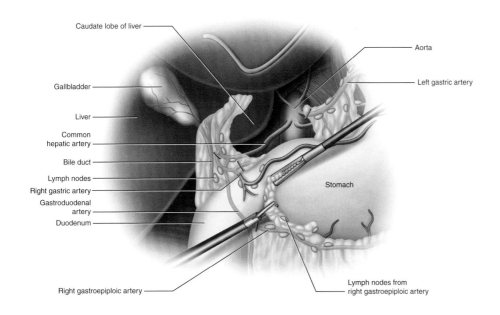

Caudate lobe of liver

Gallbladder

Liver

Common hepatic artery

Bile duct

Lymph nodes

Right gastric artery

Gastroduodenal artery

Duodenum

Aorta

Left gastric artery

Stomach

Right gastroepiploic artery

Lymph nodes from right gastroepiploic artery

Part II: Procedures for Neoplastic Disease

- Next, the duodenum is transected at the cleared point with an endo-GIA stapling device with a staple load for bowel. Only transect the duodenum after confirming with the anesthesiologist that the orogastric tube and temperature probes have been removed. During transection, take care to avoid injury to the nearby portal triad. Stapling can be done via a stapling device with or without staple line reinforcement.

Part 3: Right Gastric Vessels and Lesser Curvature Mobilization and Lymphadenectomy

- Next, identify the right gastric artery at its origin. Dissect the associated lymph nodes from the origin of the right gastric and common hepatic vessels and bring these en bloc with the specimen. The right gastric artery is ligated at its origin, usually with an ultrasonic radiofrequency device.
- Continue mobilization along the lesser curvature of the stomach to facilitate lymphadenectomy of the lesser curvature nodes. For a subtotal gastrectomy, it is important to include lymphadenectomy of the pericardial lymph nodes up to the right crus of the stomach and then include this entire lesser curvature lymph node packet en bloc by dissecting this tissue down toward the proximal transection point on the lesser curve of the stomach. This will remove all of the perigastric tissue along the lesser curve. Take care to check prior to surgery whether an accessory hepatic artery is present and preserve if possible (Fig. 18.4).
- Identify the left gastric artery and vein which will be along the posterior wall of the lesser curvature of the stomach and carefully dissect the lymph node bundle here, taking care to avoid injury to the celiac trunk or splenic artery. This lymph node packet should be dissected upward, toward the stomach, en bloc.
- Ligate the left gastric vessels at the level of the celiac trunk, via a vascular stapling device or with endoclips.
- After confirming that the posterior aspect of the stomach is free of tissue attachments at the level of transection, use a linear stapling device to transect the gastric wall at a point several centimeters above the marked lesion. Each staple firing should be done in a manner that avoids crossing staple lines and preserves the fundus of the stomach.
- Place the gastrectomy specimen with en bloc lymph nodes and omentum in a large endocatch bag and extract through the slightly enlarged right lower quadrant 12-mm port site. Usually the extraction site does not need to be larger than 3 cm in length.
- Send the specimen to pathology and have frozen sections performed of the proximal margin to ensure a microscopically cancer-free margin. If the margin is positive, further stomach must be resected and it may be necessary to perform a total gastrectomy. These possibilities should be discussed with the patient, prior to operation.

Part 4: Reconstruction with Roux-en-Y

Once the margin is confirmed as negative, the reconstruction can begin. When approximately half or more of the stomach is removed, a Roux-en-Y reconstruction is performed.

- **First Stage**
  - Position the patient in Trendelenburg position.
  - Identify the ligament of Treitz.
  - Measure a point roughly 30 cm distal to the ligament of Treitz that will allow for best mobility in an antecolic position up toward the esophageal stump.
  - Divide the jejunum at this determined point with a blue load stapling device.
  - Prepare the Roux limb by carefully transilluminating the Roux mesentery and dividing vessels that are not needed. Take care to avoid injury to the vascular arch.
  - Measure 60 to 65 cm of length along the Roux limb and choose this spot for construction of the jejunojejunostomy.
  - Align the two anti-mesenteric limbs of the biliopancreatic limb and Roux limb, make an enterotomy in both limbs of jejunum, fire the linear gastrointestinal load

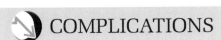

stapler, and close the resultant enterotomy with a running 2-0 silk suture from bottom to top. Additional reinforcing interrupted sutures can be used if needed. Reapproximate the mesenteric defect with an absorbable running suture.

- Next bring the Roux limb to the gastric remnant and return the patient to steep reverse Trendelenburg position.
- Create gastrotomy at a point roughly 1 cm away from the transection point on the anterior stomach wall with an ultrasonic device. Confirm that the stomach has been entered (as the gastric wall is thick). Next approximate the Roux limb parallel to the gastrotomy site. A stay stitch may be used but is not necessary. An enterotomy is created in the end of the Roux limb at a point about 2 cm from the transected jejunum and entry is confirmed. Care must be taken to assure that the limb has not been twisted around the mesentery and that there is no tension or kinking observed in the proposed anastomotic site. Hemostasis in both sites is assured as well.
- The endo-GIA stapler is fired with a 6-cm load to create a large anastomotic opening, confirming that the posterior wall of the stomach and the mesentery of the Roux limb are not compromised. As the stapler is removed, examine the anastomosis for any bleeding and confirm hemostasis.
- The anastomotic defect that remains is then approximated with a running 2-0 silk suture. A second layer may be used if necessary. The anastomosis is carefully examined.
- After creating the gastrojejunal anastomosis, a water-bubble test may be performed via an endoscopy to both visualize the anastomosis from the inside to confirm patency, hemostasis, and secure anastomosis.
- Close the 12-mm port site fascia, remove the liver retractor, deflate the abdomen, and close the incisions.

POSTOPERATIVE CARE AND FOLLOW-UP

The patient is extubated in the operating room prior to transfer to the recovery room. It is not necessary to leave a nasogastric tube in place. Intraabdominal drains are not routinely used. Postoperative analgesia is administered by patient-controlled analgesia or by an epidural. Typically, the patient may go to the floor after about 4 to 6 hours of stable monitoring in the recovery room, and if stable overnight, the patient may begin taking ice chips and sips of water the next morning and should begin ambulating and use an incentive spirometer.

Postoperative day 2, full liquids may be started assuming the patient is doing well and tolerating sips of clears.

Postoperative days 3 to 5, a postgastrectomy diet may be introduced. A nutritionist will see the patient to discuss dietary recommendations.

Patients are seen 1 to 2 weeks postoperatively and patients are then seen for follow-up at roughly 3-month intervals for a year followed by 6-month intervals and then yearly thereafter. In addition to measuring weight and examining the patient, CT scans of the chest, abdomen, and pelvis, alternating with endoscopy, are performed after surgery at ~6- to 12-month intervals.

COMPLICATIONS

Early Postoperative Complications

The main complications that may occur early after operation include postoperative bleeding, atelectasis, pneumonia, wound infection, deep venous thrombosis, and urinary tract infection. The most important early postoperative complications are esophagojejunal anastomotic leak/obstruction, jejunojejunal anastomotic leak/obstruction, or duodenal stump leak. Leak is one of the most serious complications after total gastrectomy and should be the first complication considered for any deviation of postoperative course. Manifestations of leak include early fever on postoperative day 2 or 3, tachycardia that is not otherwise well explained, or pain with swallowing in the epigastric region as well as wound infection. Management of a leak depends on the site and clinical stability of the patient. NPO and IV antibiotics with interventional guided radiology drainage are first steps for otherwise clinically stable patients who have been found to have a leak by Gastrografin swallow study or CT scan. For patients who are or become clinically unstable, return to the operating room for irrigation and placement of multiple drains in the area of the leak may be necessary.

Late Complications

Late complications are rare but may include delayed gastric emptying or anastomotic stricture. This may be relieved by endoscopic balloon dilation.

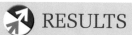 RESULTS

The only randomized, prospective series in the Western hemisphere is from Italy. In this study, the surgeon randomized all stages of surgically resectable gastric cancer into laparoscopic or open approaches. He then followed these patients for survival over a 5-year period. In this study, there were many benefits that are typically associated with the laparoscopic approach of decreased length of stay and decreased analgesia use; however, the most important finding was that there was no difference in disease-specific survival at 5 years. This landmark study demonstrated that this procedure is safe, beneficial for the patients' recovery, and most importantly oncologically equivalent to the open approach.

The largest published series of laparoscopic subtotal gastrectomy in the United States comes from Memorial Sloan-Kettering Cancer Center and City of Hope Cancer Center. In the Memorial Sloan-Kettering Cancer Center experience, a total of 60 patients were evaluated, including 30 minimally invasive gastrectomies (MIG) and 30 open gastrectomies (OG) procedures. Median operative time for the laparoscopic approach was 270 minutes (range 150 to 485) compared to 126 minutes (range 85 to 205) in the open group ($p < 0.01$). The length of hospital stay after laparoscopic gastrectomy was 5 days (range 2 to 26) compared to 7 days (range 5 to 30) in the open group ($p = 0.01$). Postoperative IV narcotic use was shorter for laparoscopic patients, with a median of 3 days (range 0 to 11) compared to 4 days (range 1 to 13) in the open group ($p < 0.01$). Postoperative late complications were significantly higher for the open group ($p = 0.03$). Short-term recurrence-free survival and margin status was similar with adequate lymph node retrieval in both groups.

In the City of Hope experience, a recent review of the gastrectomy experience compared minimally invasive to open gastrectomy. A total of 78 consecutive patients were evaluated, including 30 minimally invasive and 48 open procedures. All laparoscopic patients had negative margin resections and 15 or more lymph nodes in the surgical specimen. There was no difference in the mean number of lymph nodes retrieved by MIG or OG (24 ± 8 vs. 26 ± 15, $p = .66$). MIG procedures were associated with decreased blood loss (200 vs. 383 mL, $p = .0009$) and length of stay (7 vs. 10 days, $p = .0009$) but increased operative time (399 vs. 298 minutes, $p < .0001$). Overall complication rate following MIG was lower but statistical significance was not achieved.

In summary, this chapter demonstrates the technique of laparoscopic subtotal gastrectomy with modified D2 lymphadenectomy for the treatment of gastric carcinoma, and on the basis of data and studies so far, it appears that this technique can be recommended as a safe, oncologically equivalent operation that additionally provides many of the known benefits of the minimally invasive approach in terms of patient recovery and comfort. Additional studies will help to further confirm these initial reports.

Recommended References and Readings

Cunningham D, Allum WH, Stenning SP, et al. Perioperative chemotherapy versus surgery alone for resectable gastroesophageal cancer. *N Engl J Med.* 2006;355(1):11–20.

Guzman EA, Pigazzi A, Lee B, et al. Totally laparoscopic gastric resection with extended lymphadenectomy for gastric adenocarcinoma. *Ann Surg Oncol.* 2009;16(8):2218–2223.

Hundahl SA, Phillips JL, Menck HR. The National Cancer Data Base Report on poor survival of U.S. gastric carcinoma patients treated with gastrectomy: Fifth Edition American Joint Committee on Cancer staging, proximal disease, and the "different disease" hypothesis. *Cancer.* 2000;88(4):921–932.

Huscher CG, Mingoli A, Sgarzini G, et al. Laparoscopic versus open subtotal gastrectomy for distal gastric cancer: Five-year results of a randomized prospective trial. *Ann Surg.* 2005;241(2):232–237.

Kim YW, Baik YH, Yun YH, et al. Improved quality of life outcomes after laparoscopy-assisted distal gastrectomy for early gastric cancer: Results of a prospective randomized clinical trial. *Ann Surg.* 2008;248(5):721–727.

Macdonald JS, Smalley SR, Benedetti J, et al. Chemoradiotherapy after surgery compared with surgery alone for adenocarcinoma of the stomach or gastroesophageal junction. *N Engl J Med.* 2001; 345(10):725–730.

Siegel R, Ward E, Brawley O, Jemal A. Cancer statistics, 2011: The impact of eliminating socioeconomic and racial disparities on premature cancer deaths. *CA Cancer J Clin.* 2011;61(4):212–236.

Strong VE, Devaud N, Allen PJ, et al. Laparoscopic versus open subtotal gastrectomy for adenocarcinoma: A case-control study. *Ann Surg Oncol.* 2009;16(6):1507–1513.

19 Total Gastrectomy and Esophagojejunostomy

Andrew M. Lowy and Hop S. Tran Cao

 ## INDICATIONS/CONTRAINDICATIONS

Total gastrectomy, with subsequent restoration of alimentary tract continuity in the form of esophagojejunostomy, is an operation that can result in significant postoperative metabolic and nutritional derangements. For this reason, care must be taken to properly select and optimize the right candidate for this procedure.

The most common indication for total gastrectomy is an attempt at curative resection for gastric adenocarcinoma located within the fundus or body of the stomach. While some authors have advocated the use of subtotal gastrectomy for tumors limited to the proximal third of the stomach, this approach offers no survival advantage while being associated with greater perioperative morbidity and mortality. Instead, we reserve subtotal gastrectomies for tumors of the gastric antrum, for which distal gastrectomy has been well established as the procedure of choice as long as a generous proximal margin (5 to 6 cm) can be obtained. Linitis plastica, a diffuse form of gastric adenocarcinoma involving the entire stomach, may theoretically be treated with total gastrectomy. However, cancer cells in this disease process tend to infiltrate far beyond the visible tumor, and clear resection margins are often not achievable; surgery is therefore rarely used to treat this lethal disease.

Less common indications for total gastrectomy include the following:

- Other neoplasms of the stomach such as gastric neuroendocrine tumors, leiomyosarcomas, or lymphosarcomas
- Palliation for hemorrhagic, obstructive, or perforated gastric tumors or intractable pain. With advances in endoscopic and angiographic technologies, the need for surgical intervention in a palliative role has diminished.
- Zollinger–Ellison syndrome that has failed other attempts at symptom control. In a patient with Zollinger–Ellison, every effort should be made to identify and remove the primary gastrinoma lesion and to debulk metastatic disease when possible. Medical management should include the use of proton pump inhibitors and octreotide, a somatostatin analogue. However, when ulcer diathesis persists despite these efforts, a total gastrectomy can be offered for symptomatic relief.

Contraindications to total gastrectomy in the setting of gastric cancer include the presence of disseminated disease with peritoneal seeding and/or liver metastases and local invasion of the tumor into the aorta, celiac axis, or vena cava. On the other hand, direct extension of the tumor into adjacent structures, including the transverse colon, middle colic vessels, pancreatic body and tail, spleen, or left lobe of the liver, does not preclude resection; in this circumstance, en bloc resection of the stomach with the involved organ segment is warranted.

PREOPERATIVE PLANNING

In planning a total gastrectomy for gastric cancer, a thorough staging work-up should be undertaken. Obtaining tissue diagnosis is paramount and is achieved via upper gastrointestinal endoscopy. This modality allows visual inspection and sampling of the tumor; biopsies should be taken at multiple sites from the ulcer edges and not the base, which may be necrotic and yield false-negative results. Endoscopic ultrasound may be of value in assessing the depth of tumor invasion and nodal status, particularly in patients enrolling in neoadjuvant treatment studies.

A high-quality computed tomography (CT) scan of the chest, abdomen, and pelvis is obtained to look for metastatic disease and assess the extent of tumor invasion. Imaging of the chest is especially helpful in patients with proximal tumors when the possibility of thoracotomy is contemplated.

For the same reason, preoperative pulmonary function tests may be indicated for those patients with high proximal lesions, while a mechanical bowel preparation should be considered if the transverse colon is involved by the tumor and en bloc resection is anticipated.

Patients with gastric carcinoma often present with advanced disease and are nutritionally depleted as a result of obstructive symptoms or early satiety. Therefore, their nutritional status should be assessed and optimized if possible.

Basic blood tests, including liver function tests and coagulation parameters, are taken.

SURGERY

Pertinent Anatomy

Two major anatomical concepts should be mastered when approaching total gastrectomy. First, the blood supply to the stomach and, by extension, its lymphatic drainage must be well understood (Fig. 19.1). The stomach is supplied by an extensive vascular network formed by four major arteries stemming directly or indirectly from the celiac axis, the main vascular branch to the embryologic foregut. The lesser curvature of the stomach is vascularized by the left gastric artery, a main branch of the celiac axis, and the right gastric artery, most often a branch of the hepatic artery. The vascular supply to the greater curvature consists of the left gastroepiploic artery, a branch of the splenic artery, and the right gastroepiploic artery, which most often stems from the gastroduodenal artery. The greater curvature also receives some blood supply from short gastric arteries originating from the splenic artery near the splenic hilum.

It is also important to understand the three-dimensional relationship of the stomach with its surrounding organs (Fig. 19.2). The stomach is attached to the liver by the lesser omentum, also known as the gastrohepatic ligament. The greater omentum hangs off its greater curvature and attaches to the transverse colon along an avascular plane. The transverse mesocolon lies behind the stomach and reaches the pancreas, a retroperitoneal organ that sits directly posterior to the stomach. A tumor of the stomach may therefore encroach or directly invade any of these structures, as well as the left lobe of the liver, or the spleen.

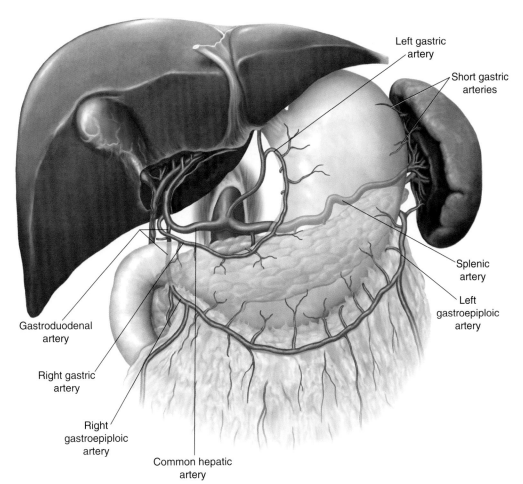

Figure 19.1 The arterial supply to the stomach originates from the celiac axis and consists of four main vessels: two along the lesser curve, the right and left gastric arteries, and two along the greater curve, the right and left gastroepiploic arteries. Lymph nodes along these vessels must be included in the specimen. A D2 lymph node dissection includes the nodes along the celiac, splenic, and hepatic arteries as well.

Left gastric artery

Short gastric arteries

Splenic artery

Left gastroepiploic artery

Gastroduodenal artery

Right gastric artery

Right gastroepiploic artery

Common hepatic artery

Part II: Procedures for Neoplastic Disease

Positioning

The patient is placed on the table in the supine position, with the bed in slight reverse Trendelenburg position. The abdomen and chest are widely prepped and draped. The arms can be abducted to allow for attachment of the Bookwalter retractor. A Foley catheter is inserted and appropriate prophylactic antibiotics administered. The patient is provided both pharmacologic and mechanical thrombophylaxis.

Incision/Exposure

When the indication for total gastrectomy is gastric cancer, we routinely start by performing a staging laparoscopy. This procedure has been shown to spare between 23 and 37% of patients with CT-occult metastatic disease an unnecessary laparotomy by detecting small peritoneal or liver deposits. Particular attention is paid to the liver surfaces, omentum, and peritoneum in the pouch of Douglas.

Even following a negative laparoscopy, we initially prefer a limited midline epigastric incision extending from the xiphoid process that allows for exploration and confirmation of resectability. Once this is accomplished, the incision is extended to or just past the umbilicus to afford adequate exposure. If the tumor involves the proximal stomach and extends to the distal esophagus, a combined thoracoabdominal approach may be necessary. A Bookwalter retractor is placed; the lateral segment of the left lobe of the liver is mobilized and is retracted anteriorly and to the right with a fan retractor.

Surgical Technique

The first step of the operation is to perform a thorough exploration of the abdominal cavity to confirm resectability.

Figure 19.2 The stomach is attached superiorly to the liver via the gastrohepatic ligament or lesser omentum. The greater omentum hangs from its greater curvature and attaches to the transverse colon along a relatively avascular plane; opening up this plane allows access to the lesser sac and evaluation of the posterior stomach, mesocolon, pancreas, and celiac axis.

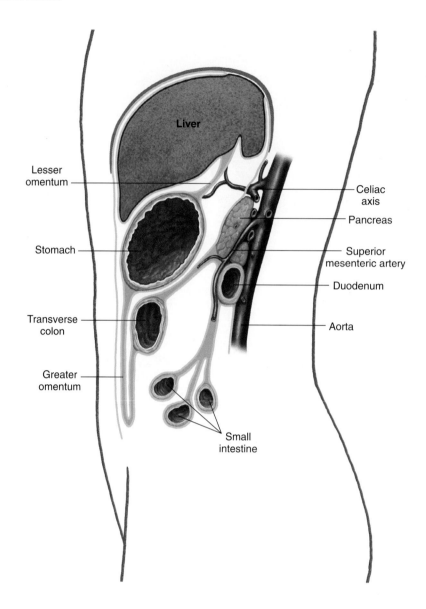

- To rule out metastatic disease, the liver is thoroughly assessed and palpated, and the peritoneal surface, especially in the pouch of Douglas, is carefully examined for tumor deposits.
- Next, the stomach is evaluated to determine the extent of local invasion. This is accomplished by manually inspecting the anterior surface of the stomach. The posterior aspect of the stomach is palpated after accessing the lesser sac to ensure that the tumor does not invade into the aorta, celiac axis, or vena cava. Such a finding should be rare as preoperative imaging is highly accurate in assessing these relationships. As previously mentioned, direct extension into the transverse colon or its mesenteric root, the pancreas, the spleen, or the left lobe of the liver does not contraindicate total gastrectomy; in such a situation, en bloc resection is indicated, although prognosis for these patients is poor.

Once the potential for surgical cure has been verified, total gastrectomy can be carried out. While there continues to be significant controversy surrounding the optimal extent of lymph node dissection, our practice is to perform a modified D2 lymphadenectomy that removes lymph nodes along the celiac, splenic, and hepatic arteries in addition to the perigastric lymph nodes. Routine splenectomy and distal pancreatectomy are not performed, as they offer no survival advantage while accounting for the majority of D2 dissection-associated complications reported in the literature. With this in mind, total gastrectomy is begun along the greater curvature and omentum.

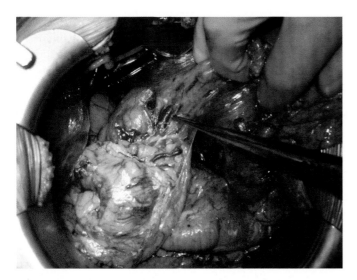

Figure 19.3 The right gastroepiploic vessels are identified along the most distal aspect of the greater omental attachment to the stomach, near the pylorus. These vessels are dissected back to the arterial origin and ligated there. The subpyloric lymph nodes are swept up and taken with the specimen.

- The transverse colon is isolated by taking down the hepatic and splenic flexures. It is then dissected away from the greater omentum along the avascular plane. The colon is then retracted inferiorly while the omentum is lifted up to expose the lesser sac, including the anterior surface of the pancreas and the transverse mesocolon.
- The greater omentum is traced up on the left side until the left gastroepiploic vessels are identified, ligated, and divided. The splenic hilum is examined; if it is involved with the tumor, a splenectomy is performed. Otherwise, the short gastric vessels are taken down as close to the spleen as possible. Vessel or tissue sealing devices can be used to complete this division rapidly with good hemostasis; likewise, they are a good option to complete the omental dissection described above.
- The distal-most gastric attachment of the greater omentum leads to the duodenum and head of the pancreas. It is there that the right gastroepiploic vessels are encountered (Fig. 19.3); these are ligated near their origins with 2-0 silk sutures and divided. Care must be taken to avoid injuring the middle colic vessels during this process. Lymphatic tissue in this area, including the subpyloric lymph nodes, is swept up toward the specimen.

Attention is next directed to the lesser omentum and the duodenum.

- First, a Kocher maneuver is performed and the duodenum is carefully separated from the anterior surface of the pancreas, making sure to ligate any bridging vessels.
- Next, with the liver retracted cephalad, the peritoneal layer covering the hepatoduodenal ligament is incised, and the right gastric vessels are identified along the superior margin of the duodenum. They are dissected to their origins, ligated, and divided. Suprapyloric lymph nodes are part of the perigastric fatty tissue here that must be swept toward the specimen.
- The duodenum can now be safely divided at a distance approximately 2 to 3 cm distal to the pylorus. This can be done with the use of a linear stapler; the staple line on the duodenal stump may be reinforced with an interrupted layer of Lembert seromuscular sutures; however, care must be taken to avoid creating excess tension. Frozen sections of the duodenum on the specimen side are obtained to ensure adequate distal margin.

With the distal stomach and duodenum having been transected, the dissection is now carried proximally toward the esophageal hiatus in order to mobilize the esophagus.

- To facilitate subsequent steps in the dissection, the triangular ligament of the left lobe of the liver is taken down with electrocautery, exposing the esophageal hiatus. The left lobe is then retracted to the right under a retractor.
- The incision in the gastrohepatic ligament, which had been initiated during the mobilization of the right gastric vessels, is now carried proximally until the inferior

phrenic vessels are encountered and divided. The peritoneal reflection overlying the esophageal hiatus is opened in continuity with the gastrohepatic ligament to expose the diaphragmatic crura. Blunt digital dissection can be performed to encircle the esophagus, facilitating placement of a Penrose drain. The left hand is then passed behind the esophagus to expose the gastrophrenic ligament, which is incised between the gastric fundus and diaphragm.

■ The common hepatic artery is identified and traced back along the superior border of the pancreas to the celiac axis; all lymphatic tissues surrounding these vessels are gently dissected toward the stomach.

■ The left gastric vessels are isolated near the origin of the artery; *prior to the ligation of the left gastric artery with 2-0 silk sutures, it is important to verify that an aberrant left hepatic artery does not originate from it.*

■ The stomach is retracted upward, and any congenital attachments are divided. The lymphatic tissue adjacent to the splenic artery can now be dissected toward the stomach for inclusion with the specimen.

■ Removing the capsule of the pancreas and the superior peritoneal leaf of the mesocolon with the specimen has been described; however, no data exist to support the necessity of this maneuver, and we do not typically perform this step.

At this time, the stomach's only remaining attachment is the esophagus, which tends to retract into the thoracic cavity once divided. Steps are taken to ensure that there remains adequate length to perform a safe anastomosis after gastrectomy and that margins are adequate (they should be at least 6 cm from the grossly detected tumor), including

■ dividing the vagus nerves between hemoclips after clearly identifying them (Fig. 19.4)

■ approximating the diaphragmatic crura posterior to the esophagus with 0 silk sutures to reduce the hiatal size

■ anchoring the esophagus to the diaphragmatic hiatus with simple interrupted sutures; the stitches are placed in a spot on the esophagus about 2 cm proximal to the site of division.

With the esophagus anchored, the stomach is retracted upward to expose the back side of the esophagus, which is then partially divided. Corner sutures are placed at the lateral edges of the esophageal opening. These are not tied down but instead tagged with hemostats. The division of the esophagus is then completed, and the specimen removed from the field (Fig. 19.5). At this time, the proximal margin of the specimen is sent for frozen section.

The next step in the operation is to proceed with reconstruction of the GI tract. Following total gastrectomy, several reconstructive methods have been described that

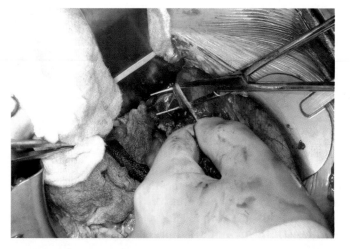

Figure 19.4 The right vagus nerve is identified along the esophagus; it is dissected free and divided between hemoclips. Division of both vagi relieves some of the upward retraction on the esophagus and facilitates construction of the esophagojejunal anastomosis.

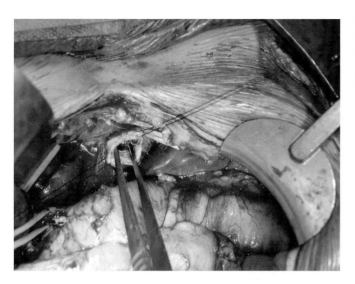

Figure 19.5 The esophagus has now been divided fully from the stomach; two corner stitches will aid in stabilizing and aligning the esophagus for esophagojejunostomy.

aim to reduce the transit time or reproduce the reservoir capacity of the resected stomach, including jejunal interposition, jejunal pouch creation, or a combination thereof. However, none of these methods have been proven to be superior to the standard Roux-en-Y reconstruction. Our preferred method is to perform a retrocolic Roux-en-Y end-to-side esophagojejunostomy, which can either be handsewn or stapled with an EEA stapler. We describe here the hand-sewn anastomosis.

- The small bowel is lifted out of the abdominal cavity and the vascular arcades inspected. The jejunum should be divided approximately 20 cm distal to the ligament of Treitz, but before doing so, this segment of bowel is tested to determine whether its mesentery can reach the diaphragm. Usually, adequate length is achieved with division of one to two arcade vessels.
- A small 4-cm incision is then made in the avascular portion of the transverse mesocolon, to the left of the middle colic artery. The Roux limb is brought up through this opening and positioned next to the esophagus, with the stapled end facing to the left, to set up the end of the esophagus-to-side of the jejunal limb anastomosis. Adequate length is once again verified. It is also important to avoid twisting or kinking the jejunal mesentery in this process.
- To avoid internal herniation, the wall of the jejunal limb is sutured to the mesocolon opening, and any remaining defect is occluded. Likewise, the free edge of the jejunal mesentery is superficially approximated to the posterior peritoneal surfaces.
- To relieve the tension on the upcoming anastomosis, the jejunal loop is suspended to the diaphragm with a row of interrupted 2-0 silk sutures placed between the diaphragm just posterior to the esophageal hiatus and the posterior wall of the jejunum near its mesentery.

At this time, the jejunal loop should be well aligned with the esophageal opening; a one-layer hand-sewn anastomosis can now be performed. The jejunal opening should be made on the antimesenteric border of the jejunum; this anticipated incision site should be scored superficially with cautery to help in the placement of the posterior seromuscular layer.

- First, two outer, posterior "seromuscular" sutures are placed at the corners of the esophageal wall and the posterior jejunum (the esophagus lacks a serosa; the bite taken on the esophageal side consists therefore of muscle only); these are tagged with hemostats. One or two simple interrupted 3-0 silk sutures are placed between these corner sutures and tied. The corner stitches are then tied down to set the Roux limb in place.
- The jejunal incision site, which should lie just anterior to this created row, is now opened with the jejunum under traction. The length of this incision should be

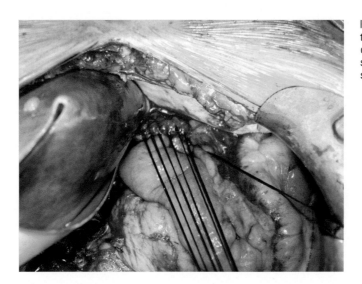

Figure 19.6 The anterior layer of the esophagojejunostomy is completed with simple interrupted sutures tied on the extraluminal side.

approximately that of the esophageal diameter. Next, the posterior anastomosis is created with the use of 3-0 silk sutures placed in an interrupted fashion, starting with a corner suture on one end and progressing toward the other. Knots are tied on the luminal side.

■ With the posterior layers now complete, a nasogastric tube is passed through the esophageal opening and guided down into the descending portion of the jejunum. The anterior layer is then closed with interrupted 3-0 silk sutures tied extraluminally; again it is best to start at one lateral edge and incrementally move toward the other end (Fig. 19.6).

Attention is now turned to the jejunojejunostomy part of the Roux-en-Y and obliteration of any newly created space to avoid internal herniation.

■ The jejunojejunostomy can be handsewn or performed with a stapler. For a handsewn anastomosis, the open end of the proximal jejunum is anastomosed to the side of the jejunal Roux limb, approximately 60 cm distal to the esophagojejunostomy; this is done in two layers using 3-0 silk sutures. Our preference is to perform a side-to-side stapled jejunojejunostomy with the use of a GIA-75 stapler. The proximal jejunal limb is lined up next to the Roux limb side-by-side, with the stapled end directed inferiorly. The antimesenteric corner of the staple line is then excised while a small incision is made in the adjoining antimesenteric border of the Roux limb. The stapler is then introduced and fired. The staple lines are checked intraluminally for hemostasis. The mucosal jejunal openings are then grasped with Allis clamps and lined up; a TA-60 stapler is fired deep to the clamps. A "crotch" stitch is placed at the end of the jejunojejunostomy staple line to take some tension off the staple line. If needed, a row of Lembert sutures may be placed to reinforce the staple line.

■ The mesenteric defects of the two jejunal limbs are then closed by reapproximating their mesenteries where possible or superficially anchoring them to the posterior parietes to prevent internal herniation.

We now proceed with abdominal closure. We typically place a standard 12-French feeding jejunostomy catheter distal to the jejunojejunostomy to provide nutritional support in the event of poor oral intake or anastomotic leak postoperatively. The peritoneal cavity is copiously irrigated with warm sterile water. Hemostasis is established. We do not generally place drains; however, if there are any concerns about the quality of the anastomoses or if the patient has significant risk factors for poor wound healing (e.g., chronic steroid use, poorly controlled diabetes, intraoperative hypotension), a Silastic drain can be placed in the surgical bed, adjacent to the duodenal stump and the esophagojejunostomy. The abdomen is then closed by reapproximating the linea alba using 1 PDS sutures, starting from opposite ends of the incision and tied in the middle. The wound is then irrigated and hemostasis verified before the skin is stapled close.

POSTOPERATIVE MANAGEMENT

At the end of the operation, the patient is extubated and admitted to the intermediate care unit where pain control is achieved with the use of either an epidural catheter or a patient-controlled analgesia (PCA) device. The Foley catheter is removed upon discontinuation of the epidural or on postoperative day (POD) 1 or 2 if the PCA is used. The patient is encouraged to exercise the lungs with the use of incentive spirometry and may require chest physiotherapy, as pulmonary complications are prevalent with gastric operations. Activity is resumed early and advanced gradually. The nasogastric tube is placed intermittent to wall suction and generally removed on POD 1 or 2. On PODs 5 to 7, a gastrografin swallow evaluation is performed to evaluate the anastomosis for a leak. If none is detected, the patient may be started on a clear liquid diet. Diet is advanced as tolerated with specific restrictions (see below). Patients in whom a feeding jejunostomy has been placed may be fed via the catheter as early as POD 1 if desired, although we tend to reserve jejunostomy feeding for those patients with poor postoperative oral intake or anastomotic leak.

A dietician is asked to see the patient early in the recovery period to provide education on the postgastrectomy diet. From a mechanical perspective, with the storage capacity of the stomach having been removed, the digestive circuitry is significantly altered, necessitating commensurate modifications to the diet in the form of smaller, more frequent meals high in protein and low in carbohydrates. From a metabolic standpoint, the stomach plays a critical role in vitamin B12 and iron absorption. The former is dependent on intrinsic factor produced by the gastric parietal cells while the latter is facilitated by hydrochloric acid, which converts dietary iron to a more readily absorbed form. Patients should therefore receive supplemental vitamin B12 and iron. Furthermore, calcium is primarily absorbed in the duodenum, which is bypassed in this operation. Hypocalcemia may ensue; calcium supplementation may be necessary as well.

 COMPLICATIONS

Following a total gastrectomy with esophagojejunostomy, nonspecific complications inherent to any major abdominal surgery may occur, including bleeding, wound infection, electrolyte imbalances, and pulmonary compromise. The latter is especially common following gastric operations due to manipulation of the diaphragm and retraction against the ribcage.

Complications specific to this operation can be categorized as surgical, unintended, complications, or expected but controllable, physiologic consequences.

Surgical complications can be dire, beginning with leakage from any suture line. The dreaded anastomotic leak at the esophagojejunostomy can be fatal if diagnosis and therapy are delayed. The same can be said of a duodenal stump blow-out or fistula formation. These problems will manifest as abdominal pain and distention, fever, and leukocytosis by POD 5 or 6. A work-up must be rapidly pursued so that corrective measures can be undertaken. While leaks from either esophagojejunostomy or jejunojejunostomy anastomoses can often be managed conservatively, a duodenal stump leak most often requires a return to the operating room. Rarely, one can get away with drainage alone, but close monitoring is required to assess adequacy of therapy. Late anastomotic complications can present as strictures that may respond to serial dilations alone or require reoperation instead. The risk for anastomotic complications is minimized when proper surgical technique is employed.

Similarly, internal herniation, which may occur through any one of several potential defects resulting from the newly reconstructed GI tract, should be avoided by mindfully tacking down the mesenteries of the bowel loops to each other or to the posterior parietes.

Physiologic consequences of total gastrectomy include dumping syndrome, which may occur early following a meal, a phenomenon attributed to rapid delivery of a hyperosmolar load to the small bowel, or late, due to a state of hypoglycemia from excess insulin production. Patients can also develop postvagotomy diarrhea and biliary stasis. Dietary modifications alone are often adequate in controlling these symptoms; still, the majority of patients will experience significant weight loss as a result of this operation. Metabolic derangements include anemia due to both vitamin B12 and iron deficiencies, as well hypocalcemia leading to bone disease (see "Postoperative Management" above).

RESULTS

Surgical resection offers the only chance at cure for gastric adenocarcinoma. A total gastrectomy with esophagojejunostomy is the procedure of choice for tumors of the gastric body and has proven to be the superior operation for proximal gastric tumors when compared to subtotal gastrectomy.

No consensus currently exists on the extent of lymph node dissection required, as conflicting data have been published. While the Japanese literature has reported improved outcomes with a more aggressive lymphadenectomy, these findings have not been reproduced in Western studies. A multicenter randomized, controlled study by the British Surgical Co-operative Group showed equivalent 5-year survival (35% for D1 dissection vs. 33% for D2 dissection). These results were corroborated in a similarly designed Dutch study, with 5-year survival rates of 45% and 47% for D1 and D2 resections, respectively, while the perioperative morbidity and mortality profile favored D1 resection. Interestingly, a 15-year follow-up of the same Dutch cohort demonstrated that while overall 15-year survival rates were not different, D2 lymphadenectomy was associated with lower locoregional disease recurrence and gastric-cancer-related death. This is counter-balanced by the significantly higher postoperative mortality and morbidity seen with D2 dissection. These worse perioperative outcomes are accounted for almost exclusively by the extraneous and unnecessary splenectomy and distal pancreatectomy, which offer no survival advantage. We now use a widely accepted approach to lymph node dissection by performing a hybrid "D1.5" resection, where D2-level lymph nodes are resected, but the spleen and pancreatic tail are preserved.

It is important to note that a review of the Surveillance, Epidemiology, and End Results (SEER) database revealed that only a third of patients undergoing curative gastrectomy in the United States receive adequate lymph node dissection, with the minimum of 15 lymph nodes being obtained, underscoring the importance of adequate lymph node resection.

Recurrence rate after curative resection remains high for gastric cancer. Both adjuvant chemoradiation and neoadjuvant chemotherapy regimens have been demonstrated to improve both disease-free and overall survival, and some form of either is now the accepted standard of care for resectable gastric cancer perioperatively.

CONCLUSIONS

Total gastrectomy with esophagojejunostomy plays a critical role in the treatment of gastric adenocarcinoma and other rare tumor types. It is a complex operation that requires a clear understanding of the anatomy and a strong grasp on sound surgical techniques.

Preoperative planning is of utmost importance and includes a history and physical examination; a thorough staging work-up consisting of endoscopic biopsy, CT scan of the chest, abdomen, and pelvis, and diagnostic laparoscopy; a realistic assessment of the patient's health risks; and nutritional optimization.

The first step of the operation should be verification of curative resectability before proceeding any further. The major steps of total gastrectomy are (1) dissection of the greater curvature with omentectomy, (2) mobilization and division of the duodenum,

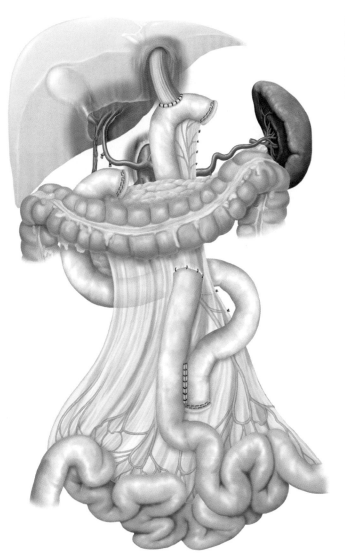

Figure 19.7 The reconstructed alimentary tract after total gastrectomy is completed by performing a retrocolic Roux-en-Y esophagojejunostomy, making sure to close any newly created space in the mesentery to avoid internal herniation.

(3) extension of the dissection along the lesser omentum toward the diaphragmatic hiatus, and finally (4) dissection and division of the esophagus. Along these steps, an appropriate lymph node dissection is performed. Proximal and distal margins should be assessed with frozen sections.

Our preferred approach for reconstruction is the creation of a retrocolic, end-to-side, Roux-en-Y esophagojejunostomy (Fig. 19.7). Anastomoses can be handsewn; alternatively, stapling devices can be used in this task.

The early postoperative course should be spent in a monitored setting. Enteral feeding can be commenced after the anastomosis has been investigated. Nutritional counseling is indispensable for these patients, and a conversation with the dietician prior to the operation should have been initiated. The patient should be monitored for nutritional deficiencies on a regular basis.

Overall, total gastrectomy with esophagojejunostomy can be performed safely and with good results if all these critical elements are assiduously addressed.

Recommended References and Readings

Baxter NN, Tuttle TM. Inadequacy of lymph node staging in gastric cancer patients: A population-based study. *Ann Surg Oncol.* 2005;12:981–987.

Bonenkamp JJ, Hermans J, Sasako M, et al. Extended lymph-node dissection for gastric cancer. *N Engl J Med.* 1999;340:908–914.

Cunningham D, Allum WH, Stenning SP, et al. Perioperative chemotherapy versus surgery alone for resectable gastroesophageal cancer. *N Engl J Med.* 2006;355:11–20.

Cuschieri A, Weeden S, Fielding J, et al. Patient survival after D1 and D2 resections for gastric cancer: Long-term results of the MRC randomized surgical trial. Surgical Co-operative Group. *Br J Cancer.* 1999;79:1522–1530.

Espat NJ, Karpeh M. Reconstruction following total gastrectomy: A review and summary of the randomized prospective clinical trials. *Surg Oncol.* 1998;7:65–69.

Glasgow RE, Rollins MD. Stomach and duodenum. In: Norton JE, Barie PS, Bollinger RR, Chang AE, Lowry SF, Mulvihill SJ, Pass HI, Thompson RW, eds. *Surgery: Basic Science and Clinical Evidence.* New York: Springer Science+Business Media, LLC; 2008:841–874.

Grabowski MW, Dempsey DT. Concepts in Surgery of the Stomach and Duodenum. In: Scott-Conner CE, ed. *Chassin's Operative Strategy in General Surgery. An Expositive Atlas.* 3rd ed. New York: Springer Science+Business Media, LLC; 2002: 225–233.

Lowy AM, Mansfield PF, Leach SD, et al. Laparoscopic staging for gastric cancer. *Surgery.* 1995;119:611–614.

Macdonald JS, Smalley SR, Benedetti J, et al. Chemoradiotherapy after surgery compared with surgery alone for adenocarcinoma of the stomach of gastroesophageal junction. *N Engl J Med.* 2001; 345:725–730.

McCulloch P, Nita ME, Kazi H, et al. Extended versus limited lymph nodes dissection technique for adenocarcinoma of the stomach. *Cochrane Database Syst Rev.* 2004;4:CD001964.

Mercer DW, Robinson EK. Stomach. In: Townsend CM, Beauchamp DR, Evers MB, Mattox KL, eds. *Sabiston Textbook of Surgery.* 17th ed. Philadelphia, PA: Elsevier Saunders; 2004:1265–1321.

Noguchi Y, Imada T, Matsumoto A, et al. Radical surgery for gastric surgery. A review of the Japanese experience. *Cancer.* 1989;64: 2053–2062.

Parikh AA, Mansfield PF. Gastric Adenocarcinoma. In: Cameron JL, ed. *Current Surgical Therapy.* 8th ed. Philadelphia, PA: Mosby; 2004:95–100.

Songun I, Putter H, Kranenbarg EM, et al. Surgical treatment of gastric cancer: 15-year follow-up results of the randomized nationwide Dutch D1D2 trial. *Lancet Oncol.* 2010;11:439–449.

20 Laparoscopic Total Gastrectomy and Esophagojejunostomy

Brant K. Oelschlager and Rebecca P. Petersen

Introduction

Over the past decade, minimally invasive surgery is being performed more frequently for the treatment of gastric cancer. As with other laparoscopic procedures, the intent of this approach is to reduce surgical morbidity while achieving similar cancer-free and overall survival rates as with conventional open surgical resection. The majority of studies comparing open and laparoscopic approaches for gastric cancer in regards to morbidity and oncologic efficacy have been for subtotal gastrectomies, mostly because it is technically easier to perform. More recently, however, laparoscopic total gastrectomy (LTG) has become a more feasible approach for many surgeons. This is due to improvements in technology as well as advancing expertise with laparoscopic surgical technique. However, LTG is considerably more complex than partial gastrectomy and requires careful patient evaluation and planning to ensure that efficacy and safety are not being compromised compared to a standard open approach.

Background

Laparoscopic gastrectomy for the treatment of gastric cancer was initially described in the early 1990s, and early experiences were limited to partial gastrectomy. To date, the majority of studies have evaluated the outcomes of laparoscopic distal gastrectomies, and in general this has become an established approach for the treatment of limited gastric cancer. Early experiences with LTG were limited by technical difficulty in performing the esophagojejunostomy anastomosis and prolonged operative times compared with the open approach. As a result, LTG was not favored by even the most experienced minimally invasive surgeons. However, advances in stapling technology have enabled totally laparoscopic intracorporeal esophagojejunostomy anastomosis to be performed.

The first LTG was reported by Umaya and colleagues in 1999, where they performed a laparoscopy-assisted total gastrectomy with a distal pancreatosplenectomy and a D2 lymphadenectomy. In the same year, Azagra and colleagues also reported performing a minimally invasive total gastrectomy in 12 patients, but in the majority of these patients a laparoscopy-assisted approach was used. Now, there are several case studies which have demonstrated the feasibility of a "totally" LTG in experienced hands. While there has not been a controlled trial comparing LTG to open gastrectomy and it is not clear whether or to what degree there is a benefit over open resection, the benefit of a laparoscopic approach has appeal due to the broader experience with laparoscopic techniques. Importantly, LTG is a technically challenging operation; thus the surgeon must carefully and thoughtfully consider patient-specific details before performing these operations and be facile with laparoscopic techniques.

Patient Selection

Patient-specific selection criteria for LTG are not well established as there are very few studies and the majority of these are small case series evaluating only the technical feasibility of LTG. Therefore, until larger long-term outcome comparative trials are performed, patient selection criteria should be focused on general principles of minimally invasive surgery and should consider the technical challenges of the operation. As with any laparoscopic procedure, eligible patients should be without significant cardiac, pulmonary, or renal disease where prolonged pneumoperitoneum with carbon dioxide will not result in increased perioperative morbidity and/or mortality. Patients who have musculoskeletal or neurodegenerative disease and/or injuries which would preclude them from being placed in a modified lithotomy position in reverse Trendelenburg required to perform a LTG should be excluded as well. Multiple prior fore- or midgut operations is a relative contraindication to LTG and this is mainly practical since taking down adhesions from prior surgery can be time consuming and potentially risky (depending on the surgeon's experience). Obesity is not necessarily a contraindication to TLG as these patients are likely to benefit in regard with decreased wound complications from a laparoscopic as compared to an open approach, but it is another factor that increases the technical difficulty of the procedure. LTG should only be attempted in conjunction with or by an experienced minimally invasive surgeon at a high-volume hospital given its overall technical complexity (Table 20.1).

Preoperative Evaluation, Treatment, and Procedure Selection

All gastric cancer patients should undergo a comprehensive preoperative evaluation which includes upper endoscopy, physical examination focusing on the abdomen and lymph nodes, appropriate noninvasive imaging to stage the tumor, assess size, and evaluate response to chemotherapy, and appropriate nutritional and cardiac screening (Table 20.2).

TABLE 20.1	**Patient Selection Criteria**

Indications for LTG
- Experienced surgeon in minimally invasive techniques, resections for gastric cancer, and laparoscopic Roux-en-y reconstructions

Contraindications for LTG (Absolute & Relative)
- Patients with severe cardiac, pulmonary, and/or renal disease intolerable to prolonged pneumoperitoneum (absolute)
- Unable to tolerate a modified lithotomy/split leg position in reverse Trendelenburg due to a musculoskeletal/neurodegenerative disease or injury (absolute)
- Patients with multiple prior fore- or midgut surgeries (relative)
- Morbid obesity (relative)

TABLE 20.2	Preoperative Assessment

- Upper endoscopy for diagnosis and to properly localize the exact location of the tumor and its boundaries. This will determine the type of resection and inaccuracy can lead to excessive or inadequate resection. This should be repeated by the surgeon if there is any doubt.
- Complete physical examination focusing especially on the abdomen and the lymph nodes
- CT scan of the chest, abdomen, and pelvis to assess for distant nodal or visceral metastases
- Endoscopic ultrasound to provide accurate tumor and nodal staging with biopsies when indicated
- All patients undergoing chemotherapy or chemoradiation therapy prior to surgery should undergo repeat staging studies (CT scan with or without FDG–PET) to rule out metastatic progression
- A comprehensive medical evaluation should be performed to determine whether further diagnostic studies such as a cardiac stress test, echocardiogram, pulmonary function tests, etc. are necessary for risk stratification prior to surgery
- Nutritional status should be assessed and optimized prior to surgery

The majority of patients with gastric cancer in the United States present with locally advanced disease, and as a result, the majority undergo multimodality therapy as outcomes have been shown to be superior to surgery alone for patients with stage II or III disease. In our center the most common regimen is perioperative chemotherapy before and after surgery as described in the MAGIC trial.

The type of gastric resection for the treatment of gastric cancer should be selected based on the anatomic site of the tumor, stage, histology, and prognostic factors. Therefore, all patients should undergo appropriate staging studies prior to considering surgical treatment. The first step is to perform an upper endoscopy with gastric biopsy to establish the diagnosis. Subsequently, a staging evaluation may include endoscopic ultrasound and CT scan of the chest, abdomen, and pelvis with or without a FDG–PET to determine the clinical stage. Some centers routinely perform staging laparoscopy as approximately 20% of patients with locally advanced tumors have peritoneal carcinomatosis.

The type of surgery should be based on the ability to achieve 5 cm gross surgical margins, clinical stage, and histology type. For patients with distal tumors, we recommend a subtotal gastrectomy. For patients with tumors located in the middle third of the stomach or in patients with infiltrative disease such as linitis plastica, we recommend a total gastrectomy and consider LTG. We also consider LTG for Siewert III gastroesophageal junction (GEJ) tumors when good esophageal margins are possible. However, most GEJ tumors (Siewert I-II) require esophagogastrectomy. Finally, the laparoscopic approach must not in any way compromise the type of gastric resection or lymph node dissection that is required.

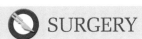

SURGERY

The following is the approach used at the University of Washington.

Set-up and Patient Positioning

Operating Room Set-up

The laparoscopic tower is placed at the patient's left shoulder or wherever facilitates placing the monitor over the head of the bed. At the beginning of the case, the surgeon operates by standing between the patients legs with an assistant at the left side of the operating room table (surgeon preference), as this facilitates the greater curve and esophageal mobilization. The scrub technician and Mayo stand are positioned above the assistant on the left side (Fig. 20.1). The patient is placed in a supine position prior to performing the Roux-en-Y reconstruction; at this point the surgeon and assistant move to the right and left side of the operating room table, respectively.

Figure 20.1 Operating room set-up.

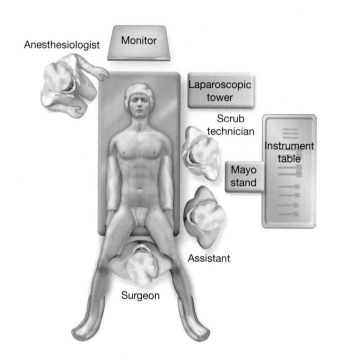

Patient Positioning

Following induction of general anesthesia after prophylactic antibiotics and heparin has been administered, the patient is initially placed in a low-lithotomy position on a bean bag which has been secured to the operating table to prevent the patient from slipping when placed in steep reverse Trendelenburg for the beginning of the operation. An alternative is a split leg table. This position allows the surgeon to comfortably stand facing the hiatus and use a left upper quadrant port for mobilizing the greater curve and especially the esophagus. Bilateral sequential compression devices are placed on the lower extremities and a Foley catheter with a temperature probe is placed for monitoring. Prior to the Roux-en-Y reconstruction, the patient is repositioned into a supine position (if desired) on the operating room table and taken out of steep reverse Trendelenburg to avoid nerve compression from long periods of time in stirrups.

Technique

Trocar Placement

Pneumoperitoneum is established by using a Veress needle technique approximately 2 cm inferior to the left costal margin. Following this, access is obtained under direct visualization with a 12-mm optical entry trocar at the same site. A 10-mm, 30° laparoscope is introduced and a 10-mm trocar is subsequently placed superiorly and to the left of the umbilicus. Three additional trocars are then placed: a 5-mm left flank trocar, a 5-mm right subcostal trocar, and a 12-mm trocar placed superior and to the right of the umbilicus. A total of five ports are placed: two 5 mm (surgeon/assistant ports), one 10 mm (camera), one 12 mm (surgeon), and one 12 mm port (this should be 15 mm if a 4.8-mm linear stapler is required) (Fig. 20.2). A Nathanson retractor is placed through a 5-mm opening just left of the midline and inferior to the subxiphoid process to retract the left lateral segment of the liver and secured to a table-mounted "strong arm".

Following placement of the camera port and prior to placing the three remaining trocars, a diagnostic laparoscopy is performed to rule out metastatic disease.

Omentectomy and Duodenal Division

The dissection begins by dividing the gastrocolic ligament just above the colon, starting at the midpoint of the transverse colon where the lesser sac is entered while reflecting

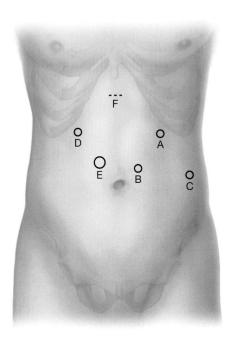

Figure 20.2 Trocar configuration: (**A**) 12 mm left subcostal (EEA stapler/surgeon), (**B**) 10 mm superior and left to the umbilicus (camera/assistant), (**C**) 5 mm left flank (assistant), (**D**) 5 mm right subcostal (surgeon), (**E**) 12 mm superior and right to the umbilicus (linear stapler/surgeon), and (**F**) Nathanson liver retractor placed through a 5-mm incision.

the greater omentum over the stomach. The omentum should be kept en bloc with the stomach. The dissection is carried out laterally to the pylorus. The right gastroepiploic artery and vein are then divided at their origins with a 2.5-mm linear stapler.

Next, the first portion of the duodenum and pylorus are dissected circumferentially, and the duodenum is divided just beyond the pylorus with a 3.5-mm linear stapler (Fig. 20.3). The right gastric artery can be divided before or after the duodenum with clips or stapler. The rest of the gastrocolic ligament is divided to the left until meeting with the short gastric vessels which are divided with an appropriate energy source.

Mobilization of the Esophagus
The hiatus is dissected by initially dividing the phrenoesophageal membrane at the left crus and carried anteriorly over the esophagus. Next, the gastrohepatic ligament and

Figure 20.3 Division of the duodenum.

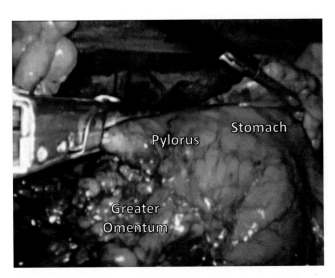

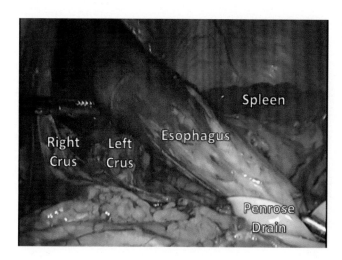

Figure 20.4 Mobilization of the esophagus.

subsequently the phrenoesophageal membrane on the right are divided. At this point a 0.5-inch wide Penrose drain is encircled around the esophagus just above the GEJ to provide downward retraction when circumferentially freeing the esophagus from its mediastinal attachments distally to lengthen the intra-abdominal esophagus (Fig. 20.4). Both the anterior and the posterior vagal nerves are dissected free distally off the esophagus and divided. The point of this division and clearing of the esophagus depends on the tumor location. For proximal gastric cancers that involve the cardia, part of the esophagus needs to be divided. The more esophagus that is included in the specimen, the more the esophagus should be mobilized, and the more difficult the reconstruction. Surgeons unfamiliar with these resections should realize that an esophagojejunostomy is substantially more difficult than a gastrojejunostomy (such as is done for a gastric bypass in obesity surgery), and every centimeter that the resection goes proximally the more difficult it becomes. This is very important to consider during patient selection.

Division of the Left Gastric Vessels

The Penrose drain is then retracted up toward the abdominal wall to provide exposure of the left gastric vessels. The vessels are circumferentially dissected at their origin and divided with a 2.5-mm linear stapler, taking the entire nodal bundle (Fig. 20.5).

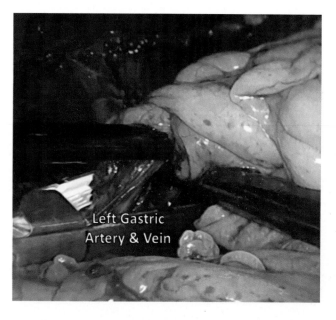

Figure 20.5 Division of the left gastric vessels.

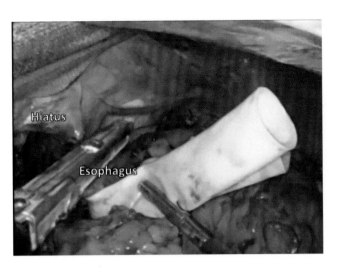

Figure 20.6 Division of the esophagus.

Part II: Procedures for Neoplastic Disease

Division of the Esophagus

The esophagus is divided above the GEJ with a 3.5-mm linear stapler in a slight oblique orientation. The level of division above the GEJ is dependent upon the position of the tumor, and the oblique orientation allows for a 25-mm end-to-end anastomosis (EEA) anvil to be placed even in a relatively small diameter esophagus. Prior to division, two stay sutures are placed for retraction just above the projected staple line (Fig. 20.6). A small esophagotomy is made at the middle of the staple line and an OrVil™ orogastric tube (tubing attached to an anvil) is then passed transorally into the esophagus by an experienced anesthesiologist. The end of the OG tube is then directed through the esophagotomy and grasped with a laparoscopic instrument and pulled gently into the peritoneal cavity until the anvil (25 mm) is visible at the esophageal stump (Fig. 20.7). Next, a pursestring suture is placed around the anvil entry site to prevent inadvertent tearing when performing the anastomosis with the circular stapling device. Alternatively a linear stapling technique or hand-sewn approach can be used, though the EEA, in our opinion, simplifies the anastomosis when performed laparoscopically (especially the greater the esophageal component of resection).

Roux-en-Y Esophagojejunostomy Anastomosis

The ligament of Treitz is identified, and the jejunum is divided approximately 30 cm distally with a 3.5-mm linear stapler. It is important that a deep division of the mesentery is performed to provide adequate mobility for the jejunum to reach the hiatus. The

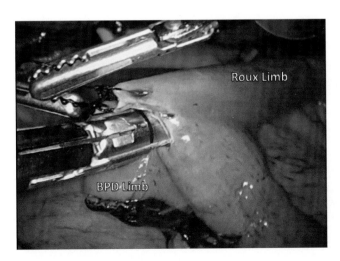

Figure 20.7 Jejunojejunostomy.

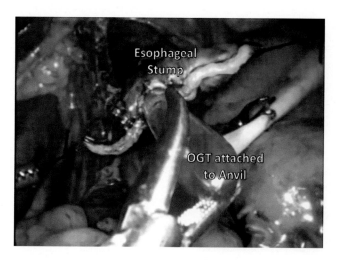

Figure 20.8 Esophageal stump and transorally placed anvil.

jejunum is then measured distally for another 60 cm and a side-to-side functional end-to-end stapled anastomosis is performed with a 3.5-mm, 60-mm in length linear stapler (Fig. 20.8). The common enterotomy is then closed with another 3.5-mm linear stapler following placement of stay sutures. The mesenteric defect is closed with interrupted sutures. Prior experience with laparoscopic bariatric surgery greatly facilitates the learning curve for this portion of the procedure; however, it is important to again emphasize the increased complexity of this more proximal anastomosis. The Roux limb is then brought up in a retrocolic fashion and placed next to the esophageal stump without tension. It should be emphasized that the retrocolic route should be performed, rather than the longer antecolic route as the extra length is important for esophagojejunostomy. The end of the Roux limb is opened and the circular stapler is then placed transabdominally at the site of the left subcostal 12-mm trocar (following lengthening of the incision and fascia with sharp and blunt dissection). The opened Roux limb is directed onto the circular stapler and the spike is brought through the antimesenteric side of the bowel. The anvil and the circular stapler are then connected, and the anastomosis is created after firing the stapler (Figs. 20.9 and 20.10). The opened end of the Roux limb is then divided and closed with a linear 3.5-mm stapler.

Next, the integrity of the anastomosis is tested with an air leak test by placing a bowel clamp across the jejunum distally and performing an endoscopy. The Roux limb is then identified at the retrocolic junction and reduced and secured to the transverse mesocolon with three mattress sutures. Our preference is to leave a drain at the site of the esophagojejunostomy within the mediastinum. If a leak occurs, this can simplify

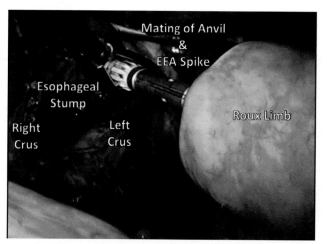

Figure 20.9 Creation of esophagojejunostomy.

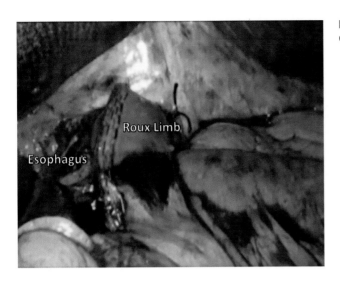

Figure 20.10 Completed Roux-en-Y esophagojejunostomy.

management, as there is little chance of being able to place a percutaneous drain to manage a leak should it occur, as drainage would then require a thoracotomy.

Removal of the Specimen En Bloc

The resected stomach with the attached surrounding tissue, greater, and lesser omentum is placed into a plastic specimen bag or the port site covered by a wound protector and removed from the left subcostal incision after slightly widening the port site. The fascia is then closed following pathology confirmation that the surgical margins are free of tumor.

Placement of Jejunostomy Feeding Tube

Selected patients may require placement of a jejunostomy feeding tube. Specifically, patients whose nutritional status is compromised as a result of their disease or by chemotherapy prior to surgery, elderly patients, or patients with significant comorbidities may require feeding tube placement. In the postoperative setting, if a patient requires prolonged enteral tube feeding due to poor nutrition or a complication, we will place a jejunostomy feeding tube laparoscopically. This can be done with relative ease given LTG does not result in a significant amount of adhesions.

 ## POSTOPERATIVE MANAGEMENT

Postoperatively, patients without significant comorbidities are admitted to the surgical floor. The Foley catheter is removed the following morning if urine output is adequate. An upper gastrointestinal study with Gastrografin followed by barium is performed around postoperative day 3 or 4. A clear liquid diet is started if there is no clinical or radiographic evidence of an anastomotic leak. The drain at the site of the esophagojejunostomy is removed following initiation of a liquid diet. Patients are typically discharged on postoperative day 5 or 6 on a postgastrectomy diet regimen if there are no complications. Physiologically they often could be discharged sooner but given the higher risk, anastomosis monitoring for complications is important. If the patient lives close and is reliable, this can be shortened. All patients with gastric cancer, in our practice, are discharged home on low-molecular weight heparin for DVT prophylaxis for 4 weeks.

 ## COMPLICATIONS

Total gastrectomy is considered a high-risk procedure, and perioperative morbidity and mortality vary widely depending on the study, surgical technique, and extent of resection.

TABLE 20.3	Immediate and Long-term Complications

Immediate
- Bleeding
- Anastomotic leak
- Duodenal stump leak
- Perioperative death
- Pulmonary embolism
- Pneumothorax
- Wound infection

Long-term
- Dumping syndrome (early and late)
- Anastomotic stricture
- Internal hernia
- Vitamin B12 deficiency

Complications specific to a laparoscopic approach theoretically include an increased risk of a pneumothorax from a more aggressive mediastinal mobilization of the esophagus and inadvertent injury to the pleura, thromboembolism (DVT/PE) due to prolonged lithotomy position, and internal herniation due to lack of adhesions as compared to an open approach. In contrast, patients undergoing a LTG would be expected to have less blood loss, wound infections, and incisional hernias. Other immediate and long-term complications include gastrojejunostomy or jejunojejunostomy anastomotic leak, duodenal stump leak, perioperative death, dumping syndrome, anastomotic stricture, and nutritional deficiencies (Table 20.3).

In the few case series of "totally" LTG which have been conducted to date, there were no reports of pneumothoraces, duodenal stump leaks, wound infections, or incisional hernias. Also, there were no major bleeding events despite a splenectomy and D2 lymphadenectomy being performed in over half the patients in one of the largest series. The esophagojejunostomy and jejunojejunostomy anastomotic leak rates ranged from 0% to 5% and 0% to 3%, respectively. Perioperative death (30-day) ranged between 0% and 2.6% where one patient died in a series of 33 patients due to cerebral hemorrhage which was presumably unrelated to the surgery. Postoperative small bowel obstruction, requiring reoperation due to internal hernias occurred in 0% to 8% of patients.

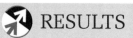 RESULTS

Over the past few years there have been several reports of "totally" laparoscopic total gastrectomies with varying surgical techniques (Table 20.4). Kachikwu and colleagues reported performing an intracorporeal esophagojejunostomy with the OrVil™ device and circular stapler, but the jejunojejunostomy was completed extracorporeally through the specimen extraction site. One of the largest case series reported by Shinorhara et al. in Japan evaluated outcomes in 55 patients undergoing LTG with D2 lymphadenectomy where more than half of the patients with T2-T4 gastric cancer underwent a concomitant splenectomy and in three patients a distal pancreatectomy. The investigators in this study performed a functional side-to-side intracorporeal esophagojejunostomy using a 45-mm linear stapler. Despite concomitant splenectomies and extended lymphadenectomies being performed in the majority of patients, there were no conversions to open procedure or perioperative deaths. Only two patients (4%) experienced minor late anastomotic leaks at the esophagojejunostomy. In another study where the outcomes of 38 patients undergoing LTG were compared to 22 patients undergoing an open approach, the authors identified patient's medical condition and surgeon expertise to be predictors of outcome as opposed to surgical approach. The surgical morbidity was higher in this series as six patients (16%) undergoing LTG required reoperation:

TABLE 20.4	Case Series Evaluating the Feasibility of Totally Laparoscopic Total Gastrectomy						
Author	F/U	N	LOS (days)	Death 30-day	Conversion to open surgery	Anastomotic leak	Other complications
Kachikwu et al. 2010	7 mos	16	8	0	0	0 (0%)	3 (19%), anastomotic stricture
Guzman et al. 2009 (subset)	47 mos	4	NA	0	NA	0	None
Shinohara et al. 2009	16 mos	55	17	0	0	2 (4%), EJ	7 (13%), pancreatic fistula 3 (5%), abdominal abscess 3 (5%), SBO-internal hernia
Topal et al. 2008	NA	38	11	1(2.6%)ᵃ	0	2 (5%), EJ 1 (3%), JJ	3 (8%), SBO-internal hernia 1 (3%), necrotizing pancreatitis 1 (3%), pulmonary empyema

EJ, esophagojejunostomy; JJ, jejunojejunostomy; F/U, follow-up (median); LOS, length of hospital stay (median); SBO, small bowel obstruction; NA, not available.
ᵃDeath from cerebral hemorrhage.

three for small bowel obstruction due to an internal hernia, one for necrotizing pancreatitis, one for a small bowel fistula at the jejunojejunostomy site, and one for a pulmonary empyema. In addition, two patients (5%) and one patient (3%) experienced esophagojejunostomy and jejunojejunostomy leaks, respectively.

Despite the varying surgical techniques and extent of resections, these case series support that a LTG is feasible and can be performed with relatively low morbidity and mortality.

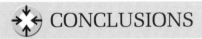 CONCLUSIONS

Although the majority of studies comparing laparoscopic to open gastrectomy in regards to surgical morbidity and oncologic outcomes have been for distal resections, there have been several studies demonstrating the feasibility of a laparoscopic approach for total gastrectomy. Totally LTG has the potential to result in reduced morbidity, shortened hospitalization, and more expedient patient recovery while adhering to oncologic principles. Although LTG is technically feasible and safe in experienced hands, it is a complex operation that should be reserved for surgeons with advanced laparoscopic skills and substantial experience with gastric resection; especially laparoscopic partial gastric resections and Roux-en-Y reconstructions.

Recommended References and Readings

Birkmeyer JD, Stukel TA, Siewers AE, et al. Surgeon volume and operative mortality in the United States. N Engl J Med. 2003; 349:2117–2127.

Brower V. Laparoscopic versus open surgery in cancer: New studies add data to debate. J Natl Cancer Inst. 2009;101:982–983.

Cuschieri A. Laparoscopic gastric resection. Surg Clin North Am. 2000;80:1269–1284.

Huscher CG, Mingoli A, Sgarzini G, et al. Laparoscopic versus open subtotal gastrectomy for distal gastric cancer: Five-year results of a randomized prospective trial. Ann Surg. 2005;241:232–237.

Kachikwu EL, Trisal V, Kim J, et al. Minimally invasive total gastrectomy for gastric cancer: A pilot series. J Gastrointest Surg. 2011; 15:81–86.

Kodera Y, Fujiwara M, Ohashi N, et al. Laparoscopic surgery for gastric cancer: A collective review with meta-analysis of randomized trials. J Am Coll Surg. 2010;221:677–686.

Ott K, Lordick F, Blank S, et al. Gastric cancer: surgery in 2011. Langenbecks Arch Surg. 2011;396:743–758. [Epub ahead of print.]

Shinohara T, Kanaya S, Taniguchi K, et al. Laparoscopic total gastrectomy with D2 lymph node dissection for gastric cancer. Arch Surg. 2009;144:1138–1142.

Song K, Park C, Kang H, et al. Is totally laparoscopic gastrectomy less invasive than laparoscopy-assisted gastrectomy? Prospective, multicenter study. J Gastrointest Surg. 2008;12:1015–1021.

Topal B, Leys E, Ectors N, et al. Determinants of complications and adequacy of surgical resection in laparoscopic versus open total gastrectomy for adenocarcinoma. Surg Endosc. 2008;22: 980–984.

Part II: Procedures for Neoplastic Disease

21 Robot-assisted Gastrectomy with Lymph Node Dissection for Gastric Cancer

Woo Jin Hyung, Yanghee Woo, and Kazutaka Obama

Introduction

Robotic surgery for gastric cancer is increasing. Many surgeons have adopted robotic surgery to facilitate the technically challenging procedure of gastrectomy with D2 lymphadenectomy. With robotic gastric cancer surgery training, experienced laparoscopic surgeons can safely provide the advantages of minimally invasive surgery to their patients. Adherence to the oncologic principles of gastric cancer treatment ensures that the long-term survival benefits of surgery will not be compromised.

INDICATIONS/CONTRAINDICATIONS

The indications for robotic surgery are similar to those of the conventional laparoscopic approach to gastric cancer. Early gastric cancer patients without perigastric lymph node (LN) involvement are ideal candidates for robotic gastrectomy with limited lymphadenectomy. Locally advanced gastric cancer without evidence of distant metastases is a generally accepted indication for robotic gastrectomy and D2 lymphadenectomy.

Indications for robotic gastrectomy with limited lymphadenectomy:

- $cT_1N_0M_0$
- Mucosal and submucosal tumors not eligible for endoscopic resection
- Failed endoscopic mucosal resection or endoscopic submucosal dissection

Indications for robotic gastrectomy requiring D2 lymphadenectomy:

- $cT_1N_1M_0$
- $cT_2N_0M_0$; $cT_2N_1M_0$

Currently, there is no evidence to support robotic surgery for gastric cancer with serosal involvement (T4a) or invasion of adjacent organs (T4b), or for palliative intent. Intolerance to pneumoperitoneum is a contraindication.

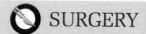

PREOPERATIVE WORK-UP

The preoperative work-up of patients undergoing robotic surgery for gastric cancer requires complete evaluation of the patient's clinical status, confirmation pathologic diagnosis, and estimation of the location and extent of disease. The preoperative work-up will guide each step of the surgical decision-making process.

■ Upper endoscopy with biopsy and with or without clipping proximal to the lesion
■ Endoscopic ultrasound
■ CT scan of the abdomen

SURGERY

Pertinent Anatomy

Robotic gastrectomy and lymphadenectomy requires the knowledge of gastric vessels and the accompanying nodal stations as defined by the Japanese Gastric Cancer Association. The operative procedure is described relative to the dissection of the LN stations in D2 lymphadenectomy.

Operating Room Configuration

The operating room configuration is centered on the patient and the da Vinci Surgical System (Sunnyvale, CA, USA). Relative position of the operating table, the surgeon console, the anesthesia cart, the surgical cart, the assistant, the monitors, and the robot during robotic gastrectomy are described.

■ The robot system is positioned cephalad to the patient.
■ The patient-side assistant is positioned to the lower left side of the patient on the opposite side of the scrub nurse, scrub table, and the main assistant monitor.
■ The vision systems rack is placed at the foot of the operating table.
■ The surgeon's master console is positioned to grant the surgeon a view of the patient.

Patient Positioning, Port Placement, Robot Docking, and Preparation of the Operative Field

The patient is placed under general anesthesia, positioned supine with both arms tucked to the patient side, and urinary catheter is placed. The abdomen is prepared from the nipple line to the suprapubic region and draped in the standard sterile fashion. Five ports, two 12 mm and three 8 mm, are used for robotic gastrectomy (Fig. 21.1). Port placements may require minor adjustments for the patient's body habitus. Once the ports are placed, the robot surgical cart is brought in from the head of the patient, and the robot arms are docked.

■ The camera arm is docked to the infraumbilical port (C)
■ The first arm holds the curved bipolar Maryland forceps
■ The second and the third arms hold the ultrasonic shears or a monopolar device and the Cadiere forceps, interchangeably.

Liver Retraction
The self-sustaining retraction of the left lobe of the liver is required during robotic gastrectomy as in other upper abdominal surgeries. Adequate liver retraction is a prerequisite for complete dissection of the suprapancreatic lymphadenectomy and along the lesser curve of the stomach. Several methods have been described.

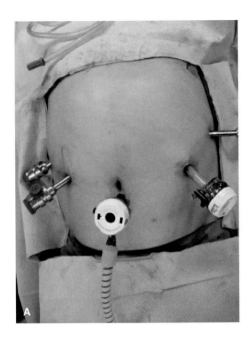
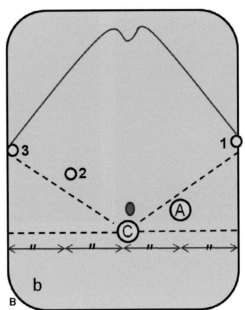

Figure 21.1 Patient preparation. **A:** Port placement. After the 12-mm infraumbilical port is placed using the Hasson technique, the patient is placed in 15° reverse Trendelenburg position for the insertion of the three 8-mm ports and the 12-mm assist port under direct visualization. **B:** Docking of the robot arms. The robot arms should be docked as indicated by the numbers.

Intraoperative Tumor Localization to Determine the Resection Extent

Intraoperative tumor localization is required to determine the appropriate margin of resection during robotic subtotal distal gastrectomy. Since robotic surgery is performed for lesions without serosal involvement, the lesion cannot be readily detected during the operation. Intraoperative tumor localization has been achieved by several different methods including dye injection, intraoperative endoscopy, or laparoscopic ultrasound. A successful technique using preoperatively placed endoclips and an intraoperative abdominal x-ray is a simple and effective method.

Procedure of D2 LN Dissection During Distal Subtotal Gastrectomy

Five Steps and Associated Anatomic Landmarks

1. Partial omentectomy and left side dissection of the greater curvature: left gastroepiploic vessels
2. Right side dissection of the greater curvature and duodenal transection: head of pancreas and right gastroepiploic vessels
3. Hepatoduodenal ligament dissection and approach to suprapancreatic area: right gastric artery, proper hepatic artery (PHA), portal vein (PV), and celiac axis
4. Exposure of the root of the left gastric artery (LGA) and skeletonization of the splenic vessels
5. Lesser curvature dissection: esophageal crus and cardia; proximal gastric resection

Partial Omentectomy and Left Side Dissection of the Greater Curvature

The exposure of the omentum can be achieved by creating a draping of the greater omentum for safe division and retrieval of LN stations 4sb and 4d (Fig. 21.2A).

- Divide the greater omentum from the midtransverse colon toward the lower pole of the spleen.
- Carefully identify, ligate, and divide the left gastroepiploic vessels at their roots. (Fig. 21.2B).
- Clear the greater curvature of the stomach from the proximal resection margin to the short gastric vessels.

Right Side Dissection of the Greater Curvature and Duodenal Transection

Attention is directed to the right side of the patient for mobilization of the distal stomach from the head of the pancreas and dissection of the soft tissues containing LN

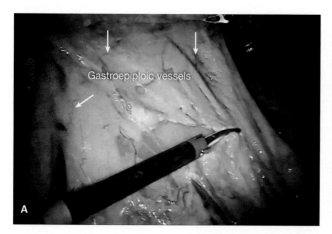
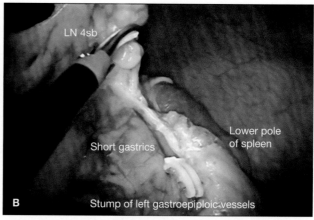

Figure 21.2 Left side dissection of the greater curvature. **A:** Partial omentectomy begins from the distal greater curvature 4 to 5 cm from the gastroepiploic vessels. **B:** The dissection is continued toward the lower pole of the spleen where the left gastroepiploic vessels are divided and the short gastric vessels are encountered.

station 6 which is bordered by right gastroepiploic vein (RGEV), anterior superior pancreaticoduodenal vein (ASPDV), and the middle colic vein (Fig. 21.3).

- Release the connective tissues between the pancreas and the posterior stomach and the duodenal attachments to the colon.
- Dissect the soft tissues on the head of the pancreas to identify, ligate, and divide the RGEV as it joins the anterior superior pancreaticoduodenal vein. (Soft tissues anterior to and superior to the ASPDV and superior to the middle colic vein should be retrieved on either side of the RGEV.)
- Identify, ligate, and divide the right gastroepiploic artery as it branches from the gastroduodenal artery (GDA).
- Release the attachments between the duodenum and the pancreas along the GDA until the common hepatic artery (CHA) is reached.
- Insert 4″ × 4″ gauze anterior to the head of pancreas to prevent injury to the GDA and proceed to the suprapancreatic region.
- Clear the supraduodenal area and divide the duodenum approximately 2 cm distal to the pylorus using an endo-linear stapler.

This completes the intrapyloric dissection.

Dissection of the Hepatoduodenal Ligament and Suprapancreatic Dissection

The en bloc retrieval of the suprapancreatic LNs is achieved by meticulous dissection along the PHA, the PV, and the CHA after the ligation of the right gastric artery.

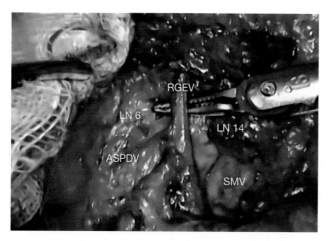

Figure 21.3 Right side dissection at the head of the pancreas. The soft tissues containing lymph nodes from station 6 have been removed to reveal the bordering vessels, the right gastroepiploic vein (RGEV), anterior superior pancreaticoduodenal vein (ASPDV), and the middle (MCV) colic vein. The area of the 14v lymph node station has also been dissected with the superior mesenteric vein (SMV) exposed.

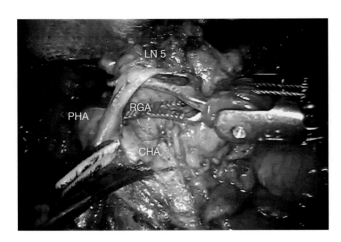

Figure 21.4 Dissection of the right gastric artery. The root of the right gastric artery (RGA) has been isolated after soft tissues containing lymph nodes from station 5 have been dissected. CHA, common hepatic artery; PHA, proper hepatic artery (PHA).

■ Dissect the anterior surface of the PHA to identify, ligate, and divide the right gastric artery at its origin for retrieval of LN station #5 (Fig. 21.4).

■ Clear the soft tissues anterior and medial to the PHA until the PV is exposed medially for LN station 12a (Fig. 21.5A).

■ The soft tissues around CHA contain LN station #8a.

■ Proceed to identify, ligate, and divide the left gastric vein as it drains into the PV. (In some patients the left gastric vein drains into the splenic vein and must be identified anterior to the splenic artery.)

■ Skeletonize the CHA toward the celiac axis to retrieve the soft tissues around the celiac artery, which contain LN station #9 (Fig. 21.5B).

Exposure of the Left Gastric Artery and Skeletonization of the Splenic Vessels

The dissection of the soft tissues along the LGA and splenic vessels ensures the retrieval of LN station 7 and 11p, respectively. (Fig. 21.6)

■ Divide the retroperitoneal attachments to the lesser curvature of the stomach to improve access to the root of the LGA.

■ Expose the root of the LGA by clearing the surrounding soft tissues and securely ligate and divide it.

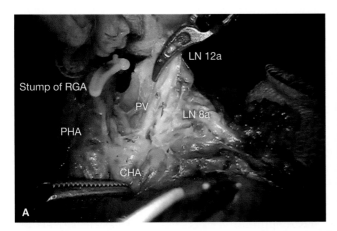
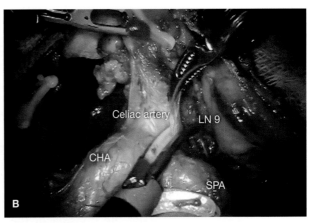

Figure 21.5 Approach to the suprapancreatic lymph node dissection. **A:** En bloc LN dissection along PHA and CHA. Soft tissues anterior to and medial to the PHA and medial to the portal vein (PV) are dissected en bloc with the soft tissues around the CHA to retrieve the lymph nodes in stations 12a and 8a, respectively. **B:** Skeletonization of the CHA toward celiac artery. The dissection continues along the proximal CHA and splenic artery to clear the soft tissues surrounding the celiac artery for soft tissues containing lymph node station 9.

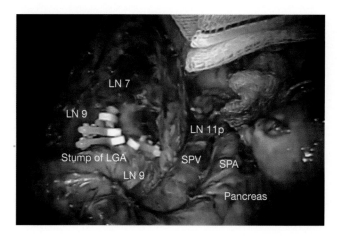

Figure 21.6 Root of the left gastric artery (LGA) and skeletonized splenic vessels. The soft tissues along the celiac axis are cleared to identify the root of the LGA and retrieve lymph nodes from station 7. Dissection along the splenic vessels continues half way toward the spleen to retrieve the soft tissues containing lymph nodes from station 11p. SPA, splenic artery; SPV, splenic vein.

■ Skeletonize the anterior surface of the splenic artery and expose the anterior surface of the splenic vein. (Dissection of LN station 11p is complete once the half-way point on the splenic vessels or until the posterior gastric artery is reached.)

Lesser Curvature Dissection and Proximal Resection

The lesser curvature of the stomach is freed from the retroperitoneum until the esophageal crus is reached. The soft tissues along the intraabdominal esophagus, the right cardia, and the lesser curvature of the stomach, which contain LN stations 1 and 3, are cleared to prepare for the proximal resection.

■ Perform the truncal vagotomy at this time by dividing the anterior and posterior branches of the vagus nerve.
■ After the stomach is fully mobilized, transect the stomach using a 60-mm blue load endo-linear stapler ensuring sufficient proximal margin (additional load for the stapler may be required.)

This completes the procedure of robotic D2 lymphadenectomy for distal subtotal gastrectomy.

Procedure of D2 Lymphadenectomy During Total Gastrectomy

For advanced gastric cancer located in the upper body of the stomach, total gastrectomy with D2 lymphadenectomy is recommended. D2 lymphadenectomy for proximal tumors require the retrieval of the soft tissues encasing the splenic hilum, which contain LN station 10. Two options exist for retrieval of lymph station 10: a total gastrectomy with splenectomy and a spleen-preserving total gastrectomy. While splenectomy-related postoperative complications, such as subphrenic abscesses and postsplenectomy syndrome, are well known, complete dissection of the splenic hilum during spleen-preserving total gastrectomy is a very complex procedure. Spleen preservation is recommended for experienced surgeons.

Spleen-Preserving Total Gastrectomy

Robotic spleen-preserving total gastrectomy requires three additional steps: the dissection of the distal splenic vessels (LN station 11d), the splenic hilum (LN station 10), and the division of the short gastric vessels (LN station 2) (Fig. 21.7).

■ After the division of the left gastroepiploic vessels, the short gastric vessels are divided until the esophagophrenic ligament is reached and released.
■ Approach the splenic hilum by identifying the distal splenic vessels behind the distal pancreas and skeletonizing the vessels toward the spleen.
■ Completely remove the soft tissues encasing the splenic hilum.

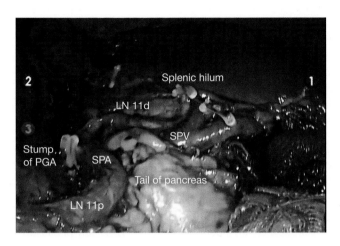

Figure 21.7 Completed dissection of the splenic vessels and splenic hilum. D2 lymphadenectomy during spleen-preserving total gastrectomy for proximal lesions requires the complete dissection of the soft tissues along the entire length of the splenic vessels for retrieval of lymph nodes 11d and the splenic hilum for lymph node station 10.

- The remaining soft tissues along the distal splenic artery and vein can be approached by completing the dissection from the proximal splenic vessels.

Total Gastrectomy with Splenectomy

Total gastrectomy with splenectomy requires the full mobilization of the distal pancreas and the spleen.

- Free the splenic vessels from the distal pancreas.
- Release the remaining splenic attachments by dividing the splenophrenic and splenorenal ligaments.
- Divide the splenic vessels behind the pancreas, approximately 5 to 6 cm from the celiac artery.

Reconstruction

After robotic gastric resection and complete LN dissection, several methods for the creation of an intracorporeal or extracorporeal gastrointestinal anastomosis have been described. The advantages and disadvantages to each approach exist. The appropriate selection of the gastrointestinal reconstruction after robotic gastric cancer surgery depends on the resection extent and remains a surgeon's preference. In general, stapled anastomoses are preferred but sutured anastomosis using robot assistance is also an option. Regardless of the method and approach used, patient-side assistance is required for the application of the stapler. Therefore, many methods used during laparoscopic gastroduodenostomy, gastrojejunostomy, and esophagojejunostomy can be applied after robotic gastric resections.

- Gastroduodenostomy, gastrojejunostomy, or Roux-en-Y gastrojejunostomy
- Intracorporeal or extracorporeal
- Linear or circular staplers including transoral anvil placement

 ## POSTOPERATIVE MANAGEMENT

Postoperative management of patients who have undergone robotic gastrectomy involves determination of when to resume oral intake, appropriate fluid maintenance, pain control, DVT prophylaxis, perioperative antibiotics, and blood work.

- Return of gastrointestinal function is expected in 3 to 5 days in patients without complications.
- Oral intake is resumed on postoperative day (POD) 2 and advanced as tolerated usually to liquid diet (POD 3), soft diet (POD 4), and regular diet (POD 5).
- Median length of hospital stay is usually 5 days without complications.

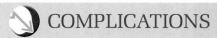

COMPLICATIONS

The reported complication rates for robotic gastrectomy vary. The largest series evaluating the short-term outcomes of robotic and laparoscopic gastric cancer surgery report wound-related issues, intraluminal bleeding and anastomotic leakage to be the most common complications encountered after robotic gastrectomies. These complications are not directly related to robot assistance since the port placements and anastomoses are not performed using the robot.

In general the morbidity and mortality associated with radical gastrectomies depend on the extent of resection, LN dissection, experience of the surgeon, and the experience of the institution where the surgery is being performed. Many of the complications are related to the extent of LN dissection and expectedly are higher with D2 lymphadenectomy than for D1. Improved surgical outcomes have been reported with spleen-preserving total gastrectomies when compared to total gastrectomy with splenectomy. No differences in complication rates have been found between laparoscopic and robotic gastric cancer surgeries.

Other possible complications are as follows:

- Intra-abdominal fluid collections/abscesses
- Intraluminal and intra-abdominal bleeding
- Pancreatitis/pancreatic leak/pancreatic fistula
- Anastomotic leak/stricture
- Gastroparesis or ileus
- Obstruction

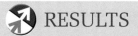

RESULTS

Robotic surgery for gastric cancer treatment is a relatively novel field. Many studies have studied laparoscopic versus open gastric cancer surgery and demonstrated many benefits of minimally invasive surgery without the loss of oncologic standards. Comparison of robotic approach to laparoscopic approach is scarce, but preliminary evidence suggest that robotic gastric cancer surgery has more benefits than laparoscopic and open surgery for the patient and the surgeon. The short-term results of the robotic gastrectomy from four major publications are shown in Table 21.1.

Benefits for the patient:

- Less pain
- Shorter length of hospital stay

TABLE 21.1 **Perioperative Factors**				
	Study A (*n* = 236)	**Study B (*n* = 24)**	**Study C (*n* = 16)**	**Study D (*n* = 7)**
Open conversion	None	None	None	None
Resection extent				
Distal subtotal gastrectomy	172	13	16	7
Total gastrectomy	62	11	0	0
Completion total	2	0	0	0
D2 lymphadenectomy	105	24	14	7
Operative time (min)	220 ± 47	268 (255–305)	259 ± 39	420 (390–480)
Estimated blood loss (cc)	92 ± 153	30 (0–100)	30 ± 15	300 (100–900)
Number of LN retrieved	42.4 ± 15.5	28 (23–34)	41.1 ± 10.9	24 (17–30)
Median LOS (days)	5	6	5	4

Study A (1), Study B (2), Study C (3), Study D (4).

- Decreased blood loss
- Faster gastrointestinal recovery
- Faster physical recovery
- Better quality of life after surgery
- Better cosmesis

Benefits for the surgeon:

- Ergonomics
- 3D view
- Control of four arms
- Accuracy of dissection
- Shorter learning curve

Disadvantages:

- Longer operative time
- Initial cost of robot for hospital
- Financial burden to patient
- Limited training opportunities

 CONCLUSIONS

Robotic surgery for gastric cancer is a safe and feasible operation. The short-term benefits of robotic gastrectomy parallel that of laparoscopy. Surgical oncologists who treat gastric cancer patients can readily adhere to the oncologic principles of gastric cancer treatment including no touch technique, negative margins, adequate LN dissection, and so on. The adoption of robotic surgery for the treatment of gastric cancer patients may improve the quality of surgery for the patient and offer a shorter learning curve for the surgeon.

Acknowledgments

This work was supported by a grant of the Korea Healthcare technology R&D project, Ministry of Health, Welfare, & Family Affairs, Republic of Korea (1020410).

Recommended References and Readings

Anderson C, Ellenhorn J, Hellan M, et al. Pilot series of robot-assisted laparoscopic subtotal gastrectomy with extended lymphadenectomy for gastric cancer. *Surg Endosc.* 2007;21(9):1662–1666.

D'Annibale A, Pende V, Pernazza G, et al. Full robotic gastrectomy with extended (D2) lymphadenectomy for gastric cancer: Surgical technique and preliminary results. *J Surg Res.* 2011;166(2):e113–e120.

Hartgrink HH, Jansen EP, van Grieken NC, et al. Gastric cancer. *Lancet.* 2009;374(9688):477–490.

Hur H, Kim JY, Cho YK, et al. Technical feasibility of robot-sewn anastomosis in robotic surgery for gastric cancer. *J Laparoendosc Adv Surg Tech A.* 2010;20(8):693–697.

Hyung WJ, Lim JS, Song J, et al. Laparoscopic spleen-preserving splenic hilar lymph node dissection during total gastrectomy for gastric cancer. *J Am Coll Surg.* 2008;207(2):e6–e11.

Hyung WJ, Song C, Cheong JH, et al. Factors influencing operation time of laparoscopy-assisted distal subtotal gastrectomy: Analysis of consecutive 100 initial cases. *Eur J Surg Oncol.* 2007;33(3):314–319.

Kim MC, Heo GU, Jung GJ. Robotic gastrectomy for gastric cancer: surgical techniques and clinical merits. *Surg Endosc.* 2010;24(3):610–5.

Kim HH, Hyung WJ, Cho GS, et al. Morbidity and mortality of laparoscopic gastrectomy versus open gastrectomy for gastric cancer: An interim report–a phase III multicenter, prospective, randomized Trial (KLASS Trial). *Ann Surg.* 2010;251(3):417–420.

Kim HI, Hyung WJ, Lee CR, et al. Intraoperative portable abdominal radiograph for tumor localization: a simple and accurate method for laparoscopic gastrectomy. *Surg Endosc.* 2011;25(3):958–963.

Patriti A, Ceccarelli G, Bellochi R, et al. Robot-assisted laparoscopic total and partial gastric resection with D2 lymph node dissection for adenocarcinoma. *Surg Endosc.* 2008;22(12):2753–2760.

Pugliese R, Maggioni D, Sansonna F, et al. Outcomes and survival after laparoscopic gastrectomy for adenocarcinoma. Analysis on 65 patients operated on by conventional or robot-assisted minimal access procedures. *Eur J Surg Oncol.* 2009;35(3):281–288.

Song J, Kang WH, Oh SJ, et al. Role of robotic gastrectomy using da Vinci system compared with laparoscopic gastrectomy: Initial experience of 20 consecutive cases. *Surg Endosc.* 2009;23(6):1204–1211.

Song J, Oh SJ, Kang WH, et al. Robot-assisted gastrectomy with lymph node dissection for gastric cancer: lessons learned from an initial 100 consecutive procedures. *Ann Surg.* 2009;249(6):927–932.

Woo Y, Hyung WJ, Pak KH, et al. Robotic gastrectomies offer a sound oncologic surgical alternative for the treatment of early gastric cancers comparing favorably with laparoscopic resections. *Arch Surg.* 2011;146(9):1086–1092.

Part II: Procedures for Neoplastic Disease

22 Laparoscopic Resection of Gastrointestinal Stromal Tumors

R. Matthew Walsh

Gastrointestinal stromal tumors (GISTs) represent 1% of all primary gastrointestinal tumors and are the most common gastrointestinal tumor of mesenchymal origin. This group of neoplasms represents an interesting aspect of cell biology as an early example of a single gene mutation-induced neoplasm. The specific mutation occurs in the intracellular domain of the c-KIT proto-oncogene which is present in 80% to 95% of these neoplasms. This allows the neoplasms to be distinguished from leiomyomas of the stomach which are positive for desmin and negative for KIT.

GISTs occur anywhere in the gastrointestinal tract but are most common in the stomach (50%) and small bowel (25%). They account for half of the submucosal lesions seen on upper endoscopy because they arise from the muscular layer of the intestine (Figs. 22.1 and 22.2). The median size at presentation is 5 cm and symptomatic patients in general present a decade earlier than asymptomatic patients with an overall median age of 66 to 69 years. The most common presenting symptom is gastrointestinal bleeding which occurs in one-third of patients and could be occult or overt bleeding. The next most common symptom is abdominal pain in 20% of patients. Additional presentations include an abdominal mass or incidental gastric mass on radiologic imaging or endoscopy. The presence of multiple GISTs can suggest familial GIST. The endoscopic view can include a well circumscribed submucosal mass that may include a deep ulceration for those presenting with gastrointestinal bleeding. And while this endoscopic finding is sufficient in symptomatic patients to proceed with resection, it is not specific.

Surgical resection is indicated for symptomatic GISTs, and biopsy is not required when tumor dissemination may be a risk. One tenet of treatment centers around the knowledge that all GISTs have malignant potential. Risk stratification is important to consider both for the indication for resection and for adjuvant therapy. Risk stratification for resection centers on size. Autopsy series demonstrate a high prevalence (22%) of small GISTs (<10 mm) in individuals over 50 years. Most of these small GISTs do not progress rapidly into large macroscopic tumors despite the presence of a KIT mutation. It is currently recommended that in acceptable risk patients, any GIST >2 cm should be resected. Contraindications to resection from a tumor biology perspective

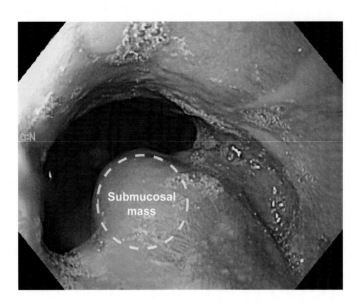

Figure 22.1 Endoscopic view of a submucosal mass. The endoscopic view is typical but not specific for a GIST. The growth pattern can be intraluminal, exophytic to the stomach or both.

include patients with known metastatic disease or unresectable tumor due to size or extended organ involvement that would lead to unacceptable morbidity or functional deficit. This latter group is amendable to neoadjuvant imatinib mesylate to downsize the tumor. This therapy typically lasts for 6 to 12 months with maximal response defined as no further improvement between two successive CT scans.

PREOPERATIVE PLANNING

A component of preoperative planning involves a consideration of the accuracy of the preoperative diagnosis for GIST. The differential diagnosis includes other submucosal masses such as lipoma, carcinoids, and leiomyomas or sarcomas, and nongastric masses which originate from the liver, pancreas, or spleen, as well as lymphoma or germ cell tumors. The diagnostic yield of endoscopy with biopsy is 35%, endoscopic ultrasound with fine needle aspiration (FNA) 84%, abdominal computed tomography 74%, and magnetic resonance imaging 91%. Endoscopic ultrasound is valuable in assessing the gastric layer from which the lesion arises as well as providing access for biopsy if that is required.

Once an accurate diagnosis of GIST has been determined, preoperative planning will be guided by size, location, and relative intra/extra gastric configuration. The interplay of all of these factors will determine the ultimate operative approach. A large lesion that is very exophytic or pedunculated on the anterior wall of the gastric body

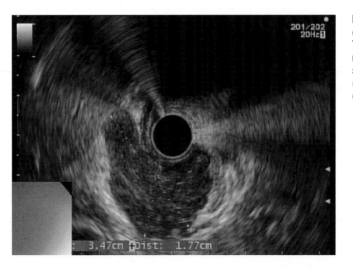

Figure 22.2 Image obtained from endoscopic ultrasound (EUS). These tumors arise from the muscularis propria as demonstrated. They can have a dumbbell configuration which is not always evident on EUS.

is a straight-forward laparoscopic resection and would be an entirely different operative approach from the same size lesion of the posterior antrum with an appreciable intragastric component which may require a standard distal gastrectomy. A posterior location may extend into the retroperitoneum requiring a pancreatic resection for complete removal. Transgastric or intragastric procedures should be considered for posterior wall or gastroesophageal junction tumors with an intragastric component. A wide variety of minimally invasive techniques are appropriate for GIST tumors which defies the concept of a single best approach for all patients. The integration and assessment of intraoperative endoscopy by the surgeon and diagnostic laparoscopy should guide operative decisions regardless of the preoperative plan.

Preoperative planning does require consideration of special equipment for many laparoscopic resections. A video endoscope, angled laparoscope, specimen retrieval bags, and endoscopic linear staplers are standard fare. Intragastric procedures where the operation occurs in an insufflated stomach with intragastric ports is a special operation which should be planned. It behooves the surgeon to be prepared with the following equipment if an intragastric approach is being contemplated.

Endoscopy Equipment

- Diluted epinephrine
- Sclerotherapy needle
- Over-tube
- Biopsy forceps
- Endo-snare
- Roth-net

Laparoscopic Equipment

- Balloon stabilized 5-mm trocars
- Needle drivers
- Ultrasonic shears
- Hook cautery
- Dual channel inputs for picture-in-picture

Robotic-assisted laparoscopy can also be performed for all manner of laparoscopic resections of GISTs including intragastric procedures. Use of robotic techniques will be determined by equipment availability and expertise.

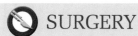

SURGERY

Regardless of the specific operative approach, laparoscopic versus open, intragastric versus transgastric, formal resection versus wedge resection, the same surgical objective should be obtained: complete resection without tumor disruption. The principle goal of resection is obtaining macroscopically negative margins. The need to achieve microscopically negative margins is uncertain, since outcomes are likely determined by biologic tumor behavior and not the microscopic margin. The presence of a positive margin may be falsely interpreted based on specimen retraction, and re-excision is not advised for a microscopically positive only (R1) resection. Radical resection that would include lymphadenectomy is not required to ensure good outcomes, but a formal resection may be required based on size and location to achieve the best functional outcome. Extended resection should be done for contiguous organ involvement only to the degree that an RO or R1 resection is accomplished. A laparoscopic approach to resection is feasible, providing the same principles of traditional surgery are upheld: complete resection without tumor disruption. It was due to concern for tumor disruption by manipulation of the tumor that laparoscopy was initially discouraged, but its utility has been borne out in many series.

Part II: Procedures for Neoplastic Disease

Positioning

Routine supine positioning is employed with video monitors at the head of the bed. Rarely will the monitors be at the feet if an intragastric resection is entertained for an antral lesion. Access to the mouth should be available for intraoperative endoscopy. Use of a split-leg bed is purely based on surgeon preference.

Technique

There are multiple techniques used for laparoscopic resection of gastric GISTs due to the varied locations of the lesions. It also points to the ingenuity of techniques fostered by minimal access surgery. General approaches will be discussed that are adaptable to specific situations.

Laparoscopic Wedge Resections

In this general scenario, wide access to the abdominal cavity is required with trocars positioned in a lazy "U" as used for most upper abdominal surgery (Fig. 22.3). This involves typically five trocars, all 5-mm except for a 12-mm at the umbilicus for endo-GIA stapler and extraction site. This approach is acceptable for all anterior wall masses of any location and many posterior wall lesions accessible via transgastric approach or via the lesser sac. There is a common misconception that a wedge resection requires elevating the lesion and its gastric wall attachment using a stapler to transect both walls of the stomach in a single firing (Fig. 22.4), and this technique is used most often by the laparoscopic novice and is really useful for only the most exophytic of GISTs. The resection of a spherical mass with a linear stapler will typically require a long staple line (use and expense of multiple cartridges) resulting in an unnecessarily large gastric deformity. It is typically a better option to resect the mass with a rim of normal stomach with any energy source (cautery, endoscopic shears; Figure 22.5A) and reconstruct the defect. The closure of the defect can be accomplished with a stapler (Fig. 22.5B) or suturing which will result in a better functional result. The specimen should be placed in a retrieval bag.

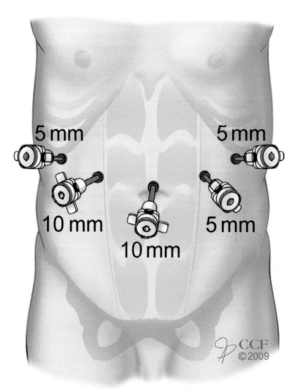

Figure 22.3 Typical trocar positioning for most laparoscopic gastric procedures (excluding intragastric techniques).

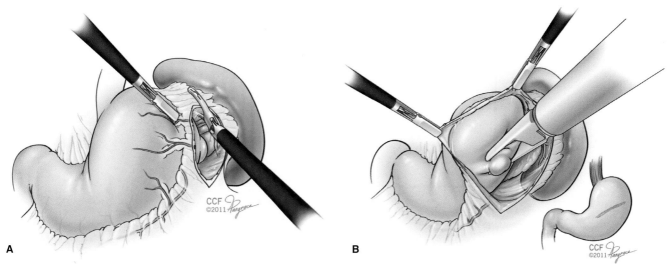

Figure 22.4 A: Laparoscopic approach to a posterior wall GIST. The gastrocolic omentum is divided with endoshears to expose the posterior wall. A transgastric approach can reach the same lesion but does not allow assessment for extragastric, retroperitoneal extension and thus is reserved for posterior wall lesions with dominant intragastric component. **B:** A stapled excision of the gastric wall containing a GIST often requires a long staple line and multiple firings to excise a spherical mass. This is ideal for exophytic and small lesions without causing excessive deformity.

Intragastric Resection

Resection of gastric GISTs can be performed while operating within the gastric lumen. This requires trocar placement directly into the gastric lumen and insufflation with CO_2 to distend the lumen. Endoscopic skills are important to allow trocar placement, suture passage, and specimen retrieval. The best candidates for this approach are those with lesions that are near the gastroesophageal junction or on the posterior wall of the proximal stomach. The lesion should be predominantly intragastric with realization that lesions can have a "dumbbell" configuration that may be seen on endoscopic ultrasound or preoperative CT. A full-thickness resection of the gastric wall is feasible with the intragastric approach as well as an enucleation that involves partial depth removal.

The operative sequence is as follows:

- Patient is in supine position and under general anesthesia.
- Endoscopy is performed to confirm position, particularly whether anterior or posterior wall, and selection of trocar location by digital indentation.

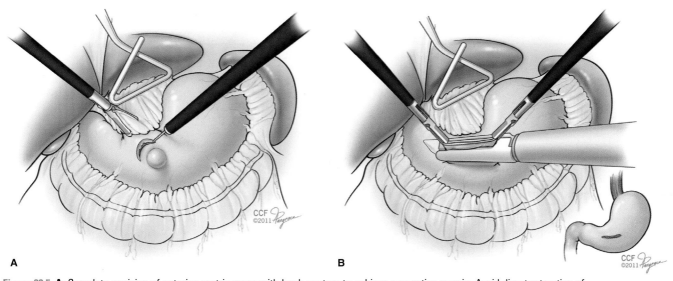

Figure 22.5 A: Complete excision of anterior gastric mass with hook cautery to achieve a negative margin. Avoid direct retraction of lesion to prevent disruption. **B:** Closure of a gastric wall defect after excision of an anterior wall GIST. The closure can be done in a transverse fashion as well and compromises the lumen minimally. Sutures can also be used to elevate the corners of the defect.

Part II: Procedures for Neoplastic Disease

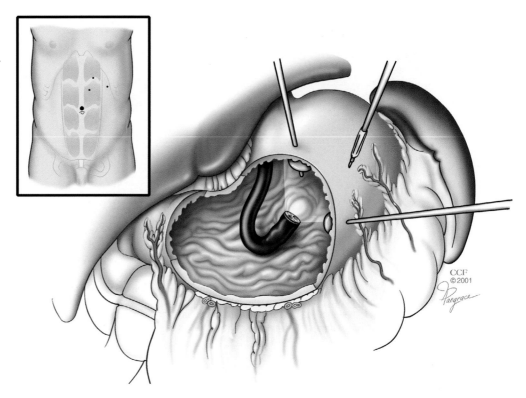

Figure 22.6 Endoscopic guidance of balloon-tipped trocars into the stomach with maximal triangulation. Typical trocar positions (inset).

- General abdominal laparoscopy to look for exophytic component and metastases.
- 5-mm balloon tipped trocars into the stomach with the stomach maximally distended with air under endoscopic visualization (Fig. 22.6). Three trocars are placed with maximal triangulation secure with balloon insufflation so trocars do not migrate from the stomach inadvertently.
- CO_2 insufflation into stomach.
- Endoscopic injection with a sclerotherapy needle of dilute epinephrine for hydrodissection and improved hemostasis. The hydrodissection allows for identification of the precise border of the GIST if enucleation is anticipated. The delineation of the lesion is clearly visible in all cases (Fig. 22.7).

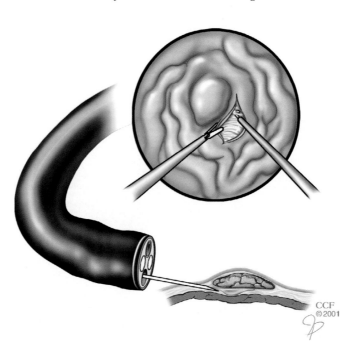

Figure 22.7 Endoscopic injection of the submucosa with epinephrine for hemostasis and hydrodissection.

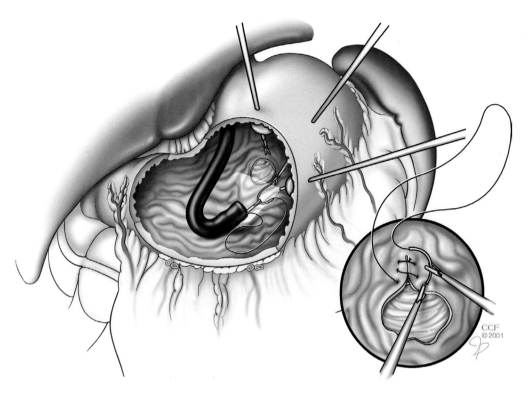

Figure 22.8 Laparoscopic closure of gastric wall defect with sutures introduced by endoscopically passed sutures.

- 5-mm instruments and camera for laparoscopic intragastric dissection. Typically the hook cautery works well for fine dissection.
- Following excision the lesion is placed in the stomach and the gastric wall defect repaired in all cases.
- The endoscope is re-inserted with an over-tube. Vicryl sutures of 4 inches length are passed into the stomach with an endoscopic biopsy forceps.
- The gastric wall defect is closed with laparoscopic needle drivers and endoscopically passed sutures (Fig. 22.8).
- The needles are removed orally. Any needed number of sutures can be passed as necessary to complete the closure.
- The GIST is removed orally after endoscopic capture with a Roth-net or snare.
- The balloon trocars are deflated and withdrawn from the stomach into the peritoneal cavity. The anterior gastric wall puncture sites are closed with standard laparoscopic suturing (Fig. 22.9).

Laparoscopic Formal Gastric Resection

A standard type of gastric resection is rarely required for resection of a GIST. It is not necessary from an oncologic perspective. This may be necessary for the size and compromising position of a GIST, typically an antral lesion whose resection and reconstruction would result in luminal compromise and outlet obstruction. An antrectomy with either Billroth I or II reconstruction is easier to accomplish as a planned excision rather than following excision where the subsequent large defect needs to be reconstructed.

The laparoscopic approach to antrectomy or distal gastrectomy is similar to the technique for a gastric cancer except that lymphadenectomy is not required. Should this be undertaken due to tumor size it must be done with the consideration of not disrupting the tumor. Many lesions that require a standard type of resection or extended resection due to tumor size are best done with open resection to avoid tumor disruption since this is of greater consequence than a laparotomy incision.

Robotic Excision

All of the aforementioned laparoscopic techniques can be performed with robotic assistance. Robotic partial gastric resection can be utilized with robotic endoscopic shears or

Figure 22.9 Laparoscopic closure of trocar sites with balloon catheters removed from the stomach into the abdominal cavity.

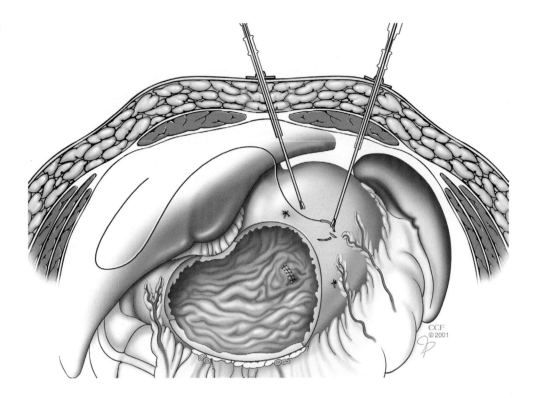

hook cautery. The defect can be easily sutured closed in two layers using robotic needle drivers, thus avoiding any staplers (Fig. 22.10A and B). This robotic suturing is effective regardless of the defect size or location and is a particularly good training procedure for residents and fellows. The degrees-of-freedom of the robotic instruments is what makes the defect size and location a straight-forward repair and is best demonstrated for intragastric suturing. The intragastric repair of the gastric wall defect is the most tedious and time-consuming aspect of the intragastric operative approach which is greatly improved with the robotic instruments. The standard 5-mm robotic trocars can be placed intragastricly without need for balloon-stabilized ports due to the robotic instrument recognition platform. A standard gastric resection is also well described robotically for early gastric cancer and can be used in this similar situation. The use of robotics in the resection of gastric GISTs is limited by the availability of the device, surgical training, and one's imagination.

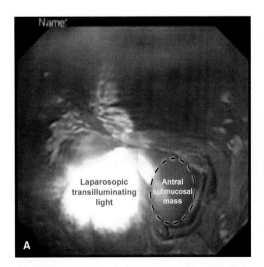

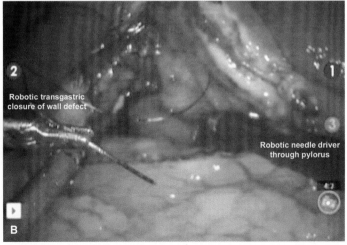

Figure 22.10 A: Endoscopic view of antral lesion that is posterior and intragastric. The light from the laparoscope shines through the anterior gastric wall. **B:** Robotic closure of the excised defect that was approached transgastrically. The right robotic needle driver is being passed through the pylorus to avoid outlet obstruction.

POSTOPERATIVE MANAGEMENT

The typical course of patients following laparoscopic GIST resection is notable for brief hospitalizations and rapid recovery. The length of stay is typically less than 5 days. A nasogastric tube is not routinely utilized nor is routine Gastrografin studies to interrogate for a leak. Patients are begun on a liquid diet the first postoperative day and advanced as tolerated. Antibiotic prophylaxis is used for 24 hours. A proton pump inhibitor is used routinely for the 2 months to aid gastric mucosal healing and reduce hemorrhage at the excision site. Any patient undergoing intragastric enucleation is surveyed yearly, to include endoscopic ultrasound, for 5 years to identify local recurrence should that occur.

 COMPLICATIONS

Procedure-specific complications are very infrequent, with many series reporting no complications. Potential morbidity would include hemorrhage, leak, and inlet or outlet obstruction.

- Hemorrhage can occur at the site of the resection if a partial thickness resection was done at an anastomosis or through a staple line. These bleeding complications can be reduced with fibrin glue for a staple line, mucosal approximation of gastric wall defects, and use of postoperative acid-suppressive medications. Bleeding complications can be diagnosed and managed with endoscopic techniques and rarely reoperation.
- Staple or suture line leaks are technical complications that are best avoided by maintaining meticulous technique. They should be suspected in a patient who is not following the anticipated recovery path, is septic, unusually tender on examination, or exhibiting delayed gastric emptying. It can be documented by oral contrast-enhanced CT scan (perigastric abscess with or without contrast extravasation) or Gastrografin swallow. Contained leaks can be managed with percutaneous drainage and antibiotics; the others with reoperation.
- The lumen can be operatively compromised at both the gastroesophageal junction and the antrum (pylorus). This can occur for lesions at both locations due to a large excision or from the reconstruction. Usually this is a consequence of poor operative selection or unsuspected narrowing with staplers. Symptoms are typically based on precise location: dysphagia or gastric outlet obstruction. Reoperation with resection and reconstruction is often required.

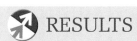 RESULTS

The patient outcome is typically a consequence of tumor biology, provided the basic surgical tenets of GIST excision are maintained. There does not appear to be an inherent disadvantage to laparoscopic resection. Small retrospective comparative trials have shown no adverse outcome from laparoscopic outcomes relative to resection, margin status, morbidity, or tumor recurrence. The length of stay can be favorably impacted by laparoscopic approaches.

Survival after surgery alone for GIST is favorable when compared to other intra-abdominal sarcomas. The overall outcome for patients who undergo complete resection with negative margins shows a 5-year disease-specific survival rate of 54% with a median survival of 66 months. The two most important prognostic features of the primary tumor are its size and mitotic index, which provides for a consensus approach to risk stratification.

An important consideration should be the use of imatinib mesylate in the adjuvant setting. A seminal trial has been published that randomized patients with >3 cm

KIT-positive GISTs to 1 year of 400 mg imatinib following complete resection. At a median follow-up of 20 months a clear improvement in recurrence-free survival was noted with imatinib, and the trial was stopped due to this interim analysis. There as yet has been no improvement in overall survival. This study clearly demonstrates that empiric adjuvant imatinib reduces rates of early recurrence, yet it is not clear whether this strategy improves overall survival, whether longer therapy beyond 1 year is warranted, and what patient selection criteria for therapy would be used.

CONCLUSIONS

Laparoscopic approaches to resection of gastric GISTs are reasonable, providing complete resection without violation of the tumor is achieved. There are a variety of operative approaches available to achieve this goal. The specific operative approach should be tailored to the patient's specific size and GIST location to obtain the optimal functional and oncologic outcomes.

Recommended References and Readings

Agaimy A, Wunsch PH, Hofstaedter F, et al. Minute gastric sclerosing stromal tumors (GIST tumorlets) are common in adults and frequently show c-KIT mutations. *Am J Surg Pathol.* 2007;31(1):113–120.

Bonvalot S, Eldweny H, Pechoux C, et al. Impact of surgery on advanced gastrointestinal tumors (GIST) in the imatinib era. *Ann Surg Oncol.* 2006;13(12):1596–1603.

Catena F, DiBattista M, Fusaroll P. Laparoscopic treatment of Gastric GIST: Report of 21 cases and literature's review. *J Gastrointest Surg.* 2008;12:561–568.

DeMatteo RP, Baliman KV, Antonescu CR, et al. Adjuvant imatinib mesylate after resection of localized, primary gastrointestinal stromal tumour: a randomized, double-blind, placebo-controlled trial. *Lancet.* 2009;373(9669):1097–1104.

DeMatteo RP, Lewis JJ, Leung D, et al. Two hundred gastrointestinal stromal tumors: Recurrence patterns and prognostic factors for survival. *Ann Surg.* 2000;231(1):51–58.

Demetri GD, Benjamin RS, Blanke CD, et al. NCCN Task Force Report: Optimal Management of Patients with Gastrointestinal Stromal Tumor (GIST) – Update of the NCCN Clinical Practice Guidelines. *JNCCN.* 2007;5(Suppl 2):51–79.

Demetri GD, von Mehren M, Antonescu CR, et al. NCCN Task Force report: Update on the management of patients with gastrointestinal stromal tumors. *J Natl Compr Canc Netw.* 2010;8(Suppl 2):51–41.

Dholakia C, Gould J. Minimally invasive resection of gastrointestinal stromal tumors. *Surg Clin N Am.* 2008;88:1009–1018.

Everett M, Gutman H. Surgical management of gastrointestinal stromal tumors: Analysis of outcome with respect to surgical margins and technique. *J Surg Oncol.* 2008;98:588–593.

Giasco G, Velo D, Angriman I, et al. Gastrointestinal stromal tumors: Report of an audit and review of the literature. *Eur J Cancer Prev.* 2009;18:106–118.

Kim MC, Heo GU, Jung GJ. Robotic gastrectomy for gastric cancer: Surgical techniques and clinic merits. *Surg Endosc.* 2010;24(3):610–615.

Learn PA, Sicklick JK, DeMatteo RP. Randomized clinical trials in gastrointestinal stromal tumors. *Surg Oncol Clin N Am.* 2010;19:101–113.

Matthews BD, Walsh RM, Kercher KW. Laparoscopic vs. open resection of gastric stromal tumors. *Surg Endosc.* 2002;16(5):803–807.

Miettinen M, Lasota J. Gastrointestinal stromal tumors: pathology and prognosis at different sites. *Semin Diagn Pathol.* 2006;23(2):70–83.

Nishimura J, Nakajima K, Omori T, et al. Surgical strategy for gastric gastrointestinal stromal tumors: Laparoscopic vs. open resection. *Surg Endosc.* 2007;21:875–878.

Novitsky YW, Kercher KW, Sing RF. Long-term outcomes of laparoscopic resection of gastric gastrointestinal stromal tumors. *Ann Surg.* 2006;243(6):738–745.

Raut CP, Ashley SW. How I do it: Surgical management of gastrointestinal stromal tumors. *J Gastrointest Surg.* 2008;12:1592–1599.

Rosen MJ, Heniford BT. Endoluminal gastric surgery: The modern era of minimally invasive surgery. *Surg Clin N Am.* 2005;85:989–1007.

Salem TB, Ahmed I. Gastrointestinal stromal tumour-evolving concepts. *Surgeon.* 2009;7(1):36–41.

Scarpa M, Bertin M, Ruffolo C, et al. A systematic review on the clinical diagnosis of gastrointestinal stromal tumors. *J Surg Oncol.* 2008;98:384–392.

Walsh RM, Ponsky J, Brody F, et al. Combined endoscopic/laparoscopic intragastric resection of gastric stromal tumors. *J Gastrointest Surg.* 2003;7(3):386–392.

23 Surgery for Gastrinoma

E. Christopher Ellison

INDICATIONS

Gastrinoma, also known as the Zollinger–Ellison syndrome (ZES), is a rare cause of ulcer disease. The incidence is about one case per million per year. The disease usually occurs between the ages of 30 and 70, although cases in children and the elderly have been reported. Sporadic cases dominate, accounting for 75% of all cases. Familial cases occur in 25% of patients and are usually part of the multiple endocrine neoplasia type 1 (MEN1) syndrome. It is very important to establish whether the patient has sporadic gastrinoma or MEN1, as the surgical treatment is different.

The diagnosis of gastrinoma is suggested by fasting hypergastrinemia off proton pump inhibitors (PPIs) in a patient with refractory ulcer disease, gastroesophageal reflex, or diarrhea. The most common causes of hypergastrinemia are achlorhydria associated with atrophic gastritis and chronic use of PPIs. PPIs induce achlorhydria, and hence, in the absence of negative feedback on the G cells in the gastric antrum, more gastrin is released. To establish that the fasting hypergastrinemia is caused by gastrinoma, it is necessary to check for the presence of gastric acid. If the patient has a gastric pH of 7 off PPIs, then ZES is excluded. If the patient has acid in the gastric aspirate, then a secretin provocative test is indicated. In a patient with gastrinoma, secretin will cause an increase in the gastrin. A positive test is defined as an increase of gastrin greater than 110 pg/mL over the baseline value (Fig. 23.1).

The contemporary surgical approach to gastrinoma is directed at tumor excision, and no gastric procedure is performed. Surgery is recommended only after the diagnosis is clearly established and imaging has localized the tumor.

PREOPERATIVE PLANNING

Two-thirds of gastrinomas are located in the gastrinoma triangle shown (Fig. 23.2). This applies to both sporadic and MEN1 patients. In sporadic gastrinoma, the tumors are located either in the duodenum (about half the cases) or the pancreas (nearly half the cases), or both. Gastrinomas may also occur primarily in lymph nodes. About one half of sporadic patients have tumors in both the duodenum and the pancreas. In those with MEN1, there is a propensity for multiple tumors, and duodenal tumors are found in

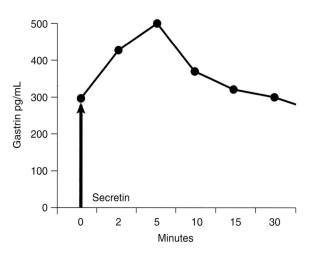

Figure 23.1 Secretin stimulation test for gastrinoma.

nearly all of these patients. The gastrin-producing pancreatic tumors are usually in the head of the pancreas. Although many patients have tumors in the body and tail of the pancreas, most of these are nonfunctional.

Preoperative localization tests should be performed. Somatostatin scintigraphy and CT scan are the initial tests. This may be supplemented with endoscopic ultrasound, MRI, and selective arterial secretin stimulation. In one-third of cases these tests will be negative. Exploration is clearly warranted in patients with positive localization tests. An individualized approach is recommended for those with negative localization tests and for patients with MEN1.

Outline of the Surgical Procedure

The operative procedure is divided into three unique major steps and is based on the principle of the gastrinoma triangle: step 1 is pancreatic exposure and management of pancreatic tumors; step 2 is assessment for and resection of duodenal tumors; and step 3 is sampling of lymph nodes in the gastrinoma triangle.

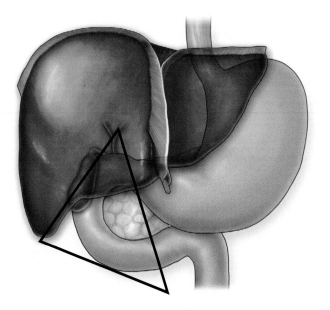

Figure 23.2 The gastrinoma triangle.

Step 1: Pancreatic Exposure and Management of Pancreatic Tumors
The operation begins after entering the abdomen through a midline incision and performing a manual exploration. The surgeon next performs a wide Kocher maneuver to fully expose the duodenum and allow palpation of the head of the pancreas. Next is the exposure of the pancreas through the lesser sac. This is followed by bimanual palpation of the pancreas and then by intraoperative ultrasound. Next is local excision of any pancreatic tumors. Pancreatic resection, either distal pancreatectomy or pancreaticoduodenectomy, is sometimes needed depending on the location and size of the tumor and in particular if the pancreatic duct is involved.

Step 2: Assessment for Duodenal Tumors and Resection
Intraoperative esophagogastroduodenoscopy and transillumination of the duodenum may be done to try to localize a duodenal tumor. However, the preferred technique is creation of a longitudinal duodenotomy to permit palpation of the duodenal mucosa. This is the most reliable method to identify duodenal tumors. If a tumor is found then it is removed by either enucleation or a full thickness local resection of the duodenal tumor if it is located in the lateral duodenum.

Step 3: Sampling of Lymph Nodes in the Gastrinoma Triangle

Details of Surgery for Gastrinoma

The operation is usually done as an open procedure; however, with improved preoperative localization a laparoscopic or robotic technique may be suitable for some patients.

Positioning
The patient is placed in the supine position. The left arm is tucked and the right arm is placed on an arm board.

Patient
A peripheral IV is started. Central venous access is used in selected cases. After induction of general endotracheal tube anesthesia, a nasogastric tube and Foley catheter are placed.

Equipment
In addition to a general laparotomy set, the following equipment should be available:

1. Intraoperative ultrasound transducer (10 MHz) and an ultrasound unit
2. An endoscopy cart and an adult upper endoscope
3. A bipolar coagulating device

Incision
A midline incision is made, and the abdomen is manually explored. The round ligament is divided. A self-retaining retractor is placed.

Pancreatic Exposure and Management of Pancreatic Tumors

Kocherization of the Duodenum
The peritoneum along the second portion of the duodenum is incised sharply. Medial retraction on the duodenum by the assistant facilitates the mobilization. The Kocher maneuver is complete when the left renal vein is seen. The duodenum and head of the pancreas are palpated (Figs. 23.3 and 23.4).

Exposure of the Pancreas
The lesser sac is entered by sharply dividing the omentum from the transverse colon. This is carried widely (Fig. 23.5).The body and tail of the pancreas are exposed. The attachments between the posterior wall of the stomach and the anterior surface of the pancreas are incised with electrocautery. The neck and anterior surface of the head of

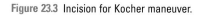
Figure 23.3 Incision for Kocher maneuver.

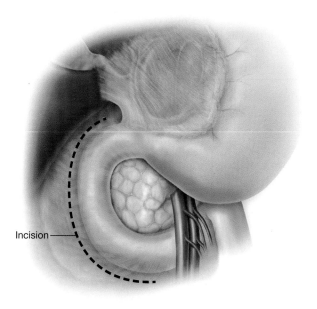
Incision

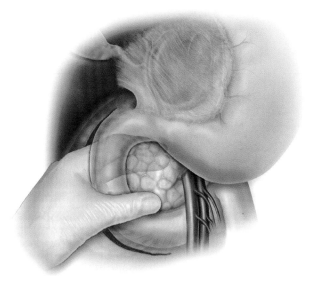
Figure 23.4 Duodenum and head of pancreas lifted by surgeons left hand.

Figure 23.5 Division of omentum to enter the lesser sac and expose the pancreas.

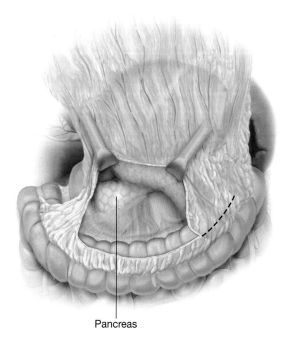
Pancreas

Figure 23.6 Pancreas exposed in the lesser sac.

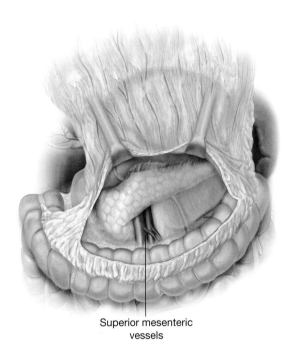

Superior mesenteric
vessels

the pancreas are exposed by continued dissection of the omentum in order to expose the vascular groove and the anterior portion of the superior mesenteric vein (Fig. 23.6). In some cases to provide enhanced exposure the gastroepiploic vein is ligated with 2-0 silk and divided. Bimanual palpation of the pancreas is performed.

Ultrasound of the Pancreas

The ultrasound transducer is placed in a sterile covering, and gel is applied to the tip of the probe. Transducers are designed to produce ultrasound waves of different frequencies. The higher the frequency of the waves, the greater the resolution of the image on the screen. Thus a 10-MHz transducer will produce a clearer image than a 5-MHz transducer. Saline is instilled into the lesser sac to cover the pancreas. The pancreas is examined for hypoechoic lesions (Fig. 23.7).

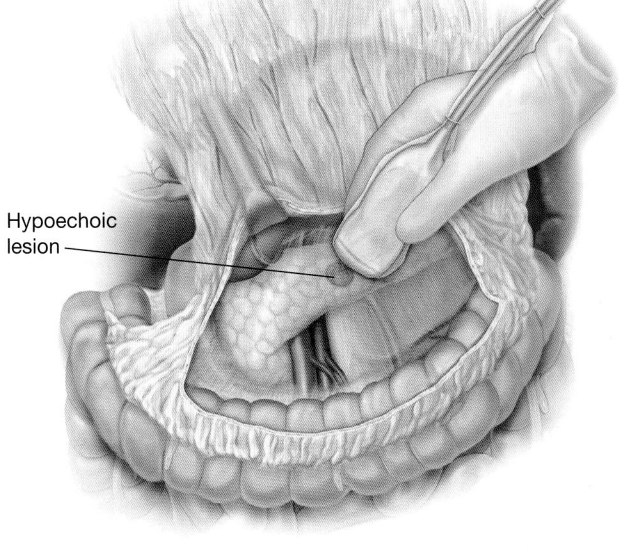

Figure 23.7 Intraoperative ultrasound of the pancreas.

Hypoechoic
lesion

Figure 23.8 Division of gastrosplenic ligament.

Resection of Pancreatic Tumors

Lesions in the tail of the pancreas are best removed by a distal pancreatectomy, usually combined with splenectomy for oncologic staging and tumor control. The pancreas is exposed as previously described. The gastrosplenic omentum is divided. This may be done using a coagulating device, or clamps and ties (Fig. 23.8). The spleen is next mobilized by dividing the splenorenal ligament. The surgeon cups the spleen gently in the left hand. With the right hand, the ligament is divided using electrocautery. Sometimes it is easier to have the assistant divide the ligament as the surgeon retracts the spleen medially (Fig. 23.9). Dividing the ligament allows blunt dissection in the retropancreatic space. The spleen and pancreas are brought together to the midline. The most superior short gastric vessel may be more easily divided at this portion of the procedure. The tail and body of the pancreas are mobilized using electrocautery for dissection. The splenic artery and vein are identified (Fig. 23.10). The artery is encircled with a vessel loop and divided with an articulated endoscopic stapler (Fig. 23.11). The neck of the pancreas is exposed and a blunt right angled instrument is used to dissect the space between the neck of the gland and the portal vein (Fig. 23.12). The neck of

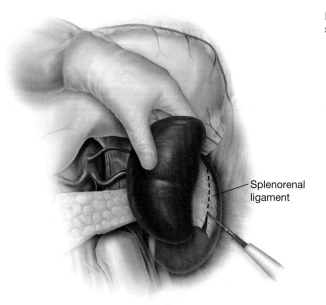

Figure 23.9 Mobilization of the spleen and tail of the pancreas.

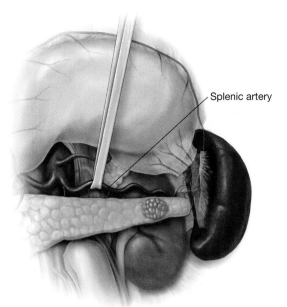

Figure 23.10 Splenic artery encircled with a vessel loop.

Splenic artery

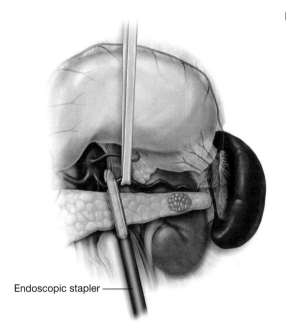

Figure 23.11 Stapling the splenic artery.

Endoscopic stapler

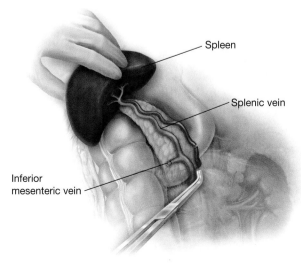

Figure 23.12 Dissection of the neck of the pancreas.

Spleen

Splenic vein

Inferior mesenteric vein

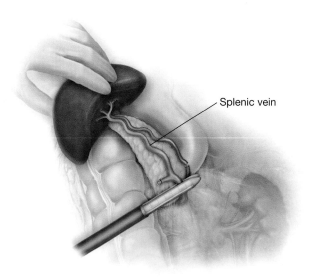

Figure 23.13 Isolation of the splenic vain and division using an endoscopic stapling device.

Splenic vein

the pancreas is encircled with a vessel loop or a ¼-inch Penrose drain. This facilitates the identification of the splenic vein. The splenic vein is encircled with a vessel loop and then divided with an articulated endoscopic stapler (Fig. 23.13). Further dissection with electrocautery allows complete mobilization of the pancreatic tail and a portion of the body of the pancreas. Next, the pancreas is divided. The pancreas may be stapled using the 3.5- or 4.8-mm staple load endoscopic stapler. The larger staple size is more frequently used. The staple line may be secured with a bioabsorbable staple line reinforcement constructed from polyglycolic acid : trimethylene carbonate, a medically proven biocompatible copolymer (Figs. 23.14 and 23.15). In some cases, the pancreas is thick and division with a stapling device would be considered inappropriate. In this case the pancreas is divided with electrocautery. It is preferable to create a fish-mouth–type incision in the pancreas to facilitate closure. The pancreatic duct is directly ligated with a 4-0 monofilament suture. In order to compress the divided pancreas, the cut end of the pancreas is closed with horizontal mattress sutures of 3-0 silk and then a layer of simple sutures of 3-0 silk to obtain finer approximation of the cut edges of the pan-

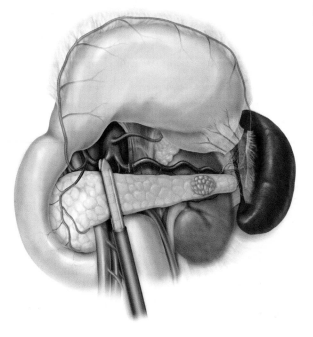

Figure 23.14 Division of the pancreas with an endoscopic stapler.

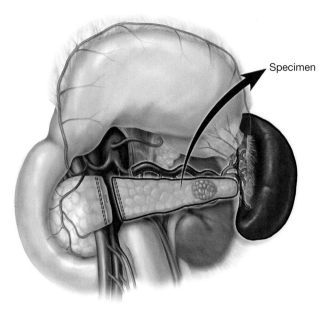

Figure 23.15 The pancreas divided and the specimen ready to be passed off the field.

Specimen

creas. Prior to closure, a closed-suction drain is inserted and placed near the cut end of the pancreas.

Tumors in the head of the pancreas (Fig. 23.16) should be locally excised by enucleation if they are less than 2 cm in greatest dimension and if the pancreatic duct is not in close proximity or compressed by the tumor. If the tumor is greater than 2 cm and/or involves the pancreatic duct, a pancreaticoduodenectomy is indicated. The enucleation technique requires excellent exposure of the pancreas. The surgeon controls the head of the pancreas and duodenum with the left hand positioned posterior to the head of the pancreas. As these tumors are highly vascular, the dissection is facilitated by the use of bipolar coagulating instrument (Fig. 23.17). As the dissection proceeds a traction suture may be placed in the tumor to permit it to be lifted away from the pancreatic parenchyma as the dissection proceeds (Fig. 23.18).

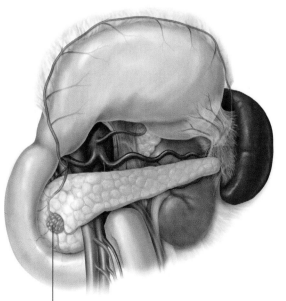

Figure 23.16 A gastrinoma in the head of the pancreas.

Tumor (gastrinoma)

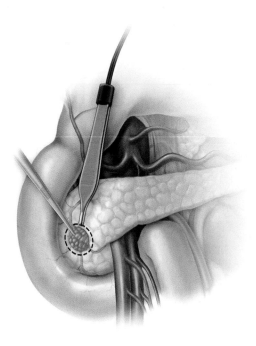

Figure 23.17 Initial steps in the enucleation of a pancreatic head gastrinoma using bipolar cautery.

Duodenal Tumors

Intraoperative Endoscopy

Upper endoscopy may be done to try to localize a duodenal tumor. Transillumination of the duodenum can identify lesions in the wall that otherwise might be missed. It is difficult to localize a duodenal tumor by this technique.

Duodenotomy

The most reliable way to identify a duodenal primary is by opening the duodenum and performing manual exploration. Duodenal tumors will be present in 50% of patients with sporadic ZES and in nearly 100% of those with MEN1. Stay sutures are placed on the lateral surface of the second portion of the duodenum, and a longitudinal incision is fashioned (Fig. 23.19). The duodenal mucosa is visually inspected and palpated. In sporadic ZES, the tumors are usually located in the first portion of the duodenum. They

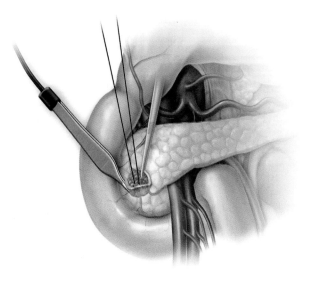

Figure 23.18 Traction stitch in gastrinoma facilitates dissection.

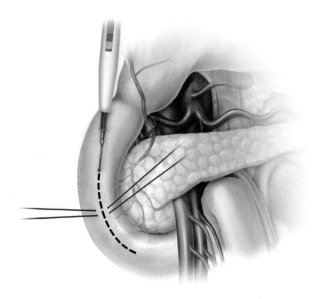

Figure 23.19 Longitudinal incision in the duodenum. Stay sutures have been placed.

may be in the pyloric channel as well. The tumors will feel rubbery in nature and protrude into the lumen.

Excision of Duodenal Tumors

The surgeon needs to be aware of the location of the ampulla of Vater so as not to confuse this structure with a medially located duodenal gastrinoma (Fig. 23.20). The medial placed tumor may be removed with an enucleation technique using monopolar cautery (Fig. 23.21). If the ampulla is difficult to visualize, then the gallbladder may be removed and the cystic duct cannulated with a 4 French biliary Fogarty catheter. This is threaded into the duodenum and the balloon insufflated with 0.5 cc of saline. The ampulla is then easily identified. As the lesions are encapsulated, resection of the duodenal wall is usually unnecessary. The duodenal mucosa is closed with interrupted 4-0 absorbable suture (Fig. 23.22). In cases of tumors on the lateral side of the duodenum, the lesion is excised with a full-thickness segment of duodenal wall. The duodenum is closed as a single layer with 3-0 silk in the longitudinal direction.

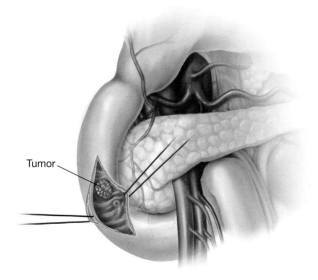

Figure 23.20 The duodenum is open and a tumor is visible just proximal to the ampulla of vater.

Tumor

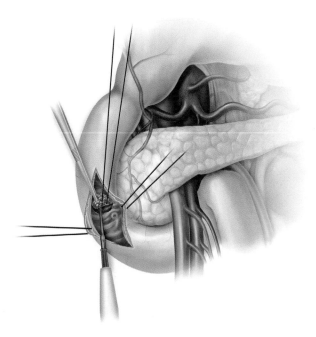

Figure 23.21 Local excision of a duodenal gastrinoma using a traction stitch and monopolar electrocautery.

Sampling of Lymph Nodes in the Gastrinoma Triangle

Lymph nodes along the porta hepatis are removed. The peritoneum lateral to the common bile duct is incised, and the bile duct retracted medially (Fig. 23.23). There are usually large nodes posterior to the bile duct, from the cystic duct to the top of the pancreas. These are removed with sharp dissection, with hemostasis achieved by hemoclips or 2-0 silk ligatures. The specimens are sent for frozen section. If the nodes are positive, then this could indicate a lymph node primary or metastasis from a duodenal or pancreatic primary.

Management of Liver Metastases

Localized liver lesions should be excised. If extensive metastases are identified the exploration should be aborted as treatment of the primary lesion will not be of benefit to the patient.

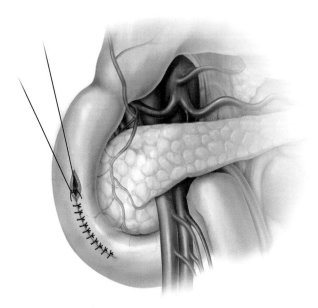

Figure 23.22 Closure of the mucosal incision made to remove the submucosal mass.

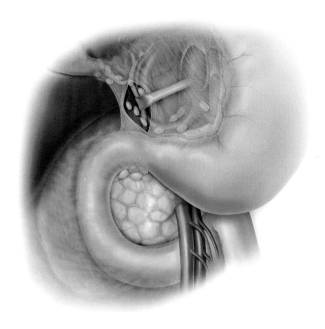

Figure 23.23 Sampling of lymph nodes in the gastrinoma triangle.

 POSTOPERATIVE MANAGEMENT

Intravenous fluids are administered. Urine output is monitored. The PPI should be administered intravenously even if a tumor was found as there is hyperplasia of the parietal cell mass and there will be continued excess gastric secretion for up to 3 months after surgery. The nasogastric tube is removed on postoperative day 1, unless the output exceeds 300 mL per shift. Diet is resumed the day after the nasogastric tube is removed. The drain is removed after the drain amylase is lower than the upper limit of normal for serum amylase. A fasting gastrin is obtained prior to discharge. Discharge medications should include a PPI.

 COMPLICATIONS

The surgeon should be aware of the problem of pancreatic fistula. If the drain amylase is elevated over serum, the drain should not be removed. The patient may be fed and discharged with a pancreatic fistula. Weekly drain fluid is sampled for amylase, and when it normalizes the drain is removed. Leakage from the duodenum is rare and would be evidenced by bilious nature of the drain output. In this case the patient should be made NPO, provided parenteral nutrition, and observed until closure. Reoperation for either of the aforementioned complications is rarely required.

Follow-up

About 30% of sporadic gastrinoma patients are cured and have normal postoperative gastrin levels after what is thought to be a complete resection. This indicates the problem with microscopic disease. Only 5% of patients with MEN1 and gastrinoma are cured after resection. However, complete resection of all visible gastrinoma in the duodenum and/or pancreas is associated with a survival advantage in both sporadic gastrinoma and MEN1 patients. The recommended testing protocol for patients with initial surgical cure, defined as a normal postoperative serum gastrin concentration, is as follows:

1. Fasting gastrin each year
2. Secretin provocative test for elevated gastrin

3. Screen for MEN1 each year
   a. Calcium
   b. Parathyroid hormone
   c. Prolactin
4. Imaging for an increasing serum gastrin concentration or an abnormal secretin test
   a. Octreotide
   b. MRI
   c. CT

For patients not cured by initial surgery, the follow-up is individualized depending on the stage of the disease and clinical evaluation at yearly visits. If disease progression is identified decision for re-exploration is made on an individual basis.

CONCLUSIONS

Exploration for gastrinoma is targeted by preoperative imaging. The intraoperative plan should be directed by the concept of the gastrinoma triangle. The goal of surgery is to resect all visible tumors. In the standard patient no gastric procedure is performed as was required in the past. This has been replaced by effective treatment of acid secretion by PPI. Exceptions are patients refractory to PPI (which is rare) and those rare patients with serious complications of peptic ulcer disease such as gastrojejunocolic fistula. Total gastrectomy may be warranted in such patients.

Recommended References and Readings

Ellison EC, Johnson JA. The Zollinger-Ellison syndrome: A comprehensive review of historical, scientific, and clinical considerations. *Curr Probl Surg* (Review). 2009;46(1):13–106.

Ellison EC, Sparks J, Verducci JS, et al. 50-year appraisal of gastrinoma: Recommendations for staging and treatment. *J Am Coll Surg.* 2006;202:897–905.

Isenberg JI, Walsh JH, Passaro E, et al. Unusual effect of secretin on serum gastrin, serum calcium, and gastric acid secretion in a patient with suspected Zollinger-Ellison syndrome. *Gastroenterology.* 1972;62:626–631.

McGuigan JD, Trudeau WL. Immunochemical measurement of elevated levels of gastrin in the serum of patients with pancreatic tumors of the Zollinger-Ellison variety. *New Engl J Med.* 1966;298:1308–1315.

Norton JA, Warren RS, Kelly MG, et al. Aggressive surgery for metastatic liver neuroendocrine tumors. *Surgery.* 2003;134(6):1057–1063.

Oberhelman HA, Nelson TS. Surgical considerations in the management of ulcerogenic tumors of the pancreas and duodenum. *Am J Surg.* 1964;108:132.

Wermer P. Genetic aspects of adenomatosis of the endocrine glands. *Am J Med.* 1954;16:363.

Zollinger RM, Ellison EH. Ulcerations of the jejunum associated with islet cell tumors of the pancreas. *Ann Surg.* 1955;142:709–728.

24 Bile (Alkaline) Reflux Gastritis

Daniel T. Dempsey

 ## INDICATIONS/CONTRAINDICATIONS

Alkaline or bile reflux gastritis is an unusual clinical syndrome consisting of chronic abdominal pain, bilious vomiting, and gastric mucosal inflammation associated with an "abnormal" amount of bilious duodenal contents in the stomach. Primary bile reflux gastritis is thought to be due to the presence of excess duodenal fluid in the stomach, perhaps because of abnormal motility patterns in the antrum, pylorus, and/or duodenum. More common is secondary bile reflux gastritis which occurs after pyloroplasty or gastrectomy with either Billroth I or Billroth II reconstruction. Since many dyspeptic patients (as well as many asymptomatic postsurgical patients) have both histologic gastritis and bilious duodenal contents in the distal stomach, the diagnosis of bile reflux gastritis must be made with care and circumspection. Prior to operation for bile reflux gastritis, an attempt should be made to quantitate enterogastric reflux, and to rule out other possible causes of the patient's symptoms.

Indications for operation in bile reflux gastritis are intractable chronic symptoms, particularly bilious vomiting (with or without abdominal pain), which are unresponsive to medical treatment including proton pump inhibitors and promotility agents. There should be good evidence of both excessive enterogastric reflux and gastric mucosal inflammation. *Relative contraindications* to operation are inanition, narcotic addiction, and excessive use of NSAIDs or tobacco. Care should also be exercised in patients with severe gastroparesis, and in asthenic patients. It is prudent for the surgeon contemplating operation for bile reflux gastritis to ask, "how would this patient look 10 to 15 pounds lighter?", because that is what often happens when an ill-conceived operation is done for this poorly understood functional GI malady.

 ## PREOPERATIVE PLANNING

The *differential diagnosis* of bile reflux gastritis includes peptic ulcer disease, gastroparesis, mechanical gastric outlet obstruction, gastric remnant carcinoma, partial small bowel obstruction, afferent loop syndrome, and other upper abdominal disorders.

Other causes of gastritis such as helicobacter pylori, alcohol, and NSAIDs should also be considered. Unrecognized marginal ulceration is common in distal gastrectomy patients who are reoperated on for bile reflux gastritis, so retained antrum and gastrinoma should be ruled out; serum gastrin levels consistently above two times the upper limit of normal should prompt a secretin stimulation test. It is important to recognize that some patients sent for surgical evaluation of bile reflux gastritis will have more than one diagnosis, e.g., bile reflux gastritis and gastroparesis; or recurrent peptic ulcer disease and afferent loop syndrome.

In patients considered to be surgical candidates for primary or secondary bile reflux gastritis, the *minimum preoperative evaluation* should include the following:

- upper gastrointestinal series with small bowel follow-through
- esophagogastroduodenoscopy with biopsy
- HIDA scan
- gastric emptying scan
- abdominal CT scan
- serum gastrin level
- review of previous operative notes

An important part of the preoperative management in patients with bile reflux gastritis is the *management of postoperative expectations* with the patient, family, and referring physician. It is helpful to remind patients that there are expected ups and downs during the recovery period, and that the success of the operation cannot be judged until the 3-month postoperative visit at the earliest. Many patients are unable to take their full nutritional requirements by mouth during the first few postoperative weeks, and it is rare to render patients with bile gastritis asymptomatic with an operation. Though the operations discussed below are quite effective in eliminating bilious vomiting, persistent pain is reported in up to 30% of patients, and 20% of patients develop postoperative delayed gastric emptying. It is important that these patients be managed both preoperatively and postoperatively by a *multidisciplinary team* including a gastroenterologist, surgeon, dietitian, psychologist/psychiatrist, and pain management specialist.

Choice of Operation

The rare patient with *primary bile reflux gastritis* (no previous gastroduodenal surgery) should be considered for duodenal switch and highly selective vagotomy (Table 24.1). The duodenal switch operation is inherently ulcerogenic, so it is reasonable to add a parietal cell vagotomy. Alternatively proton pump inhibitors are continued indefinitely after the duodenal switch operation. Cholecystectomy should be considered because after duodenal switch, ERCP may be impossible and cholecystectomy difficult. The duodenal switch operation should be avoided in patients with primary gastroparesis. Success with biliary diversion alone (choledochojejunostomy) has been reported and may be considered in patients with a history of primary common duct stones or sphincter of Oddi dysfunction. If the patient with primary bile gastritis has a significant history of peptic ulcer disease, consideration should be given to vagotomy and hemigastrectomy, with Roux-en-Y gastrojejunostomy, or Billroth II gastrojejunostomy with Braun reconstruction. The latter may be the preferable reconstruction in patients with delayed preoperative gastric emptying.

In patients with secondary bile reflux gastritis after Billroth II gastrectomy, the operations to consider are

- Roux-en-Y gastrojejunostomy (60 cm Roux limb)
  - Tanner 19 modification
- Braun gastrojejunostomy
- Henley loop (40 cm isoperistaltic jejunal interposition between the gastric remnant and duodenum)

Conversion of Billroth II to Billroth I gastroduodenostomy alone is not helpful though success has been reported when combined with Roux choledochojejunostomy.

TABLE 24.1	Choice of Operation for Bile Reflux Gastritis	
Previous Operation	**Surgical Options**	**Special Considerations**
None (primary enterogastric reflux)	Duodenal switch procedure (consider parietal cell vagotomy and cholecystectomy)	Avoid if primary gastroparesis present
	Roux choledochojejunostomy (if history of primary CBD stones or ampullary dysfunction)	Does not prevent enterogastric reflux of non-bile duodenal contents
Pyloroplasty	Distal gastrectomy with Roux reconstruction	Subtotal gastrectomy if significant gastroparesis
	Duodenal switch procedure (to avoid difficult duodenal stump)	Avoid if primary gastroparesis present
Loop gastrojejunostomy	Takedown gastrojejunostomy (if pyloric channel patent)	
	Subtotal gastrectomy with Roux reconstruction or Henley loop	If gastroparesis exists
	Distal gastrectomy with Billroth II and Braun reconstruction	If gastroparesis does not exist
Billroth I distal gastrectomy	Re-resection with Roux or Henley loop reconstruction	Subtotal gastrectomy if gastroparesis exists
Billroth II distal gastrectomy	Roux-en-Y gastrojejunostomy (+/− Tanner 19 modification)	Subtotal gastrectomy if gastroparesis exists
	Braun enteroenterostomy (+/− uncut Roux modification)	May not completely eliminate enterogastric reflux
	Henley loop (isoperistaltic jejunal gastroduodenal interposition)	Subtotal gastrectomy if gastroparesis exists

CBD, common bile duct.

In patients with bile reflux gastritis after Billroth I gastrectomy, conversion to Roux-en-Y gastrojejunostomy or Henley loop interposition should be considered.

The choice of operation for bile reflux gastritis depends on whether there are associated problems such as peptic ulcer disease, outlet stricture and/or gastroparesis. If not, patients with pure *secondary bile reflux gastritis following gastric surgery* are most easily treated by conversion of Billroth I or II to a Roux-en-Y gastrojejunostomy or Billroth II with Braun enteroenterostomy. Substantial re-gastrectomy is unnecessary. In patients with uncomplicated bile gastritis following loop gastrojejunostomy to an intact stomach, consideration should be given to takedown of the anastomosis if the pylorus and duodenum are patent.

Postgastrectomy and postpyloroplasty patients with *bile reflux gastritis* and *recurrent peptic ulcer disease* should be treated with subtotal gastrectomy (70%) and Roux-en-Y gastrojejunostomy. Patients with *postsurgical bile reflux gastritis and gastroparesis* may benefit from near total gastrectomy with Roux reconstruction. In this difficult subgroup of patients, if the left gastric artery remains intact, construction of a small (5% to 10%) vertically oriented proximal gastric pouch with resection of the fundus and remaining stomach may minimize persistent gastric stasis.

Operations that prevent buffering bile and duodenal contents from entering the stomach tend to be ulcerogenic. Anastomosis of a large gastric remnant to a Roux limb or Henley loop should be avoided since marginal ulceration is likely and gastroparesis common. While truncal vagotomy may prevent the former, it may also predispose to the latter complication. Vagotomy should be avoided in patients with clinically significant gastroparesis. In the current era, perhaps it is prudent to avoid truncal vagotomy when operating for bile reflux gastritis, relying instead on chronic proton pump inhibitor treatment. Thoracoscopic vagotomy is an option for the rare patient who develops marginal ulceration despite a small gastric remnant and acid suppression.

Part III: Operations for Postgastrectomy Syndromes

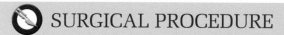

SURGICAL PROCEDURE

Positioning and Other Considerations

Operations for bile reflux gastritis can be done via a midline or transverse incision, or laparoscopically. Epidural infusion should be considered for postoperative analgesia. The patient is secured to the operating table in the supine position with the arms extended. Urinary catheter and nasogastric tube are inserted. Prophylactic antibiotics and DVT prophylaxis is initiated prior to incision. Sometimes intraoperative upper endoscopy is helpful. It must be remembered that in the postsurgical patient with chronic bilious vomiting, partial small bowel obstruction can be missed in the preoperative evaluation. If the proximal small bowel is distended, lysis of adhesions should be performed in addition to the remedial planned operation. Feeding jejunostomy should be considered since many patients with bile reflux gastritis are malnourished; ideally this would be placed distal to new anastomoses.

Braun Enteroenterostomy

This is the simplest operation for postsurgical bile reflux gastritis (Fig. 24.1). A hand sewn or stapled side to side anastomosis is performed between the afferent and efferent limbs of the gastrojejunostomy in the patient with a Billroth II. The anastomosis should be placed on the efferent limb at least 45 cm distal to the gastrojejunostomy to minimize reflux. The afferent limb may be occluded in continuity between the new Braun enteroenterostomy and the stomach with a TA stapler (5 cm away from the enteroenterostomy). This creates an "uncut Roux" arrangement which may not be durable but it minimizes gastric bile exposure for a while. Obviously it is imperative

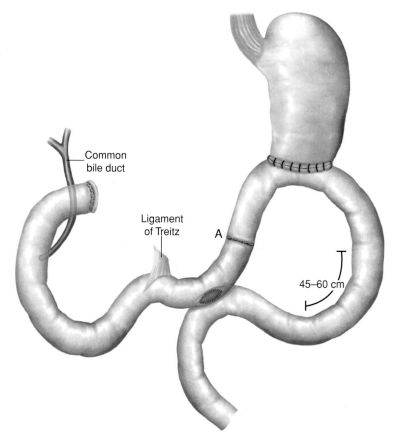

Figure 24.1 Addition of Braun enteroenterostomy to Billroth II gastrojejunostomy. The Braun anastomosis between the afferent and efferent limbs of the gastrojejunostomy is placed on the efferent limb at least 45 cm distal to the gastrojejunostomy. If the afferent limb is stapled in continuity with a TA stapler 5 cm distal to the Braun anastomosis (A), an uncut Roux is created.

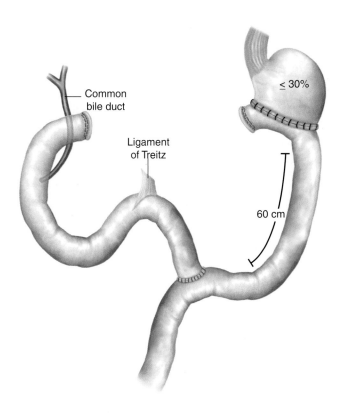

Figure 24.2 Roux-en-Y gastrojejunostomy. The enteroenterostomy is placed 60 cm distal to the gastrojejunostomy. It is usually best to leave a small gastric remnant.

that the surgeon be certain of the afferent limb prior to the application of this occlusive TA staple line.

Roux-en-Y Gastrojejunostomy

In the patient with bile gastritis and Billroth I anatomy, the duodenum is transected with a blue stapler distal to the gastroduodenostomy and the stomach is transected with a green stapler, resecting the gastroduodenostomy and leaving a 30% to 50% gastric remnant (Fig. 24.2). The ligament of Treitz is unequivocally identified and the jejunum is transected with a blue stapler 50 cm distal to this. The distal end is brought antecolic and anastomosed to the stomach with hand sewn or stapling technique. Sixty centimeters distal to the gastrojejunostomy, the proximal jejunum is anastomosed to the Roux limb completing the operation. If it is necessary to bring the Roux limb retrocolic, it should be sutured to the mesocolon with three interrupted sutures of 3-O silk.

When additional gastrectomy is unnecessary *in the patient with Billroth II anatomy,* the afferent loop is divided with a stapler just proximal to the gastrojejunostomy, and anastomosed to the efferent limb 60 cm distal to the gastrojejunostomy. If the afferent limb is unusually long, it may be used to construct the **Tanner 19 modification of the Roux operation** (Fig. 24.3) by transecting the afferent limb 30 cm proximal to the existing gastrojejunostomy. The distal end is then anastomosed to the efferent limb 20 cm distal to the gastrojejunostomy while the proximal end is anastomosed 60 cm distal to the gastrojejunostomy. The Tanner 19 arrangement putatively decreases the possibility of the Roux syndrome, i.e., postoperative gastric stasis.

Again it is mandatory that the surgeon correctly identify the afferent and efferent limbs. This is best done by finding the ligament of Treitz proximally and tracing the afferent limb to the stomach, then identifying the efferent limb and tracing in distally toward terminal ileum. When additional gastric resection is required, both afferent and efferent limbs are transected near the existing gastrojejunostomy and the short

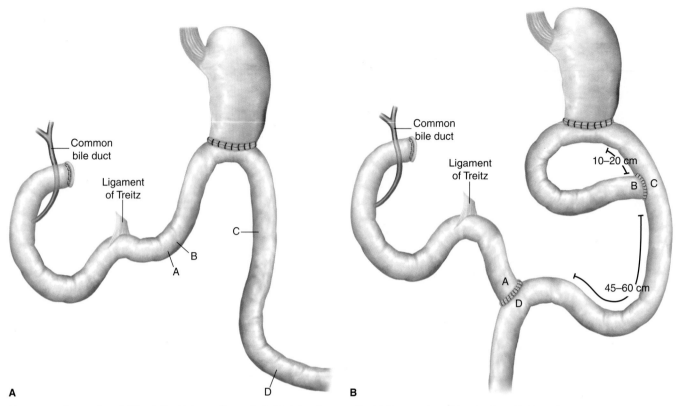

Figure 24.3 Conversion of Billroth II with long afferent limb (24-3a) to Roux-en-Y with Tanner 19 modification (24-3b). The afferent limb is divided between a-b, and b is anastomosed c, 10–20 cm distal to the gastrojejunostomy; "a" is then anastomosed to "d", 60 cm distal to the gastrojejunostomy.

perianastomotic segment of jejunum is removed with the additional gastrectomy. If possible, the left gastric artery is left intact. Reconstruction is with Roux gastrojejunostomy as above.

Motility of the Roux limb is abnormal and this leads to a functional obstruction. In some patients this results in profound gastric stasis (*the Roux syndrome*), particularly in patients with a large gastric remnant. Vagotomy may exacerbate the situation.

Henley Jejunal Interposition

The Henley loop is an isoperistaltic 40 cm segment of proximal jejunum interposed between the proximal gastric remnant and the duodenum; it is quite effective in preventing enterogastric reflux (Fig. 24.4). *If the patient has a Billroth I,* the gastroduodenostomy is taken down and the Henley loop is interposed between the gastric remnant and the duodenum. *If the patient has an isoperistaltic Billroth II* with the efferent limb coming off the lesser curvature side of the gastric remnant, it may be converted into a Henley loop by dividing the afferent limb flush with the gastrojejunostomy on the greater curvature side, and dividing the efferent limb 40 cm distal to the stomach. The latter is then anastomosed to the duodenum, and an enteroenterostomy is performed to restore small bowel continuity. If the efferent limb comes off the greater curvature side of the stomach, then the gastrojejunostomy is resected and the Henley loop fashioned from the efferent limb.

Gastric Resection

It has been suggested that total gastrectomy will cure bile reflux gastritis as well as any associated maladies like recurrent peptic ulcer disease and gastroparesis. However,

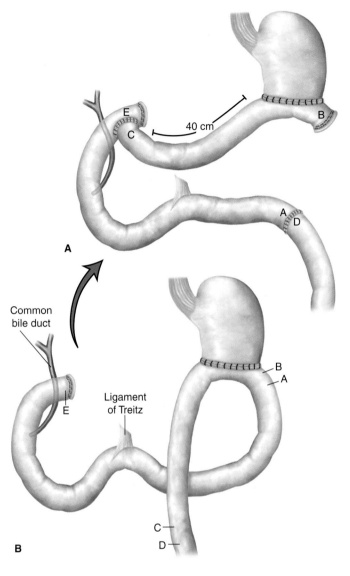

Figure 24.4 Conversion of isoperistaltic Billroth II to Henley Loop jejunal interposition. The afferent limb is divided just proximal to the gastrojejunostomy between a-b, and the efferent limb is divided 40 cm distal to the gastrojejunostomy between c-d. Then "c" is anastomosed to the duodenal stump (e), and intestinal continuity is restored by anastomosing "a" to "d".

most surgeons favor a more conservative approach. That being said, most patients requiring reoperation today for postsurgical bile reflux gastritis will benefit from additional gastrectomy, to excise an inflamed, strictured or ulcerated perianastomotic region; and/or to pare down a large gastric remnant. If preoperative evaluation shows substantially delayed solid gastric emptying in the patient with secondary bile reflux gastritis status post pyloroplasty or distal gastrectomy, and conversion to Roux-en-Y is planned, the gastric remnant should be pared down, leaving no more than a 30% gastric remnant. This may minimize symptomatic gastric stasis.

Duodenal Switch

This operation was designed to treat the rare patient with primary enterogastric reflux gastritis (Fig. 24.5). The proximal duodenum is mobilized and divided distal to the duodenal bulb. The proximal end is then anastomosed to a 60 cm Roux limb. We add a parietal cell vagotomy since there is only a short segment of proximal duodenum with Brunner's glands to buffer the acid from an intact stomach prior its entry into the uninitiated Roux limb.

We have performed a variant of this operation in several patients who developed debilitating enterogastric reflux and gastric stasis following esophagectomy and gastric

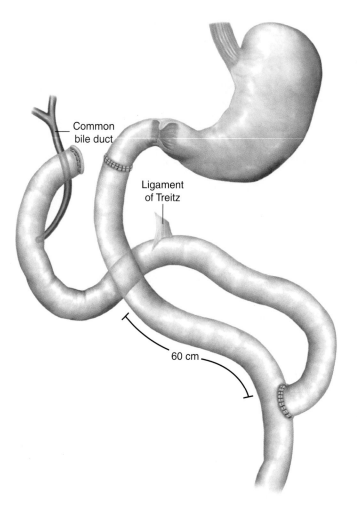

Figure 24.5 Duodenal switch for primary enterogastric reflux. The duodenum is transected distal to the bulb, and the proximal end is joined to a 60 cm Roux limb. The addition of a parietal cell vagotomy and cholecystectomy should be considered.

pull-up with pyloroplasty. At reoperation, the duodenum is divided just distal to the pylorus while care is taken not to injure the right gastroepiploic artery, the main blood supply to the gastric conduit. A 60 cm Roux limb is then fashioned and anastomosed to the distal antrum. In these cases preoperative upper GI had confirmed that the pylorus and distal antrum were below the diaphragm and accessible transabdominally.

POSTOPERATIVE MANAGEMENT

Prophylactic antibiotics are stopped within 24 hours of incision. DVT prophylaxis is continued until hospital discharge. Supplemental oxygen is administered for at least 48 hours. Foley catheter is left in place for 24 hours, or until the epidural catheter is removed. Incentive spirometry and early ambulation are strongly encouraged by nurse and physician members of the care team. A nasogastric tube is positioned in the gastric remnant intraoperatively, and left in place for 48 hours, or until bowel sounds return and drainage decreases. Reinsertion or manipulation of the nasogastric tube should be done with care since anastomotic disruption is possible.

When the patient is clinically ready to begin a liquid diet, we perform a limited upper GI series to help rule out leak and to document patency and return of effective gastrointestinal transit. Jejunostomy feedings are typically started on postoperative day 3, and plans are made upon hospital discharge for patients to receive at least half of their caloric requirements by tube over 12 hours daily. Both in hospital and after discharge, the patient should be seen by members of the multidisciplinary care team. The surgeon is wise to defer both inpatient and outpatient pain management issues to the anesthesiologist and/or pain management specialist.

COMPLICATIONS

The most frequent complications following remedial operation for bile reflux gastritis are pulmonary and wound problems. Atelectasis is common, and aspiration pneumonia is not unusual. Though most of these operations are classified as "clean contaminated," wound infection is more common than expected in these patients. Operations can be long and patients are frequently malnourished. Motility problems are common and nearly all operative candidates are on chronic proton pump inhibitor therapy. These factors conspire to increase the concentration and diversity of bacteria in any intraoperative wound inoculation, and to decrease local resistance to infection. Other possible postoperative complications include

- intraabdominal abscess
- intestinal leak or fistula
- ischemia of the gastric remnant or transverse colon
- hemorrhage
  - intraabdominal
  - anastomotic
- ileus and small bowel obstruction

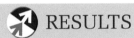

RESULTS

The operative mortality risk of remedial operation for secondary bile reflux gastritis is 2% to 10% and depends upon (inter alia)

- patient's comorbidities
- patient's nutritional status
- magnitude of operation
- difficulty of operation

If the patient and the operation are selected carefully and appropriately, long-term outcomes are as follows:

- 65% of patients are improved
- 25% of patients are unchanged
- 10% of patients are worse

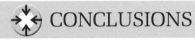

CONCLUSIONS

Bile reflux gastritis is an unusual syndrome and the diagnosis must be made cautiously. Often patients with this disorder have other problems such as recurrent peptic ulcer disease or gastroparesis, and symptoms may be more related to these concomitant maladies than to bile reflux gastritis. Multidisciplinary management is helpful, and surgeons should not be too eager to operate. While enterogastric reflux and bile in the vomitus can be eliminated by the operations discussed above, persistent symptoms and side effects are common. Carefully selected patients may benefit from operation. Primary bile reflux gastritis is treated surgically with duodenal switch. Secondary (postsurgical) bile gastritis is treated with Roux-en-Y or Braun enteroenterostomy or Henley jejunal interposition. Results may be optimized by leaving a small (30% or less) gastric remnant especially when Roux-en-Y is performed.

Recommended References and Readings

Aranow JS, Matthews JB, Garcia-Aguilar J, et al. Isoperistaltic jejunal interposition for intractable postgastrectomy alkaline reflux gastritis. *J Am Coll Surg.* 1995;180(6):648–653.

Burden WR, Hodges RP, Hsu M, et al. Alkaline reflux gastritis. *Surg Clin North Am.* 1991;71(1):33–44.

Davidson ED, Hersh T. The surgical treatment of bile reflux gastritis: A study of 59 patients. *Ann Surg.* 1980;192(2):175–178.

Eagon JC, Miedema BW, Kelly KA. Postgastrectomy syndromes. *Surg Clin North Am.* 1992;72(2):445–465.

Fiore AC, Malangoni MA, Broadie TA, et al. Surgical management of alkaline reflux gastritis. *Arch Surg.* 1982;117(5):689–694.

Hinder RA. Duodenal switch: A new form of pancreaticobiliary diversion. *Surg Clin North Am.* 1992;72(2):487–499.

Madura JA. Primary bile reflux gastritis: Diagnosis and surgical treatment. *Am J Surg.* 2003;186(3):269–273.

Mathias JR, Fernandez A, Sninsky CA, et al. Nausea, vomiting, and abdominal pain after Roux-en-Y anastomosis: Motility of the jejunal limb. *Gastroenterology.* 1985;88(1 Pt 1):101–107.

Miedema BW, Kelly KA. The Roux operation for postgastrectomy syndromes. *Am J Surg.* 1991;161(2):256–261.

Ritchie WP Jr. Alkaline reflux gastritis. Late results on a controlled trial of diagnosis and treatment. *Ann Surg.* 1986;203(5):537–544.

Ritchie WP. Alkaline reflux gastritis: A critical reappraisal. *Gut.* 1984;25(9):975–987.

Rutledge PL, Warshaw AL. Diagnosis of symptomatic alkaline reflux gastritis and prediction of response to bile diversion operation by intragastric alkali provocation. *Am J Surg.* 1988;155(1):82–87.

Sawyers JL, Herrington JL Jr, Buckspan GS. Remedial operation for alkaline reflux gastritis and associated postgastrectomy syndromes. *Arch Surg.* 1980;115(4):519–524.

Stavraka A, Madan AK, Frantzides CT, et al. Gastric emptying time, not enterogastric reflux, is related to symptoms after upper gastrointestinal/biliary surgery. *Am J Surg.* 2002;184(6):596–599; discussion 599–600.

Strignano P, Collard JM, Michel JM, et al. Duodenal switch operation for pathologic transpyloric duodenogastric reflux. *Ann Surg.* 2007;245(2):247–253.

Tu BN, Sarr MG, Kelly KA. Early clinical results with the uncut Roux reconstruction after gastrectomy: Limitations of the stapling technique. *Am J Surg.* 1995;170(3):262–264.

Van Stiegmann G, Goff JS. An alternative to Roux-en-Y for treatment of bile reflux gastritis. *Surg Gynecol Obstet.* 1988;166(1):69–70.

Vogel SB, Woodward ER. The surgical treatment of chronic gastric atony following Roux-Y diversion for alkaline reflux gastritis. *Ann Surg.* 1989;209(6):756–761; discussion 761–763.

Warshaw AL. Intragastric alkali infusion: A simple, accurate provocative test for diagnosis of symptomatic alkaline reflux gastritis. *Ann Surg.* 1981;194(3):297–304.

Wickremesinghe PC, Dayrit PQ, Manfredi OL, et al. Quantitative evaluation of bile diversion surgery utilizing 99mTc HIDA scintigraphy. *Gastroenterology.* 1983;84(2):354–363.

Xynos E, Vassilakis JS, Fountos A, et al. Enterogastric reflux after various types of antiulcer gastric surgery: Quantitation by 99mTc-HIDA scintigraphy. *Gastroenterology.* 1991;101(4):991–998.

25 Dumping Syndrome

Thomas A. Miller and Jeannie F. Savas

 ## INDICATIONS/CONTRAINDICATIONS

Dumping occurs when the pyloric sphincter mechanism has been altered so that an ingested meal is not properly processed and is discharged into the upper intestine prematurely. It may result from resection of the distal stomach that usually includes the sphincter, ablation of the sphincter (from pyloroplasty), or bypass of the sphincter (as in gastroenterostomy). The vasomotor (tachycardia, palpitations, diaphoresis, light-headedness, and flushing) and gastrointestinal (nausea, vomiting, abdominal cramping, and diarrhea) manifestations evoked by this premature emptying are collectively called the *dumping syndrome.* Both early (within 10 to 30 minutes of eating) and late (usually 2 to 3 hours after eating) forms of dumping have been identified.

While the precise mechanisms responsible for dumping are still debated, the early form is thought to be a consequence of the rapid passage of food of high osmolality into the upper small intestine from the stomach, while the late form is related to a high carbohydrate load in the intestinal lumen that evokes hyperglycemia that then induces hypoglycemia from insulin overproduction. Fortunately, both forms of dumping can be effectively managed medically by limiting the amount of liquids in a meal, avoiding hyperosmolar substances, and eliminating "trigger" foods if these can be identified. Occasionally carbohydrate gelling agents (such as pectin) or the somatostatin inhibitor, octreotide, may need to be employed as adjunctive therapy to the dietary modifications. In 99% of patients with dumping symptoms, these conservative measures will prove efficacious. Thus, surgery is truly a "last resort" approach to treatment and should only be employed when non-operative management has been tried, and proven ineffective, for a sustained period of time (usually, at least a year).

 ## PREOPERATIVE PREPARATION

Once the decision has been made that non-operative therapy for dumping has proved ineffective, cineradiographic studies should be obtained. This will accomplish two things: *First,* it will determine whether dumping does in fact exist, and *second,* it will provide an anatomic "roadmap" in planning the operation to be performed. On occasion, such radiologic analysis will fail to demonstrate any significant dumping, calling into question whether the patient's symptoms have anything to do with this abnormality.

It would be tragic to subject a patient to a procedure designed to correct dumping when the disorder does not even exist.

Assuming that the cineradiographic evaluation supports the diagnosis of dumping, the remainder of the preoperative preparation concerns the basic issues that need to be addressed in any patient being considered for surgery. Thus, if the patient has a history of heart disease, cardiac clearance needs to be assured. Similarly, if some other organ dysfunction exists, such as hepatic or renal disease, such function will need to be optimized before proceeding with the operation. Once such optimization has been assured, scheduling for surgery can be safely undertaken.

Operative Therapy for Dumping

Unfortunately, no operation has emerged as being the "gold standard" for the management of the dumping syndrome. Because of the infrequency of needing surgical care for this condition, such lack of a specific operation for treatment should not be surprising. In the authors' personal experience, we have only been called upon to treat this condition surgically several times over the past two decades. As minimally invasive surgery has become more commonplace for surgery involving the upper gut, and radical ablative procedures have almost reached "anecdotal status," surgery for dumping is likely to soon be of historical interest only.

Nonetheless, of the many operations that have emerged to manage dumping, two have achieved some level of durability. The first is the placement of a jejunal segment interposed between the stomach and duodenum, and the second is a Roux-en-Y-gastrojejunostomy. The interposition operation consists of interposing a jejunal segment measuring 10 to 20 cm between the stomach remnant and the proximal duodenum. (see Fig. 25.1). Although usually placed in a reversed, antiperistaltic fashion, it may also be positioned isoperistaltically. The rationale behind this operation is that the interposition

Figure 25.1 The jejunal interposition operation which consists of interposing an antiperistaltic or isoperistaltic segment of jejunum between the gastric remnant and the duodenum.

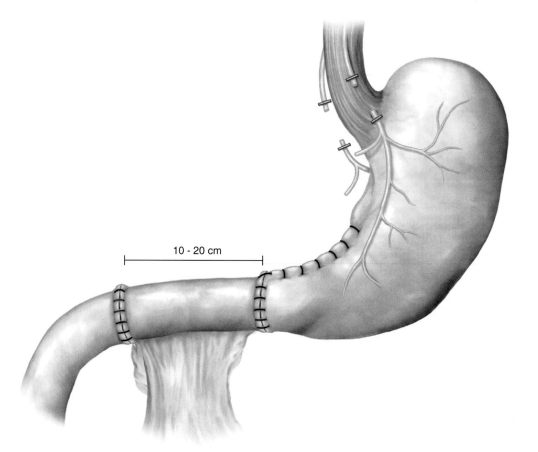

10 - 20 cm

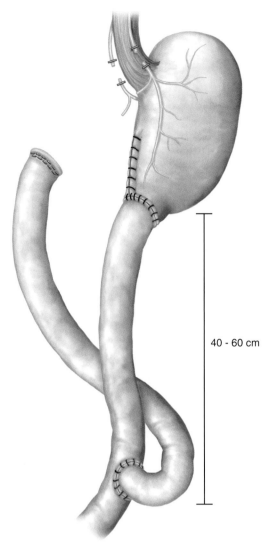

Figure 25.2 The Roux-en-Y gastrojejunostomy operation which is performed by transecting the jejunum just distal to the ligament of Treitz and anastomosing the distal portion of the jejunum to the gastric remnant. The proximal jejunum is then anastomosed to the distal jejunum 40 to 60 cm distal to the gastric pouch.

40 - 60 cm

slows down gastric emptying. Although short-term results have generally demonstrated benefit, when patients have been followed for longer periods, dumping symptoms have often returned. Less commonly, interposition procedures have initiated obstructive symptoms making reoperation necessary.

The second procedure, and the one that is more commonly employed, is the Roux-en-Y gastrojejunostomy (see Fig. 25.2). This procedure transects the proximal jejunum distal to the Ligament of Treitz. The distal limb of jejunum is then anastomosed to the gastric remnant and the proximal limb anastomosed to the downstream jejunum some 40 to 60 cm distal to the gastrojejunostomy. The procedure appears to work by delaying gastric emptying in the Roux limb through alteration in its motility. This procedure has been shown to effectively decrease dumping symptoms in a sustainable fashion. Unfortunately, some patients develop the Roux stasis syndrome which manifests itself with a variety of symptoms, including nausea, vomiting, epigastric fullness, and abdominal pain. Thus, because both procedures have their "good and bad" points, great care should be undertaken before subjecting a patient with dumping to surgical intervention.

POSTOPERATIVE MANAGEMENT

No special postoperative considerations are linked to surgery for the treatment of dumping. As with all operations involving the upper gastrointestinal tract, careful attention should be directed to adequate fluid balance, pulmonary toilet, and prevention of thromboembolic disease. Since bowel anastomoses are involved, a period of bowel dysfunction will occur in the early postoperative period. This usually resolves in 3 to 4 days allowing oral liquids to be given. Full oral alimentation can usually be commenced by days 5 or 6 with discharge from the hospital following soon thereafter.

Recommended References and Readings

Cullen JJ, Kelly KA. Gastric motor physiology and pathophysiology. *Surg Clin North Am.* 1993;73:1145–1160.

Henley FA. Experiences with jejunal interposition for correction of postgastrectomy syndromes. In: Harkins HN, Nyhus LM, eds. *Surgery of the Stomach and Duodenum.* Boston: Little Brown and Company; 1969:777–789.

Miller TA, Savas JF. Postgastrectomy Syndromes. In: Yeo CJ, et al. ed. *Shackelford's Surgery of the Alimentary Tract.* 6th ed. Philadelphia: Saunders; Volume 1, 2007:870–881.

Miranda R, Steffes B, O'Leary JP, et al. Surgical treatment of the postgastrectomy dumping syndrome. *Am J Surg.* 1980;139:40–43.

Ramus NI, Williamson RCN, Johnston D. The use of jejunal interposition for intractable symptoms complicating peptic ulcer surgery. *Br J Surg.* 1982;69:265–268.

Sawyers JL, Herrington JL Jr. Superiority of antiperistaltic jejunal segments in management of severe dumping syndrome. *Ann Surg.* 1973;178:311–321.

Vogel SB, Hocking MP, Woodward ER. Clinical and radionuclide evaluation of Roux-Y diversion for postgastrectomy dumping. *Am J Surg.* 1988;155:57–62.

26 Surgical Management of the Afferent Limb Syndrome

Carol E.H. Scott-Conner

 ## INDICATIONS

Afferent limb syndrome is a specific constellation of signs and symptoms associated with partial or complete obstruction of the afferent limb of an upper gastrointestinal reconstruction. The syndrome was first described in 1881 as a complication of partial gastrectomy with Billroth II reconstruction. The term has been used to describe obstruction of one of the limbs of other upper gastrointestinal reconstructions, such as Roux-en-Y gastric bypass, in which a jejunal limb reconnects to another limb of jejunum carrying the stream of succus. That situation is usually due to an internal hernia and will not be further discussed here.

This chapter describes the pathogenesis, prevention, diagnosis, and surgical management of afferent limb syndrome after Billroth II gastrectomy. Because gastric surgery is much less common than it used to be, the peculiarities of the Billroth II gastrectomy are not as well understood by many surgeons. This is a condition that can be prevented by attention to several details during the original operation. Those details will be outlined here, and the remainder of the chapter will describe the surgical management.

Pathogenesis

Billroth II reconstruction involves a side-to-end anastomosis of a loop of jejunum to the gastric remnant. Two limbs are thus created: the *afferent* limb, which conveys bile and pancreatic juice to the gastric remnant and hence to the stream of chime; and the *efferent* limb which conveys food from the stomach into the small intestine. Clearly, either limb can become obstructed. This obstruction may be partial or complete, acute or chronic. When the obstruction involves the efferent limb, the diagnosis is relatively straightforward because the patient vomits food and is unable to eat. When the obstruction involves the afferent limb, the diagnosis is more subtle because food may still pass through in the normal manner and an upper gastrointestinal contrast study may well fail to demonstrate the etiology of the problem.

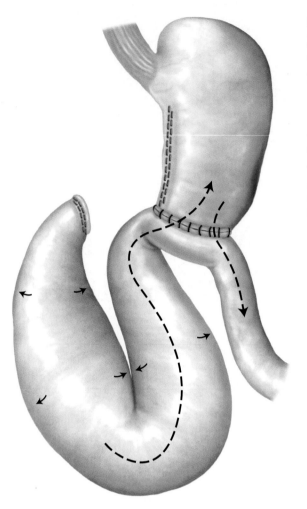

Figure 26.1 Pathogenesis of afferent limb syndrome. Afferent limb syndrome occurs when there is partial or complete obstruction of the afferent limb of a gastric reconstruction. Pressure builds up in the afferent limb and the resulting distension causes pain (and may even result in acute pancreatitis or ischemic necrosis). When the pressure in the limb is high enough to overcome the resistance at the anastomosis, a large amount of bile and pancreatic juice reflux into the gastric remnant, usually causing bilious vomiting. Because the efferent limb is not obstructed, food passes normally into the jejunum and is generally not found in the vomitus.

The term *afferent limb syndrome* is used to describe the chronic, partially obstructed situation (Fig. 26.1). Usually a problem is a kink or twist where the *afferent* limb attaches to the gastric remnant, but the obstruction can, in theory, be anywhere along the limb. Bile and pancreatic juice accumulate in the afferent limb until the pressure in the limb is sufficient to overcome the partial obstruction. During this phase, the patient typically experiences some degree of abdominal fullness or pain. When the obstruction is overcome, bile and pancreatic secretions flood the gastric remnant, often triggering bilious vomiting (and relief of pain). The vomitus generally contains little or no food, because the food has passed down the *efferent* limb without obstruction. Figure 26.1 shows some of the technical factors that contribute to the development of this syndrome: a long afferent limb, and anastomosis of the jejunum to the stomach in an isoperistalic fashion—that is, anastomosing the *afferent* limb to the lesser curvature and the *efferent* limb to the greater curvature.

When the obstruction is complete and occurs in the early postoperative period, blowout of the duodenal stump may occur. Thus, when a duodenal stump leaks, always check the afferent limb for obstruction. Complete obstruction late in the postoperative period may cause acute pancreatitis, or ischemic necrosis of the obstructed loop of jejunum.

Prevention

When creating a Billroth II reconstruction, the crucial factors to keep in mind to prevent afferent limb syndrome are these: Keep the afferent limb short, and anastomose the afferent limb to the *greater* curvature of the stomach rather than the *lesser* curvature in an antiperistaltic rather than an isoperistaltic fashion. The completed reconstruction should look like Figure 26.2A rather than Figure 26.2B.

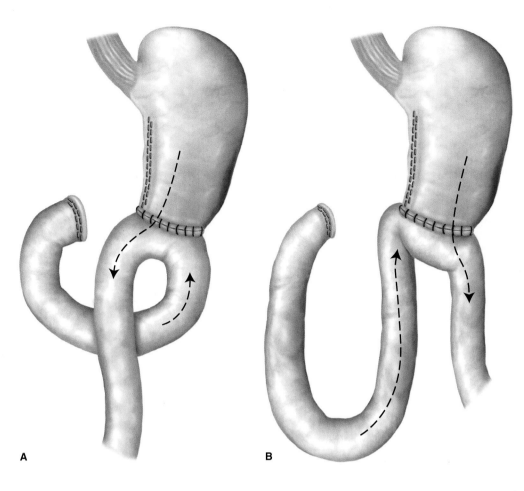

A   B

Figure 26.2 **(A)** Prevention of afferent limb syndrome. The ideal Billroth II reconstruction incorporates a short afferent limb anastomosed in an antiperistaltic fashion to the gastric remnant. The afferent limb is thus anastomosed to the greater curvature and the efferent limb to the lesser curvature. **(B)** Incorrect Billroth II geometry. If, instead, the afferent limb is anastomosed to the lesser curvature and the efferent limb to the greater, in an isoperistaltic fashion, kinking is more likely. In addition, the afferent limb generally must be longer. This longer afferent limb further contributes to the potential for kinking and obstruction.

In practice, this is easily accomplished by tracing the jejunum back to the ligament of Treitz. If you take the proximal jejunum in your two hands, flip the loop 180 degrees (by passing the distal part over the proximal part of the bowel), and then lay it against the gastric remnant, you will create the *ideal geometry* shown in Figure 26.2A. If, instead, you simply hold the loop up against the gastric remnant, you will *create* the problem shown in Figure 26.2B which predisposes to development of this syndrome. In working with residents over the years, it seems that the "flip" maneuver is counterintuitive to many inexperienced surgeons. This maneuver is, however, crucial; it allows the limb to lie comfortably without kinking.

The second important maneuver is to shorten the limb, thus placed, as much as possible without compromising the natural position in which it lies.

Retrocolic placement of the gastrojejunostomy allows the loop to be further shortened and may provide additional protection against kinking. This is the method recommended by many experienced surgeons. It introduces the potential problems of herniation or obstruction due to incomplete closure of the defect in the transverse mesocolon, and obstruction by recurrent gastric cancer in the bed of the gastrectomy (when the procedure is performed for cancer). To prevent this (if a retrocolic anastomosis is chosen), carefully close the defect in the transverse mesocolon by suturing it to the gastric remnant, so that the jejunum limbs hang free. Alternatively, if an antecolic anastomosis is performed, pull the greater omentum to the right side of the abdomen and pass the jejunum to the left of the omentum, to minimize the length of jejunum.

PREOPERATIVE PLANNING

In any reoperative situation, it is imperative to obtain and study the records from the original operation. Look particularly for details of anastomotic construction. Was the

Part III: Operations for Postgastrectomy Syndromes

gastrojejunostomy constructed in an antiperistaltic fashion (Fig. 26.2A) or an isoperistaltic fashion (Fig. 26.2B)? Was the reconstruction routed through the transverse mesocolon (retrocolic) or anterior to the colon (antecolic)? Was the operation performed for gastric cancer? Obtain the original pathology report.

The diagnosis is often suspected on clinical grounds and then confirmed by radiographic studies. A standard upper gastrointestinal series rarely demonstrates the problem, but will confirm lack of *efferent* limb obstruction. Generally the *afferent* limb will not visualize.

Use of a contrast medium excreted into the bile, such as HIDA, will allow the flow of bile to be traced into the *afferent* limb and will then show delayed transit into the rest of the gastrointestinal tract. Upper gastrointestinal endoscopy is crucial to exclude carcinoma. Obviously, this is important when the operation was originally performed for cancer. It is important to remember that carcinoma of the gastric remnant can occur after any procedure in which bile refluxes into the stomach. Upper GI endoscopy is also helpful to exclude marginal ulcers. CT or MRI scans with 3-dimensional reconstruction further help demonstrate the anatomy.

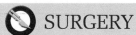 # SURGERY

As with any reoperative surgery, the correction of afferent limb syndrome must be tailored to the individual circumstance. Unless you are in a dire emergency situation, it is good to obtain the best anatomic and diagnostic information possible before going to surgery. This section will first discuss the approach in the emergency situation and will then provide an array of options for correcting the situation when it is encountered electively.

Emergency Surgery

Suspect afferent limb obstruction whenever the duodenal stump leaks. Duodenal stump leak or "blowout" is one of the most feared complications of the Billroth II. Emergency surgery will involve placement of drains and washout of the abdomen. A catheter may be placed in the duodenal stump to convert the blowout to a controlled fistula. It is important to check the afferent limb for obstruction, and to correct this obstruction by the simplest means possible. Correct any internal hernias or adhesive bands. If a kink is the problem, the simplest fix is to perform a jejuno-jejunostomy (Fig. 26.3). This can be done close to the gastrojejunostomy, as shown in this figure, or at a distance if it is too difficult to approach the gastrojejunostomy safely. It is rarely possible or advisable to attempt to redo the gastrojejunostomy.

The theoretical concern about creating a recirculating loop in which bacterial proliferation can occur has been raised. This concern would argue in favor of making the jejuno-jejunostomy close to the gastric remnant as shown in Figure 26.3, to minimize the size of any such recirculating loop. Alternatively, if the afferent limb is sufficiently redundant, a remote anastomosis to the efferent limb may be advantageous as it recreates the anatomy of an uncut Roux-en-Y (discussed below).

In the late postoperative period, the duodenal stump may remain intact, but acute pancreatitis or ischemic necrosis of the completely obstructed afferent limb may require emergency surgery for correction. In this situation, carefully inspect the entire duodenum and jejunum by mobilizing the right colon and small intestine with a Cattell-Braasch maneuver. If any necrotic areas are found, resection may be required. Pancreaticoduodenectomy has been reported in isolated severe cases when neglected complete obstruction has caused extensive ischemic duodenal necrosis.

If there is no necrosis, the simplest remedy is jejuno-jejunostomy as described above.

Elective Surgery

Jejuno-jejunostomy remains a simple straightforward remedy that is applicable to most patients, and any surgeon embarking upon reoperation for afferent limb syndrome

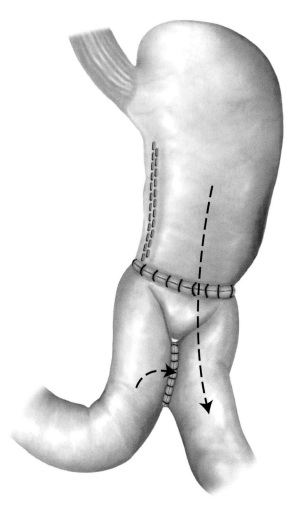

Figure 26.3 Jejuno-jejunostomy. The simplest corrective maneuver for afferent limb syndrome is jejuno-jejunostomy. Anastomose the afferent limb (shown to the left in this figure) to the efferent limb (shown to the right). Either do this close to the stomach (to minimize the potential for blind loop syndrome, as shown here) or sufficiently downstream to re-create the uncut Roux-en-Y reconstruction shown in Figure 26.5. Be careful not to cause kinking of the efferent limb.

should keep this reliable fall-back maneuver in mind. It is safe and involves the least dissection of any options.

The next simplest corrective maneuver is division of the afferent limb where it attaches to the gastric remnant and conversion to a standard Roux-en-Y reconstruction (Fig. 26.4) by anastomosing the end of the afferent limb in an end-to-side fashion to the efferent limb. This may be hand-sutured, as shown in Figure 26.4, or stapled. This conversion reliably corrects the afferent limb syndrome, and it is also used to correct alkaline reflux gastritis. Division of the afferent limb is easily accomplished with a cutting linear stapler. The new jejuno-jenunostomy should be constructed 40 to 60 cm distal to the gastrojejunostomy to prevent alkaline reflux. This is also a safe and reliable immediate remedy, but Roux-en-Y reconstruction after partial gastrectomy is associated with two characteristic problems of its own.

First, because bile and pancreatic juice no longer combine with gastric contents, acid peptic ulceration is common and this is considered an "ulcerogenic" preparation. In the past, truncal vagotomy was recommended as a routine, and this is still found in many textbooks. In the modern era of pharmacologic manipulation, the need for routine vagotomy should be critically assessed.

The second and thornier problem with Roux-en-Y reconstruction is poor gastric emptying due to diminished peristalsis in the proximal jejunum. Complete division of the proximal jejunum interrupts the conduction of pacemaker impulses from the duodenum, leading to decreased jejunal peristalsis, and truly refractory stasis can result. The so-called "uncut" Roux-en-Y provides an alternative (Fig. 26.5). The similarity to the previously described jejuno-jejunostomy is evident. The new jejuno-jejunostomy should be made 40 to 60 cm distal to the gastric remnant to prevent bile

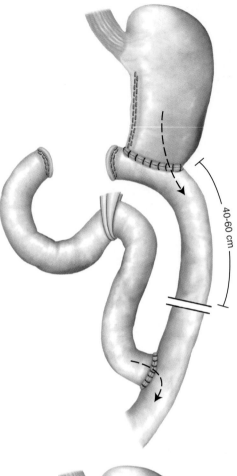

Figure 26.4 Conversion to Roux-en-Y. Another relatively simple and reliable corrective maneuver is to disconnect the afferent limb close to the gastrojejunostomy. Then anastomose this to the efferent limb 40 to 60 cm distal to the gastrojejunostomy to create a standard Roux-en-Y reconstruction.

40–60 cm

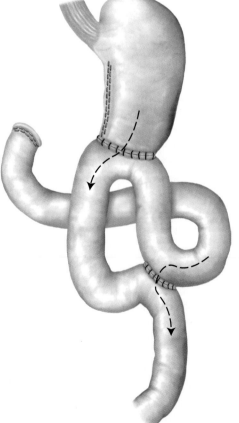

Figure 26.5 Uncut Roux-en-Y reconstruction. If there is sufficient redundancy in the afferent limb, anastomosis to the efferent limb 40 to 60 cm distal to the gastrojejunostomy will create an uncut Roux-en-Y reconstruction. This combines the complete bile diversion of the Roux-en-Y, but does not interrupt pacemaker activity from the duodenum and hence may be less likely to cause gastric emptying problems.

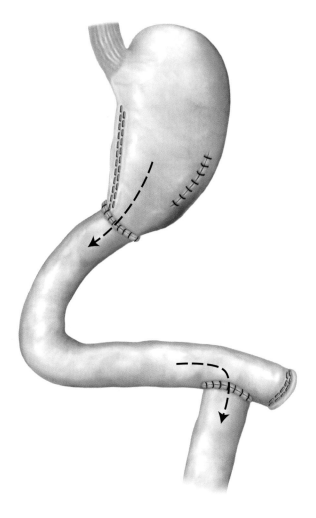

Figure 26.6 Conversion to Billroth I. The most radical solution is conversion to a Billroth I reconstruction.

reflux gastritis. Cullen et al. reported significantly less gastric stasis with this method of reconstruction.

One final alternative has been described, but should only be attempted by a highly experienced gastric surgeon. This is conversion of the Billroth II to a Billroth I reconstruction (Fig. 26.6). To accomplish this, take down the gastrojejunostomy and close the gastric incision. Tailor a smaller gastric outlet and anastomose this to the duodenal stump. Complete the reconstruction by re-establishing gastrointestinal continuity with a jejuno-jejunostomy. There is considerable intuitive appeal to this corrective maneuver, but also considerable peril. The most difficult part is likely to be dissection of the duodenal stump to a sufficient degree to allow safe creation of the gastroduodenostomy. In some situations, chronic obstruction may produce sufficient redundancy of the proximal duodenum to make this easy. The second potential issue is creation of a blind segment at the jejuno-jejunostomy. Such a blind segment may be associated with bacterial overgrowth and the blind limb syndrome.

It is important to note that stenting has been reported as an alternative to surgery and may be particularly useful when the syndrome is caused by inoperable recurrent cancer. Scattered case reports document primarily the use of the transhepatic route for this method (see recommended readings).

Recommended References and Readings

Cooperman AM. Postgastrectomy syndromes. *Surg Annu.* 1981;13: 139–161.

Delcore R, Cheung LY. Surgical options in postgastrectomy syndromes. *Surg Clin North Am.* 1991;71:57–75.

Eagon JC, Miedema BW, Kelly KA. Postgastrectomy syndromes. *Surg Clin North Am.* 1992;72:445–465.

Gwon DI. Percutaneous transhepatic placement of covered, self-expandable nitinol stent for the relief of afferent loop syndrome: Report of two cases. *J Vasc Interv Radiol.* 2007;16:157–163.

Mitty WF, Grossi C, Nealon TF Jr. Chronic afferent loop syndrome. *Ann Surg.* 1970;172:996–1001.

Mon RA, Cullen JJ. Standard Roux-en-Y gastrojejunostomy vs. "uncut" Roux-e-Y gastrojejunostomy: A matched cohort study. *J Gastrointest Surg.* 2000;4:298–303.

Vogel SB, Drane WE, Woodward ER. Clinical and radionuclide evaluation of bile diversion by Braun enteroenterostomy: Prevention and treatment of alkaline reflux gastritis. An alternative to Roux-en-Y diversion. *Ann Surg.* 1994;219:458–466.

Yoshida H, Mamada Y, Taniai N, et al. Percutaneous transhepatic insertion of metal stents with a double-pigtail catheter in afferent loop obstruction following distal gastrectomy. *Hepatogastroenterology.* 2005;52:680–682.

27 The Roux Stasis Syndrome: Diagnosis, Treatment, and Prevention

Michael G. Sarr

The Roux stasis syndrome was coined by Matthias and colleagues to explain a symptom complex of postprandial fullness, nausea, vomiting, and abdominal pain occurring after restoration of esophagoenteric or gastroenteric continuity using a Roux-en-Y reconstruction. Several other groups then studied this clinical syndrome in humans in depth. Multiple other experimental, laboratory-based, and clinical studies have investigated the incidence, etiology, pathogenesis, and treatment of this unusual disorder of gastrointestinal motility. Recent experience with bariatric procedures using a Roux-en-Y type reconstruction offers considerable insight into the pathogenesis of this disorder when considered in the context of prior Roux-en-Y reconstructions in the era of postgastrectomy/postvagotomy syndromes after duodenal ulcer surgery. The importance for the gastrointestinal surgeon of today is that operative attempts at correction of this problem are usually neither indicated nor successful; the Roux stasis syndrome is predominately a disorder of gastric or intestinal motility related to the effects of vagotomy and intestinal transection.

 ## INDICATIONS/CONTRAINDICATIONS

Clinical Recognition

The Roux stasis syndrome was much more common in the era of gastrectomy (including vagotomy) for duodenal ulcer and gastric cancer and was a well-recognized, though poorly understood, postgastrectomy syndrome that followed a Roux-en-Y type of reconstruction. This spectrum of symptomatology involves a varied constellation of five patient complaints: early satiety, postprandial fullness, nausea, vomiting of non-bile stained food, and postprandial pain. Weight loss is present inconsistently but can be a part of the spectrum of symptoms as well, and on occasion may lead to severe malnutrition requiring enteral or parenteral nutritional support. Vomiting of poorly digested food is quite common, but most notable is the lack of bile staining of the food and lack of bilious vomiting between meals or at night. The epigastric and central abdominal pain that occurs postprandially can be especially troublesome, is more visceral than somatic, but is not crampy nor characteristic of mechanical obstruction. One feature is virtually always present—the coexistence of vagotomy, either carried out as part of the therapeutic approach (i.e., acid-suppression for ulcer diathesis) or necessitated as a result of the gastric resection. The Roux stasis syndrome is extremely uncommon after a Roux-en-Y gastric bypass for morbid obesity, an operation that does not necessitate an abdominal vagotomy but involves a similar reconstruction of esophageal and gastroenteric continuity. The pain of the Roux stasis syndrome is very reminiscent of the abdominal pain of patients with idiopathic intestinal pseudo-obstruction and primary idiopathic gastroparesis.

There are two clinical presentations of the Roux stasis syndrome. One involves the presence of this symptom complex beginning immediately after the Roux-en-Y operation and persisting past the usual time period of adaptation to occur. The second more common form appears one or more years after the original Roux-en-Y reconstruction, becoming established often in an indolent fashion and with no apparent extenuating circumstances or putative cause. The symptomatology does not often wax and wane as with diabetic gastroparesis or some forms of intestinal pseudo-obstruction, but rather the symptom complex persists without much change in severity.

- Clinical presentation: early satiety, postprandial fullness, nausea, vomiting of non-bile stained food, and postprandial pain
- Occurs after Roux-en-Y reconstruction after partial or less commonly total gastrectomy accompanied by vagotomy
- Very rare (if present at all) after Roux-en-Y gastric bypass for obesity
- Two presentations: *early* with persistent symptoms immediately after Roux reconstruction, or *late*—occurring months to years postoperatively

Etiopathogenesis

van der Mijle, Vantrappen and others were the first to suggest a motor abnormality, and several groups have measured a disordered direction of contractions in the Roux limb. Normally, all contractions in the small intestine propagate distally secondary to the direction of the myoelectric "slow wave" driven by the duodenal pacemaker; this intestinal slow wave determines both the timing and the direction of contractions through the small intestine. When the small intestine is transected, this duodenal pacesetter becomes "isolated electrically" from the intestine distal to the site of transection. A new pacemaker region(s) appears distally and serves as the new site for generation of the myoelectric slow wave, but the direction of the myoelectric slow wave and thus contractions depends on the site of the new spontaneous pacemaker; the new slow wave (and the direction of contractions) then propagates both proximally and distally from this site.

Several groups have carried out a series of experimental studies in dogs examining both the direction of spread of intestinal contractions (proximal, distal) as well as the effect on the rate of gastric emptying using a standard loop gastrojejunostomy versus a Roux-en-Y type reconstruction (necessitating intestinal transection) after a hemigastrectomy (with vagotomy). After Roux reconstruction, 56% of contractions in the proximal aspect of the Roux limb were retrograde (proximal!), and gastric emptying was significantly slowed. In man, van der Mijle and colleagues were able to confirm abnormalities in the direction of spread of contractions in the Roux limb in patients with the Roux stasis syndrome. But equally and possibly more importantly, they showed an associated gastroparesis in these patients that did not appear to be correlated as closely with the extent of abnormally directed contractions as would have been expected if the major abnormality involved primarily a dysmotility of the Roux limb. Similarly, symptoms also failed to correlate closely with the contractile dysmotility of the Roux limb, suggesting to these investigators that most patients with the clinical findings of the Roux stasis syndrome had predominantly gastroparesis as the origin of their symptoms and not a functional obstruction by the Roux limb. There were only a small fraction of patients with objective "stasis" within the Roux limb of the radionuclide marker used to quantitate gastric emptying. These findings corroborated prior studies by Gustavsson and Kelly and McAlhany et al. who found the Roux stasis syndrome in only a small percentage of patients after a complete gastrectomy (~8%); note also that all of these patients by necessity of the total gastrectomy had a concomitant vagotomy.

- Roux-en-Y reconstruction disrupts the normal distal direction of contractions in the Roux limb
- Most symptomatology involves a gastroparesis more than a mechanical obstruction of the Roux limb
- All patients have had a vagotomy

PREOPERATIVE PLANNING

Diagnosis

The diagnosis of the Roux stasis syndrome is a clinical diagnosis of exclusion. First, the clinician must exclude any true mechanical obstruction, such as a stomal stricture at the gastro- or esophagojejunal anastomosis, as well as a more distal, partial small intestinal obstruction either from adhesions or internal hernia at the site of the jejunojejunostomy, the mesocolic defect (if a retrocolic orientation), or the infracolic so-called Petersen's hernia. These exclusionary investigations require both an upper endoscopy and a radiographic or computed tomography contrast study of the small intestine. A gastric emptying test using a more solid marker in the absence of any mechanical obstruction will confirm the diagnosis in the appropriate clinical setting—Roux anatomy with vagotomy. In truth, vomiting of non-bilious, partially digested food ingested hours beforehand is as sensitive as and possibly more specific than a formal, quantitative, radionuclide gastric emptying study. While transoral manometry of gastric contractions and the contractile activity of the Roux limb are possible, this test is uncomfortable for the patient, is not readily available in many/most hospitals, and usually is unnecessary, because the diagnosis is one of exclusion on the basis of symptomatology in an appropriate clinical setting.

- Roux stasis syndrome is a clinical diagnosis of exclusion
- Must rule out partial mechanical obstruction
  - At gastrojejunostomy or esophagojejunostomy
  - At potential sites of internal hernias—mesocolic defect or Petersen's hernia
  - Distal adhesive obstruction
- Radioscintigraphic gastric emptying (or vomiting of solid food eaten hours previously) confirms delayed emptying

Surgery or Non-Operative Treatment and Results

The best form of treatment is actually one of prevention. The role of a therapeutic-directed vagotomy is disappearing as we have come to better understand the etiology of duodenal ulcer disease (H. pylori and aspirin/NSAID use) and as we have access to progressively more powerful, acid, anti-secretory medications. Thus, the need for gastrectomy with vagotomy is currently a rarity for ulcer disease.

Similarly, one might envision certain techniques of gastro- or esophagoenteric resection/reconstruction that would avoid the abdominal vagotomy (such as a selective vagotomy) and the intestinal transection used classically to construct a Roux-en-Y limb. Indeed, a number of innovative techniques of an "uncut" Roux limb reconstruction have been explored experimentally in the laboratory as well as clinically.

Prevention: Experimental Studies

Because the intestinal transection required to construct a classic Roux limb leads to disordered motility, several animal models have been evaluated after creating a "functional" Roux limb, i.e., a "defunctionalizing limb," by diverting the chyme distally but without fully transecting the intestinal wall—the so-called "uncut" Roux limb first suggested by Merrill, McClusky, and Letton. Early techniques (Fig. 27.1) utilizing one application of a non-cutting linear stapler led to an unacceptable rate of staple line dehiscence; however, this technique preserved myoelectric continuity and, in doing so, maintained the direction of the slow wave (and direction of contractions) propagating across the staple line, thereby preserving the normal, distally oriented propagation of the slow wave and associated contractions. Indeed, when compared to a classic Roux drainage, gastric emptying with the uncut Roux limb was faster. Several other techniques have been introduced to attempt to prevent dehiscence of the staple line using a serosal buttress of Teflon® or other materials or techniques to provide a definitive scaffold onto which the staples will be fixed more securely. Another imaginative approach involved preserving a muscular bridge between the "afferent limb" and the proximal Roux limb but otherwise transecting the remainder of the lumen to form a modified Roux limb; this technique also preserved successfully the myoneural continuity, but although easy to create in a dog, attempts to do so in human jejunum have been largely unsuccessful (personal observation).

Attempts experimentally to treat the already-established disordered motility in a previously constructed Roux limb have involved placement of pacing electrodes on the proximal-most aspect of the Roux limb which, at least in the dog model, are able to "entrain" the slow wave in a distal direction by pacing at a frequency just greater than the inherent jejunal frequency; this directional pacing speeds gastric emptying. The use of a jejunal pacemaker is not, unfortunately, applicable in man due to the characteristics of myoelectric activity in the jejunum. Other attempts involved moving the site of the gastrojejunostomy to a more distal location in the Roux limb, hopefully to a region downstream (distal) to the site(s) of the new, spontaneous pacemaker. This approach and other similar approaches have not been successful universally. Unfortunately, the concept of taking down the gastrojejunostomy and restoring jejunal continuity by end-to-end jejunojejunostomy does not restore myoelectric continuity with the duodenal pacemaker.

Prevention: Clinical Studies

Several groups have evaluated the use of various forms of "uncut Roux" reconstructions in patients requiring a Roux-type reconstruction after subtotal or total gastrectomy. Kelly's group used a single firing of a non-cutting, linear stapler. While the postoperative clinical course was excellent, in early follow-up 5 of the 14 patients developed a dehiscence of the staple line leading to bile reflux esophagitis and need for operative repair—i.e., conversion to a classic Roux limb. Other groups have utilized two firings of a non-cutting linear stapler with or without a serosal, external prosthetic scaffold to maintain security of the stapled partition of the uncut Roux (Fig. 27.1B). Others have evaluated a Rho-shaped limb (Fig. 27.1A) or the "Noh procedure," (Fig. 27.1C) both done in an attempt to prevent the syndrome.

- Prevention of the Roux stasis syndrome involves the following:
  - Avoiding vagotomy
  - Creating various forms of "uncut Roux" procedures by using staplers, Rho-shaped limbs, or the Noh procedure

Treatment—Clinical Studies

Because the extensive clinical investigations by van der Mijle and colleagues and the lack of a clinical Roux stasis syndrome after a Roux-en-Y gastric bypass for obesity suggests that the vast majority of patients with the Roux stasis syndrome in reality probably have a postvagotomy gastroparesis as the primary disorder rather than a primary functional

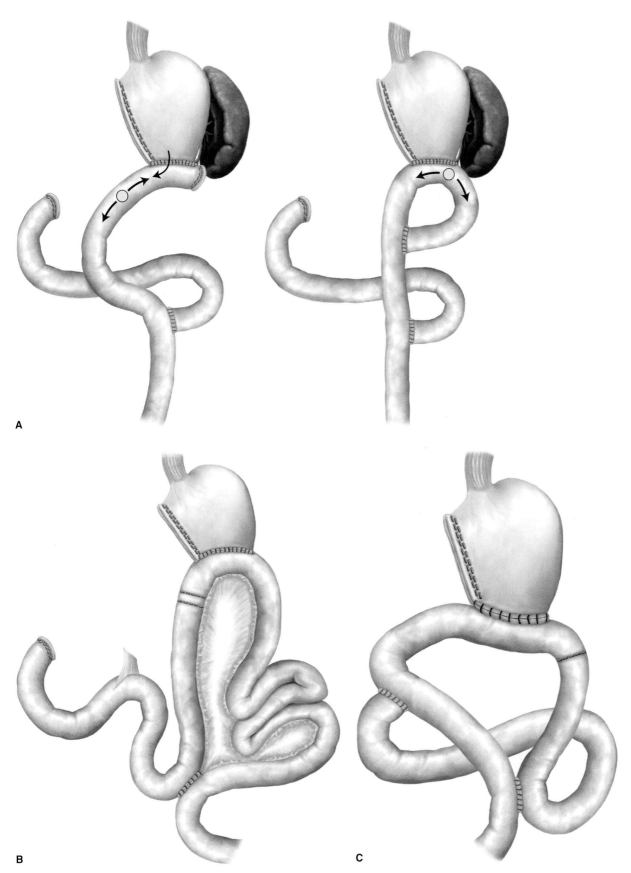

Figure 27.1 Variations of the "uncut" Roux or other configurations (Rho) to prevent Roux stasis syndrome. **(A)** Rho limb anatomy. Left panel—classic Roux anatomy. Right panel—Rho anatomy. **(B)** Two firings of a non-cutting stapler. **(C)** Noh procedure.

obstruction or "stasis" in the Roux limb. Exceptions of course include the rare patients after a total gastrectomy reconstructed with an esophagojejunostomy, but these patients have also undergone a vagotomy.

Medical Treatment

Every attempt at dietary modification and pharmacologic therapy should be exhausted before any operative therapy is undertaken. A primary strategy toward managing the patient with gastroparesis is the optimal approach. Avoidance of high roughage foods that can form bezoars is suggested. Blenderized foods and liquid supplements may allow for adequate nutritional support, but the patient may require multiple, small feedings throughout the day. In contrast, attempts at intragastric enteral feeding via gastrostomy will, of course, be unsuccessful.

Several medications have met with anecdotal success. Metoclopramide should not work, because its primary target for efficacy is the antrum; however, a short trial is warranted if for no other reason than its effect on nausea. Erythromycin, tegaserod (a partial 5-HT agonist), and cisapride are also appropriate therapeutic agents, although impressive success with trials of these agents is unusual. Tegaserod and cisapride may be difficult to obtain in the United States, because they have been taken off the market for rare but serious side effects.

- Try dietary modification with less solid foods, liquid supplements, and multiple small meals
- Medications to consider
  - Metoclopramide (primarily for nausea)
  - Erythromycin to "speed" gastric emptying
  - Cisapride or tegaserod—not available in the United States

The indications for operative treatment of the Roux stasis syndrome, unfortunately, are limited. Progressive weight loss and malnutrition would be the most common indications, while debilitating symptoms of nausea, vomiting, and postprandial abdominal pain might be considered as relative indications. Because myoelectric restoration of normal, distally oriented propagation of the slow wave and associated contractions are not possible with restoration of intestinal continuity, most attention should be directed at the gastric remnant combined with a feeding enterostomy tube; enteral feeding may prove difficult as well due to postvagotomy intestinal dysmotility.

Most patients with the "Roux stasis" syndrome have a combined postvagotomy gastroparesis and intestinal dysmotility as the primary defect. As with studies of the operative treatment of postvagotomy gastroparesis, the focus should be on removing the non-contractile gastric reservoir via a near total gastrectomy. Results are only partially rewarding with marked improvement in 45% to 75% of patients, depending on the definition of improvement. As many as 50% of patients will still require some form of enteral (and occasionally parenteral) nutritional supplementation to maintain health.

The rare patient with the (true) Roux stasis syndrome after total gastrectomy with vagotomy represents a very difficult situation. An attempt to move the esophagojejunostomy more distally along the Roux limb combined with a Rho-type revision (proximal end of the Roux limb anastomosed to the distal aspect of the Roux limb) seems rational, because the further distally, the more likely the contractions will be oriented aborally; however, there is minimal documented experience with this approach. Aside from this theoretic approach, no definitive operative therapy has proven effective in this group of patients; a primary supportive medical approach is suggested as described above—medical treatment. Avoiding narcotic treatment of the abdominal discomfort should be stressed; "treating" the discomfort with narcotics will only lead to the addition of a new problem of substance dependency and all its implications.

- There are no really good, reliable, effective operations for Roux stasis syndrome.
- If there is a sizable gastric remnant, near total gastrectomy, as for gastroparesis, may be warranted in the nutritionally crippled patient.

▓ Attempts at creating a Rho-type anatomy seem rationale, but experience is limited.

▓ A feeding enterostomy tube is mandatory, but enteral feeding may be complicated.

▓ Avoid "treating" the abdominal pain with narcotics.

Recommended References and Readings

Gujar P, Remde A, DeAntonio JR. Roux stasis syndrome: Clinical improvement with Tegaserod. *J Clin Gastroenterol.* 2005;39:550–551.

Gustavsson S, Ilstrup DM, Morrison P, et al. Roux-Y stasis syndrome after gastrectomy. *Am J Surg.* 1988;155:490–494.

Hirao M, Kurokawa Y, Fujitani K, et al. Randomized controlled trial of Roux-en-Y versus rho-shaped-Roux-en-Y reconstruction after distal gastrectomy for gastric cancer. *World J Surg.* 2009;33:290–295.

McAlhany JC Jr., Hanover TM, Taylor SM, et al. Long-term follow-up of patients with Roux-en-Y gastrojejunostomy for gastric disease. *Ann Surg.* 1994;219:451–455; discussion 455–457.

Merrill JR, McClusky DA Jr., Letton AH. Obstruction of afferent limb of gastrojejunostomy with jejunojejunostomy in treatment of alkaline gastritis. *Am Surg.* 1978;44:374–375.

Mon RA, Cullen JJ. Standard Roux-en-Y gastrojejunostomy vs. "uncut" Roux-en-Y gastrojejunostomy: A matched cohort study. *J Gastrointest Surg.* 2000;4:298–303.

Noh SM, Jeong HY, Cho JS, et al. New type of reconstruction method after subtotal gastrectomy (Noh's operation). *World J Surg.* 2003;27:562–566.

Noh SM. Improvement of the Roux limb function using a new type of "uncut Roux" limb. *Am J Surg.* 2000;180:37–40.

Petrakis J, Vassilakis JS, Karkavitsas N, et al. Enhancement of gastric emptying of solids by erythromycin in patients with Roux-en-Y gastrojejunostomy. *Arch Surg.* 1998;133:709–714.

Richardson WS, Spivak H, Hudson JE, et al. Teflon buttress inhibits recanalization of uncut stapled bowel. *J Gastrointest Surg.* 2000;4:424–429.

Speicher JE, Thirlby RC, Burggraaf J, et al. Results of completion gastrectomies in 44 patients with postsurgical gastric atony. *J Gastrointest Surg.* 2009;13:874–880.

Tu BN, Sarr MG, Kelly KA. Early clinical results with the uncut Roux reconstruction after gastrectomy: Limitations of the stapling technique. *Am J Surg.* 1995;170:262–264.

van der Mijle HC, Beekhuis H, Bleichrodt RP, et al. Cisapride in treatment of Roux-en-Y syndrome. *Dig Dis Sci.* 1991;36:1691–1696.

van der Mijle HC, Beekhuis H, Bleichrodt RP, et al. Transit disorders of the gastric remnant and Roux limb after Roux-en-Y gastrojejunostomy: relation to symptomatology and vagotomy. *Br J Surg.* 1993;80:60–64.

Van Stiegmann G, Goff JS. An alternative to Roux-en-Y for treatment of bile reflux gastritis. *Surg Gynecol Obstet.* 1988;166:69–70.

Part III: Operations for Postgastrectomy Syndromes

28 Open Bariatric Operations

J. Wesley Alexander

 ## INDICATIONS/CONTRAINDICATIONS

During the past two decades, there has been a major increase in the number of laparoscopic bariatric procedures compared to open procedures for the surgical treatment of morbid obesity. The advantages of the laparoscopic procedures have been improved cosmesis (lack of a long scar), a slightly decreased mortality rate (approximately 0.2% vs. 0.4% related somewhat to patient selection and characteristics) and a reduction in postoperative incisional hernias. However, the laparoscopic procedures have an increased leak rate, a higher rate of bleeding and small bowel obstruction and an increase in costs. The amount of long-term weight loss is similar for open vs. laparoscopic procedures as is improvement in co-morbidities and quality of life.

The selection of open vs. laparoscopic procedures depends in large part upon the experience of the surgeon and the desire of the patient. However, additional consideration for open procedures should be made in patients who are extremely obese (e.g., BMI >60), have had previous gastric procedures or prior operations in the central subdiaphragmatic region or with the need for additional intraabdominal operations or revision of prior bariatric procedures. Furthermore, there is sometimes a need for conversion of a laparoscopic to an open procedure. Therefore, it is mandatory that anyone who does laparoscopic bariatric procedures be qualified to do open procedures as well.

This chapter will discuss gastric bypass, biliopancreatic diversion, sleeve gastrectomy and revisions, but not various types of gastric banding as nearly all of these are done laparoscopically.

Indications for bariatric surgery should follow guidelines by the NIH and ASMBS which generally include a BMI >40 or >35 with significant co-morbidities.

Untreated coronary artery stenosis needs correction before any major surgical procedure, but hypertension, cardiovascular disease, severe sleep apnea, severe diabetes, advanced renal disease and thromboembolic disease should not themselves prevent the performance of needed bariatric surgery.

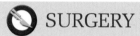 PREOPERATIVE PLANNING

- In patients who have had prior gastrointestinal surgery, obtaining and reviewing the operative report is essential.
- In patients who have had prior bariatric procedures, an upper GI series and endoscopy are needed.
- Preoperative endoscopy should be done in patients who have a history of reflux disease.
- Some surgeons perform preoperative evaluations for the presence of *H. pylori,* but this is unnecessary in patients who have no history of reflux symptoms or ulcer disease.
- Preoperative weight loss has been mandated in some programs to reduce liver size, but is unnecessary in open procedures.
- To reduce skin organisms, the patient should shower with chlorhexidine the night before as well as the morning of operation.
- A laxative is given the night before operation.
- Preoperative oral neomycin/metronidazole is helpful in reducing both gastric and intestinal organisms.
- All patients should undergo psychiatric evaluation, nutritional counseling, and physical therapy counseling preoperatively.
- All patients should attend support groups preoperatively.

SURGERY

Positioning

- Patient must be placed supine on the operating table being careful to avoid any pressure points to prevent rhabdomyolysis.
- Place both arms out being careful to prevent any stretch on the brachial plexus.

Management of the Incision and Prevention of Wound Infection

- All patients should receive preoperative systemic antibiotics. Cefazolin is used widely for this. The initial dose should be based on weight, giving 2 grams for patients under 300 pounds and 3 grams for patients weighing more than this, approximately 30 minutes before incision. A repeat dose should be given approximately 3 hours later in lengthy operations.
- For skin preparation, scrubbing with a sponge saturated with 70% alcohol is used to remove grease, desquamated skin, dirt, and debri. After this dries, paint the skin with DuraPrep®. Wait until it dries *completely* and then apply Ioban®. Press firmly over the site of the incision since this has a pressure-sensitive adhesive, and lifting of the Ioban® from the skin edge will result in an increased incidence in wound infection. Evacuate all trapped bubbles. If the Ioban® adheres well to the skin edges, there is no possibility of contamination from the skin.
- Make the incision from the xiphoid to just above the umbilicus. Incise the subcutaneous fat with a knife rather than electrocautery to minimize tissue damage. Electrocautery can be used to spot coagulate bleeders. Make the fascial incision in the center of the linea alba without cleaning off any of the attached fat.
- Closure of the fascia at the end of the operation should be done with a running #2 Prolene starting at each end and tying the sutures together somewhere in the middle with six square tightly tied knots. The ends of the suture should be cut short to avoid sharp points. To avoid the "cheese cloth" type of hernias, the bites into the fascia should be placed approximately 1 cm from the edge and 1 cm apart, making certain not to pull the sutures excessively tight. It might seem intuitive to take larger bites into the fascia, but this actually increases tension at spots where the fascia is not as strong and promotes the development of the "cheese cloth" hernias.

- The deep subcutaneous tissue is closed partly with a running suture of 3-0 Vicryl using a very large curved needle (XLH) so that the space, including the Scarpa's fascia and down to the midline fascia, is basically obliterated. The skin is closed with a subcuticular stitch using 3-0 PDS starting at each end and burying the knot in the middle using vertical rather than horizontal dermal stitches. Steri-strips are applied to the wound immediately after closure.
- Before dermal closure, place a drain from a Hemovac® into the subcutaneous space. After skin closure, infuse 20 to 80 mL of solution of gentamicin (320 µg/mL) or kanamycin (1000 µg/mL) and attach the tubing to the reservoir but do not activate suction, leaving the fluid to remain in the wound for 2 hours before removal by activation of the collection device. This allows for diffusion of the antibiotic into the tissues and will reduce the incidence of wound infections to <0.5%. The drain can be removed on the second postoperative day just before discharge.
- Some surgeons use a left subcostal approach, but this may prevent doing a cholecystectomy, and it is important to do a thorough intraabdominal examination with the initial procedure.
- If the patient has an umbilical or epigastric hernia, it should be repaired as part of the initial closure since this could be a site for a postoperative small bowel incarceration, and repair usually prevents the need for re-operation.

Cholecystectomy

A concurrent cholecystectomy may be performed if the patient has not already had one. This adds 20 to 30 minutes to the procedure, but is a safe cost-effective means to prevent the need for a subsequent cholecystectomy. An intraoperative cholangiogram is done if there are relative indications for doing so. It is important to address this since access to the duodenum by EGD is obviously not possible after GBP.

If common duct exploration is done, placement of a T-tube should be done using an additional length of the T-tube intraabdominally since it can be dislodged by excessive tension when the patient stands up because of an excessive abdominal wall thickness.

Gastric Bypass

Creation of the Enteroenterostomy

- Before performing the enteroenterostomy, the entire bowel should be examined and adhesions from prior operations lysed using appropriate treatment for any pathologic lesions that are found (e.g., ovarian mass).
- Next, the length of the alimentary, biliopancreatic and common channels limbs should be determined. A frequent choice is to make the biliopancreatic limb 80 to 100 cm and the alimentary limb 150 cm. This is sometimes modified if the mesentery is short, making it difficult to bring the end of the alimentary limb to the gastric pouch without tension. In our program, we have chosen to modify the length of the alimentary and biliopancreatic limbs to be longer as the patient's weight increases (e.g., each limb 0.5 cm × patient's weight in pounds). For a patient weighing 400 pounds, the alimentary limb would be 200 cm and the biliopancreatic limb 200 cm; for a patient weighing 500 pounds, both the biliopancreatic limb and alimentary limb would be 250 cm.
- Once the site is selected, the bowel is divided with a GIA-55 stapler and the cut ends oversewn with 3-0 Prolene. The suture on the antimesenteric side of the closure of the distal limb is cut long so that it can be identified later as the proximal end of the alimentary limb.
- The mesentery is then divided.
- A side-to-side anastomosis is then made with the bilio-pancreatic limb using a handsewn anastomosis using an inner layer of 3-0 Maxon® and outer layer of 3-0 Prolene® (Fig. 28.1). After completion of the posterior outer suture line, opposing enterotomies are made with an electrocautery to form an orifice of approximately 5 cm. It is important

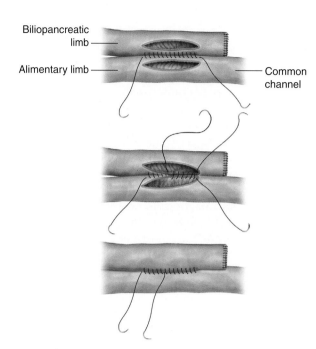

Figure 28.1 Technique for hand sewn enterostomy. Place knots for inner and outer layers at opposite end.

Biliopancreatic limb

Alimentary limb

Common channel

not to make the orifice too large as this can result in a sack that does not empty well and is prone to bacterial overgrowth. The inner suture line is placed and continued anteriorly so that there is only one knot, using a running lock stitch. This type of anastomosis is extremely stable. In approximately 1,000 patients, there has been only one patient who has had postoperative bleeding from this site, and there have been no leaks or obstructions. The mesenteric defect is closed with interrupted 2-0 silk sutures.

Creation of the Pouch

- First, make sure the alimentary limb will reach the pouch without tension. Then, the upper fundus and cardio-esophageal junction are mobilized by blunt dissection behind the upper part of the stomach. The peritoneum on the right side can then be incised to mobilize circumferentially. Care should be used not to enter the stomach by keeping the blunt dissection posteriorly.
- Bring an 18 French urinary catheter behind the stomach with the open end toward the right. Then thread the catheter onto the posterior anvil of a TA90B stapler and bring the anvil behind the stomach using the catheter as a guide (Fig. 28.2).
- Staple with three firings of the staple gun in such a way as to create a pouch of approximately 20 to 25 mL with the anterior lip of the pouch being slightly larger than the posterior side. With each firing, compression with a maximal amount of pressure that can be achieved with the hand should be maintained for at least 10 seconds. This is essential to prevent gastrogastric fistulas. Less than three firings should never be used. Be careful not to staple the nasogastric tube.
- Many surgeons create the pouch by dividing the stomach with a stapler, but this is not done with a TA90B stapler.

Creation of the Gastrointestinal Anastomosis

- The proximal end of the alimentary limb is brought through the transverse mesentery of the colon, making sure that there is no injury to the middle colic artery. It is then positioned in an antegastric fashion, placing it adjacent to the pouch. A side-to-side anastomosis is then made placing the sutures similarly to the enteroenteric anastomosis with several exceptions (Fig. 28.3). The outer running suture uses 3-0 PDS since a nonabsorbable suture sometimes erodes into the lumen and predisposes to ulcer formation. The orifice itself is made to be approximately 1.2 to 1.5 cm in diameter.

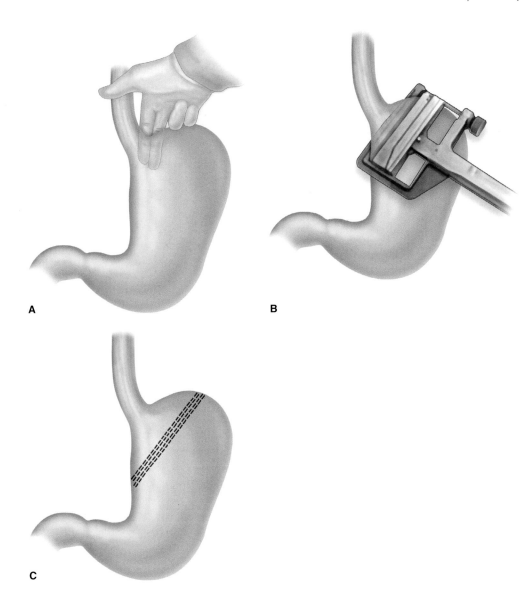

A

B

C

Figure 28.2 Creation of the gastric pouch. **(A)** The upper fundus and cardio-esophageal junction are mobilized by blunt dissection behind the upper part of the stomach. **(B)** Application of the TA90B stapler to create a pouch of approximately 20 to 25 m with the anterior lip of the pouch being slightly larger than the posterior side. **(C)** Staple with three firings of the staple gun. With each firing, compression with a maximal amount of pressure that can be achieved with the hand should be maintained for at least 10 seconds.

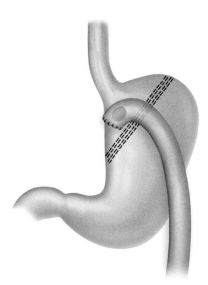

Figure 28.3 Creation of the gastroenterostomy. A side-to-side anastomosis is made. The outer running suture uses 3-0 PDS. The orifice itself is made to be approximately 1.2 to 1.5 cm in diameter. The anterior layers are placed over an 18 French nasogastric tube which is passed through the opening, thus avoiding an inadvertent incorporation of the posterior wall.

The anterior layers are placed over an 18 French nasogastric tube which is passed through the opening, thus avoiding an inadvertent incorporation of the posterior wall.

■ Once the anastomosis is completed, it is tested by occluding the alimentary limb with a vascular clamp and infusion of 8 to 10 L of oxygen/minute through the nasogastric tube while the anastomosis and staple lines are submerged in a topical antibiotic solution. After assurance that there are no leaks, the nasogastric tube is removed after application of suction.

■ The mesenteric defect in the transverse mesentery is closed with interrupted silk sutures. Petersen's defect is then closed if it can be done without tension which is often not the case. We have not seen obstructions from Petersen's hernias in our series of patients.

Sleeve Gastrectomy

Sleeve gastrectomy is gaining increased popularity because it can achieve weight loss comparable to a gastric bypass but is not malabsorptive. Improvement in diabetes is regularly achieved, and there is also a significant reduction in hunger. In some series, late benefit has lessened because of dilatation of the stomach. To prevent this, we have recently used a band of human dermis around the upper part of the stomach to decrease overeating and prevent dilatation of the gastric tube.

■ The first maneuver is to divide all of the vessels along the greater curvature down to the pylorus using a LigaSure®.

■ A 46 to 50 French bougie (sizer) is then passed down to the pylorus.

■ A stapling device used to remove the body and fundus of the stomach beginning approximately 5 to 6 cm from the pylorus and extending up to the angle of His.

■ The posterior blood vessels to the fundus are left intact until the staple line is completed to insure complete stapling of the stomach. Care is taken to provide adequate compression with stapling which is done with maximal pressure for at least 10 seconds with each firing. After removal of the specimen, the entire staple line is oversewn with a running 3-0 PDS suture.

■ The line of closure is then tested for leaks by occluding the pylorus and infusing oxygen through a nasogastric tube to create relatively high pressure within the gastric lumen while the suture line is placed under solution of topical antibiotic (gentamicin). The nasogastric tube is then removed. Placement of a drain is unnecessary.

■ Recent experience achieved good success with additional banding of the sleeve gastrectomy. A piece of preserved human dermis (Alloderm®) measuring 2.0 × 6 cm is placed around the muscular tube with the upper edge approximately 5–6 cm from the esophagogastric junction using a 38F bougie as a sizer (Fig. 28.4). This creates a pouch and prevents dilatation of the distal stomach. However, there is no long-term follow-up past two years. Since there is no malabsorption and weight loss is similar to gastric bypass, this might be a preferred procedure, especially for patients with organ transplant.

Duodenal Switch

The duodenal switch operation first employs a sleeve gastrectomy and then adds an intestinal diversion (Fig. 28.5). This has been done primarily for extremely obese patients, but the second phase is now reserved for patients who have had insufficient weight loss after the sleeve gastrectomy.

Biliopancreatic Diversion

This procedure has not been done as a primary procedure in our patients, but is shown diagrammatically in Figure 28.6. Conversion to a modified biliopancreatic diversion is sometimes used for failed primary procedures.

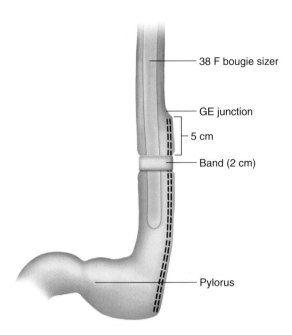

Figure 28.4 Banded sleeve gastrectomy. A piece of preserved human dermis (Alloderm®) measuring 2.0 × 6 cm is placed around the muscular tube with the upper edge approximately 5–6 cm from the esophagogastric junction using a 38F bougie as a sizer.

Revisional Surgery for Failed Bariatric Procedures

The techniques for surgical treatment of obesity have evolved enormously during the past several decades. Virtually all procedures have had failures.

Horizontal Gastroplasty

This operation was used fairly frequently during the early development of bariatric surgery. It consisted of application of a staple line across the entire stomach after removal of 1 to 2 staples or simply not stapling to the edge of the stomach so that a small gastrogastric orifice was present. Invariably, in all of these patients, the orifice became progressively larger with regain of weight. Revisional surgery consists of conversion to gastric bypass with removal of the affected portion of the stomach.

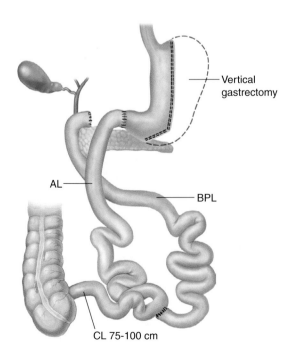

Figure 28.5 Duodenal switch. A sleeve gastrectomy with an intestinal diversion.

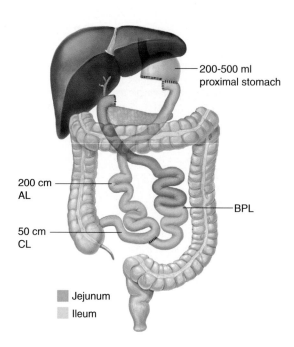

Figure 28.6 Biliopancreatic diversion.

200-500 ml
proximal stomach

200 cm
AL

BPL

50 cm
CL

Jejunum

Ileum

Vertical Banded Gastroplasty

Failure of this initially effective procedure occurred primarily because of stenosis at the outlet, development of a gastrogastric fistula in the vertical staple line or widening of the outlet. There can also be erosion or other problems with the band. It is very important to determine which of these have occurred, especially the gastrogastric fistula.

Revisional surgery usually involves resection of the band and closure of any fistulas by dividing the stomach, often with removal of the upper part of the fundus. Conversion to RYGBP is probably the best option for revision, making a vertical gastric pouch (Fig. 28.7). All staple lines should be oversewn.

Gastric Bypass

Failure of gastric bypass characteristically involves dilatation of the pouch and/or its stoma. Corrective surgery may involve revision of the pouch and/or the anastomosis, which can be technically quite difficult, or conversion to a modified biliopancreatic diversion which is much easier. This is done by disconnecting the enteroenteric anastomosis with reanastomosis of distal part of the alimentary limb to the ileum, approximately 75 to 100 cm from the ileocecal valve, depending somewhat on the length of the alimentary limb (Fig. 28.8).

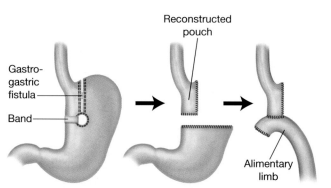

Reconstructed
pouch

Gastro-
gastric
fistula

Band

Alimentary
limb

Figure 28.7 Conversion of vertical banded gastroplasty to gastric bypass.

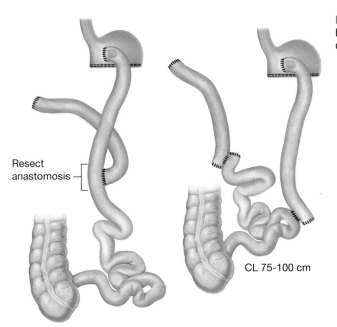

Figure 28.8 Conversion of gastric bypass to modified biliopancreatic diversion.

Resect anastomosis

CL 75-100 cm

Biliopancreatic Diversion

Malabsorption can be excessively severe in a small minority of patients, and this can be correctly by simply increasing the length of the alimentary limb at the site of the distal anastomosis—sort of the reverse of shortening the alimentary limb as just described.

Lap Band

Increasing numbers of patients have had failure of adjustable band placement. These can be treated by removal of the band and conversion to gastric bypass or sleeve gastrectomy.

Sleeve Gastrectomy

The primary cause for failure is insufficient weight loss or weight regain because of dilatation of the sleeve. The sleeve gastrectomy was used initially as a preliminary procedure before the duodenal switch operation, so the revisional procedure may be to complete the duodenal switch. However, some surgeons recommend doing a "resleeve" operation by excising the dilated outer curvature or placing an adjustable band.

Jejunoileal Bypass

Intestinal bypass operations have not been done for several decades, but there are still occasional patients that present because of persistent malnutrition. The surgical treatment is to restore some of the continuity of the excluded intestine, but this can present problems because on occasion the excluded intestine has atrophied to such a degree that there is no or a limited functional lumen. Before placing the excluded intestine into the enteric flow, one must be absolutely certain that a lumen persists. This can be done by infusion of saline down the bowel or by passage of a small catheter. Once the patent but atrophied intestine is placed back in circulation, it does rapidly grow and become functional. Care should be made to make the lumen of the anastomosis wide enough to accommodate the growth of the excluded intestine. A sleeve gastrectomy can be performed in patients with weight regain.

Postoperative Management

Appropriate postoperative management can result in prevention of most postoperative complications.

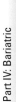

- Thromboembolic problems are a major risk after bariatric surgery. Heparin, 6,000 to 8,000 units, depending on weight, should be given every 8 hours, beginning preoperatively. Pneumatic leg compression devices should be used routinely during the operation and whenever the patient is not ambulating. For patients with a prior thromboembolic complication, warfarin should be started promptly. For most patients, 10 mg is given on the first day, 5 mg given postop day 2, and 2 mg on postop day 3. INR must be checked on a daily basis until it is stabilized. Target for INR should be 2 to 2.5. In general, there is a decrease in the dosage of warfarin that was administered preoperatively in postoperative patients after gastric bypass. Over-anticoagulation is not infrequent and will be the rule with patients who are placed on the same dosage of Coumadin as they were on preoperatively. Obviously, over-coagulation is a significant risk but can be avoided by aggressive monitoring.
- Positive pressure ventilation with BiPAP is used for patients >350 pounds. In patients with sleep apnea, CPAP or BiPAP is used routinely. Nasal O_2 is given to all patients to maintain O_2 sat >92. Incentive spirometers are used in all patients.
- Ambulation is encouraged the day of operation and is mandatory by the next morning. The more the patient walks, the quicker will be the recovery.
- Clear liquids, 30 mL/hr, are offered by mouth the day of operation and a pureed diet is offered the first postoperative day with solid food being given after four weeks.
- Pain control can be achieved by standard approaches.
- Urinary catheter should be removed on the first postoperative day unless the patient is unable to ambulate.
- Ulcer prophylaxis should be given using a proton pump inhibitor for at least 6 months.
- If the patient has been on beta blockers, these should be continued during the time of operation and afterward.
- The large majority of patients can be discharged after 48 hours. Removal of the Hemovac is done just before discharge. Patients who live more than a one-hour drive from the hospital, and/or have additional medical problems that require continued hospitalization (such as renal failure requiring dialysis), will be kept for a longer period of time.

Complications

Numerous complications can occur in both the early and late postoperative periods.

- Atelectasis is one of the more common early complications. The primary prevention for this is early ambulation and the use of an incentive spirometer.
- Pneumonia is much less common but sometimes cannot be easily distinguished from atelectasis. Antibiotic therapy is indicated if pneumonia is likely.
- Thromboembolism can be fatal. If a pulmonary embolism is suspected, a CT scan or pulmonary angiogram should be done so that appropriate therapy can be instituted promptly. A duplex scan of the lower extremities is sometimes helpful. Placement of a vena caval filter is infrequently indicated.
- Bleeding occurs in 1% to 4% of patients but is less common after open procedures. This can be from anastomotic sites, sites of surgical dissection or from ulcers. A thorough workup should include endoscopy, coagulation profiles and sometimes tagged red cell studies or angiography. On rare occasions, bleeding is associated with lesions in the excluded stomach so if no other cause is found, a transgastric endoscopy can be done, either open or laparoscopically. Death from bleeding is rare in the absence of a severe coagulopathy.
- A leak can occur from any of the procedures where the GI tract is opened, but they are less common with open procedures when all staple lines are oversewn. In general, detection measures using drain placement or upper GI contrast studies are not done routinely with open procedures. Most leaks from the stomach can be treated without reoperation.
- Wound infection is reported in 3% to 25% of patients. In general, the incidence of abdominal wound infection is approximately five times higher in obese patients than

in nonobese patients. With the use of appropriate means to prevent wound infection as described earlier, (use of an incise drape, proper preparation of the skin, systemic antibiotics just before the incision in doses which are appropriate for morbidly obese patients with redosing as necessary, use of monofilament rather than multifilament sutures, running sutures rather than interrupted sutures, and the administration of antibiotics into the wound for a short period of time), the incidence of infection can be reduced to <0.5%.

■ Gastrointestinal disturbances including cramping, bloating, diarrhea and abdominal pain are not infrequent and can be caused by bacterial overgrowth. This usually responds to treatment with probiotics (such as VSL#3) with or without prebiotics.

■ Hypoglycemia can also occur, often related to an increased production of GLP-1. Treatment usually responds to Acarbose®.

■ Nutritional deficiencies can occur with any bariatric procedure, especially related to protein, vitamin D, thiamine, B12, calcium, and iron as well as others. Careful monitoring is mandatory.

■ The incidence of kidney stones is increased and can be reduced by the administration of calcium citrate with vitamin D.

■ Intestinal obstruction can occur at any time from a variety of causes. Early obstructions often involve herniation and late obstructions often involve adhesions. Treatment should be straightforward but is beyond the scope of this communication.

■ Ulcer formation is not uncommon and prevention requires the use of protein pump inhibitors at least for several months. Ulcers at the anastomosis can involve exposure of suture material which, if present upon endoscopy, should be removed endoscopically. Nonsteroidal anti-inflammatory drugs should be avoided.

■ Stenosis of the gastrojejunal anastomosis can cause outlet obstruction with repeated vomiting. This is usually treated easily with endoscopic balloon dilatation.

RESULTS

Risks of the procedure as well as the benefits are related at least in part to the procedure being done. Of the common procedures, adjustable gastric banding is associated with a slightly improved survival, and reduced complication compared to procedures which open the GI tract, but long-term weight loss and resolution of co-morbidities such as diabetes are not nearly as good as with the more invasive procedures. Gastric bypass has been the most frequent operation, but sleeve gastrectomy is gaining in popularity and will probably replace gastric bypass as the most desirable operation. Overall mortality with the open procedures is <0.5%. The benefits include the improvement of almost all co-morbidities, a marked reduction in the health expenditure and a significant improvement in overall survival.

CONCLUSIONS

Open bariatric procedures can provide excellent results in experienced hands with equal or better outcomes than laparoscopic procedures in most situations.

Every surgeon doing bariatric procedures should be fully capable of performing these open techniques.

Recommended References and Readings

Alexander JW, Martin Hawver LR, Goodman HR. Banded sleeve gastrectomy—Initial experience. *Obes Surg*. 2009;19:1591–1596.

Christou NV, Sampalis JS, Liberman M, et al. Surgery decreases long-term mortality, morbidity, and health care use in morbidly obese patients. *Ann Surg*. 2004;240:416–424.

Deitel M. A synopsis of the development of bariatric operations. *Obes Surg*. 2007;17:707–710.

Gumbs AA, Pomp A, Gagner M. Revisional bariatric surgery for inadequate weight loss. *Obes Surg*. 2007;17:1137–1145.

Jones KB Jr, Afram JD, Benotti PN, et al. Open versus laparoscopic Roux-en-Y gastric bypass: A comparative study of over 25,000 open cases and the major laparoscopic bariatric reported cases. *Obes Surg*. 2006;16:721–727.

Larrad-Jiménez Á, Díaz-Guerra CS-C, de Cuadros Borrajo P, et al. Short-, mid- and long-term results of Larrad biliopancreatic diversion. *Obes Surg*. 2007;17:202–210.

Maggard MA, Shugaman LR, Suttorp M, et al. Meta-analysis: Surgical treatment of obesity. *Ann Intern Med.* 2005;142:547–559.

Obeid F, Falvo A, Dabideen H, et al. Open Roux-en-Y gastric bypass in 925 patients without mortality. *Am J Surg.* 2005;189: 352–356.

Puzziferri N, Austrheim-Smith IT, Wolfe BM, et al. Three-year follow-up of a prospective randomized trial comparing laparoscopic versus open gastric bypass. *Ann Surg.* 2006;243:181–188.

Sarr MG. Open Roux-en-Y gastric bypass: Indications and technique. *J Gastrointest Surg.* 2004;8:390–392.

Slotman GJ. Non-transectional open gastric bypass as the definitive bariatric procedure for 61 patients with BMI of 70 and higher. *Obes Surg.* 2010;20:7–12.

Tian HL, Tian JH, Yang KH, et al. The effects of laparoscopic vs. open gastric bypass for morbid obesity: a systematic review and meta-analysis of randomized controlled trials. *Obes Rev.* 2010; June 9 (Epub ahead of print).

Yao DC, Stellato TA, Schuster MM, et al. Gastrogastric fistula following Roux-en-Y bypass is attributed to both surgical technique and experience. *Am J Surg.* 2010;199:382–385.

29 Laparoscopic Roux-en-Y Gastric Bypass

Alfons Pomp and Mustafa Hussain

 ## INDICATIONS/CONTRAINDICATIONS

Obesity and obesity-related comorbidities, such as diabetes and heart disease, constitute a significant and increasing health problem. Currently, nearly two-thirds of the US population is overweight with one-third being classified as obese (BMI > 30 kg/m^2). Unfortunately, public health campaigns, lifestyle modifications, and medical therapy have little effect on long-term weight loss. Weight loss induced by surgical therapy, however, appears to be both significant in magnitude as well as sustainable over a long period of time. Weight loss procedures are generally classified into restrictive or malabsorbtive. Mason and Ito are credited for employing the Roux-en-Y gastric bypass (combining restriction and malabsorption) for the treatment of morbid obesity. In 1996, Wittgrove reported on the first totally laparoscopic gastric bypass, which has generally been shown to have lower rates of wound and pulmonary complications than the open procedure. Laparoscopic Roux-en-Y gastric bypass is currently the most commonly performed bariatric procedure in the United States.

In 1991, the National Institutes of Health Consensus of Conference on Obesity stated that bariatric surgery is an effective and safe method of achieving sustained weight loss in morbidly obese individuals and that the benefit that results from weight loss after surgery outweighed the risk of the surgical procedures. The procedures are indicated for those individuals who are morbidly obese (BMI > 40 kg/m^2) or with a BMI > 35 kg/m^2 and a comorbidity that would resolve if the patient had significant weight loss, such as diabetes or obstructive sleep apnea. Recently, there has been increased interest in citing type 2 diabetes as a primary indication for those patients with BMI < 35 kg/m^2. This is based on the observation of frequent diabetes resolution after gastric bypass in the morbidly obese and experimental evidence that there may be a weight-loss-independent function of gastric bypass that impacts blood glucose levels. Currently, gastric bypass is being performed in lower BMI patients only under IRB-approved protocols.

The NIH consensus also stated individuals who undergo surgery should be those who are not likely to lose weight by other means (e.g., failed prior nonsurgical techniques) and those who would comply with long-term follow-up. Many insurance companies require a medically supervised weight loss program of varying lengths of time before approving bariatric surgery. While commonplace, there is limited evidence that this appropriately selects patients for surgery and only prolongs the patient's wait time. Patients should, however, meet with a nutritionist prior to surgery in order to optimize healthy eating habits and diet choices, as well as have reasonable expectation of diet postoperatively. Any vitamin or mineral deficiencies should be diagnosed preoperatively and optimized prior to surgery.

The patients should have reasonable expectations from the surgical procedure and desire significant weight loss. Generally, preoperative psychiatric evaluation is performed to ensure that patients are prepared for what can be a life-altering event and able to comply with the life-long follow-up that is necessary for best results. Patients with untreated or undiagnosed psychiatric disorders generally should not undergo bariatric surgery. In addition, the patients should be of appropriate surgical risk from a cardiopulmonary standpoint and have an abdomen that is amenable to the surgical procedure.

These guidelines generally apply to all bariatric procedures. Laparoscopic gastric bypass is appropriate for those who meet these criteria. Currently, no set criteria define which procedure is more preferable over another. However, operations that can be performed in a shorter period of time such as sleeve gastrectomy or adjustable gastric banding may be more appropriate in cases where minimizing time under anesthesia is a consideration. In diabetics, bypass maybe preferred, as there appears to be a greater frequency of resolution after this procedure. On the other hand, bypass may be less effective in super morbidly obese patients and biliopancreatic diversion might be more appropriate. Commonly, the choice of bariatric procedure is generally left to the patient.

Indications

- BMI > 40 kg/m^2
- BMI > 35 kg/m^2 with a comorbidity (e.g., diabetes, hypertension, obstructive sleep apnea.)
- Failed attempts at nonsurgical weight loss

Contraindications

- BMI < 35 kg/m^2 (unless under IRB-approved protocol)
- Inability to comply with postoperative follow-up
- High anesthetic risk
- Hostile abdomen: Extensive foregut surgery or extensive small-bowel adhesions

PREOPERATIVE PLANNING

A thorough history and physical examination should be obtained. History should include pertinent information regarding dietary habits and diet history. There should be documentation of attempts at nonsurgical means of weight loss. Generally, counseling by a registered dietician is warranted to establish this. Any preoperative vitamin or mineral deficiencies (e.g., vitamin D, iron) should be treated. Comorbidities should be elucidated and risk stratification and optimization should be undertaken before general anesthesia. This may include stress echocardiograms, pulmonary function tests, and sleep studies. Many patients present for operation with previously undiagnosed diabetes or sleep apnea. These and other newly diagnosed conditions should be optimized prior to surgery. Patients are assessed for hypercoagulable states and history of venous thromboembolism (VTE). Some patients, particularly super-super morbidly obese patients, may require a preoperative inferior vena cava (IVC) filter. Upper endoscopy should be performed to evaluate the stomach for pathology prior to bypass. If *Helicobacter pylori* is present, it should be treated prior to surgery to reduce the risk of postoperative ulcers and stricture. Notation of a hiatus hernia should be made; an upper GI series may be helpful for this. If significant hernia is present, it should be repaired at the time of surgery in order to prevent the creation of a large gastric pouch. Patients should not be active smokers, as this not only leads to postoperative pulmonary complications but also increases the risk of later ulcer formation. Psychiatric evaluation should also be performed both to diagnose and optimize any pre-existing pathology and to assess patient's ability to cope and comply with postsurgical life and follow-up.

Pertinent points in the physical examination include abdominal fat distribution. Patient's who are "apple" shape or android tend to be more challenging to operate on than "pear" shape or gynecoid patients. Notation of prior abdominal surgery, scars, and hernias should be made. Skin folds should be examined for extensive fungal infection or cellulitis. Lower extremity edema, particularly asymmetric edema, may portend an underlying deep venous thrombosis (DVT), and this should be evaluated. The ability to ambulate and "clear a chair" should be assessed. Immobile patients are at significantly higher risk of postoperative complications.

Some surgeons require their patients to undergo a strict low-calorie, low-carbohydrate diet (e.g., Optifast) in the weeks leading up to surgery. The thinking here is not absolute weight loss per se, but the hopes it will reduce the size of the liver and amount of visceral fat. This makes access to the hiatus easier and safer and allows for easier manipulation of the mesentery. This may be particularly useful in higher BMI patients. Some surgeons also use this as a "test" to determine whether the patients have the willpower to comply with postoperative dietary restrictions. Generally, we do not feel that this is necessary or appropriate. Certainly patients should not be actively gaining weight in the weeks leading up to surgery, and such behavior should be discouraged.

Immediately prior to surgery all patients should receive appropriate antibiotic prophylaxis to limit wound infection. This is particularly the case when using transoral anvil and EEA stapling device. In addition, patients should have appropriate VTE prophylaxis. There have not been adequate studies to determine the best means of VTE prophylaxis in this patient population and it must be weighed against the risk of postoperative bleeding. There is unlikely to be such a study given the large number of patients required to measure differences. Generally, all patients should walk to the operating room if possible and ambulate hours after surgery. All patients should wear pneumatic compression devices prior, during, and after surgery while in bed. It is also generally recommend that some chemoprophylaxis be utilized. We administer 5,000 units of subcutaneous heparin prior to surgery and continue it every 12 or 8 hours. Low-molecular weight heparin administered in low doses may also be appropriate.

Preoperative Assessment

- Nutritional assessment: Diet history, expectations after surgery, and optimization of nutritional deficiencies
- Medical evaluation and optimization: Treat uncontrolled blood sugars, cardiac evaluation, assess for risk of VTE, diagnose and treat sleep apnea, and assess ambulatory status
- Endoscopy: Evaluation of pre-existing pathology and treatment of *H. pylori*
- Psychiatric: Diagnose and treat underlying psychiatric conditions if present. Assess for patient compliance and identify maladaptive behaviors
- Abdominal assessment: Predict the likelihood of successfully completing a laparoscopic gastric bypass
- Preoperative diet: Reduce liver size and intra-abdominal fat
- Preoperative antibiotics and VTE prophylaxis as appropriate

 ## SURGICAL TECHNIQUE

- **Pertinent Anatomy:** Surgeons undertaking laparoscopic gastric bypass should be well versed in foregut anatomy. Identification of the gastroesophageal junction and the anatomy of the angle of His is necessary to safely create the gastric pouch. The surgeon should be comfortable around the hiatus of the diaphragm and able to repair a hiatus hernia. The spleen lies at the superior extent of the dissection when creating the gastric pouch and may be injured during the process. The pancreas

Part IV: Bariatric

and splenic vessels run in the retroperitoneum behind the stomach. Injury here can result in bleeding or postoperative pancreatitis or fistula. Preservation of the left gastric artery and the lesser curve vasculature ensures blood supply to the gastric pouch. Identification of the ligament of Treitz is crucial in appropriately making the Roux-en-Y jejunal limbs. Generally, it can be located by its fixed attachment to the transverse colon mesentery. Often, the inferior mesenteric vein is seen just to the patient's left of the fourth portion of the duodenum as it exits the transverse colon mesentery. Appropriately orienting the proximal and distal ends of the bowel is crucial when reconnecting bowel segments and creating the gastrojejunostomy.

- **Patient positioning and equipment:** The operating room table should have the capability to withstand 800 lbs and should have split leg capabilities with right angle foot board attachments and have the ability to undergo steep reverse Trendelenburg. We prefer the Alphastar table (Maquet, Rastatt, Germany). Intubating the morbidly obese patient can be a challenge for the untrained anesthesiologist and having a dedicated bariatric team is ideal. Placing a "bump" or a "wedge" under the patient's upper back can facilitate intubation and pull away flesh from the upper chest that can hinder manipulation of the patient's airway. Once intubated, the patient should have all pressure points protected with foam padding. The arms should be out to the sides, just shy of 90 degrees. Care must be taken to assure that the arms are not hyperextended in both the cephalo-caudal and the anterior-posterior direction.

  - **French Position:** The patient is in split leg with all pressure points protected and each leg secured to boards with circumferential bandages or tape. The operating surgeon is between the legs. The first assistant stands to the patient's right and is a dedicated camera driver and liver retractor. A second assistant is on the left and assists with retraction. The scrub technician stands on the patient's left. A single high-definition screen should be positioned above the patient's head at eye level. Alternatively, the surgeon can stand on the patient's right with the camera driver between the legs.

  - **American Position:** The patient is supine with legs together. Right angle foot supports are still necessary for steep reverse Trendelenburg. The surgeon stands to the patient's right and the first assistant on the left. The scrub technician stands on either the left or the right. Two high-definition screens are required over each of the patient's shoulders. A second assistant is generally not required.

- **Trocar placement:** Peritoneal access can be quite challenging in the obese patient. Several techniques have been described. We feel the safest method is to cut-down at the umbilicus. This site can serve as an optical port and all subsequent ports are placed under direct vision. Other techniques include the blind insertion of a Veress needle to establish pneumoperitoneum with blind placement of the first trocar and optical non-bladed trocar placement. If these techniques are used, it is generally recommended that they be placed in the left upper quadrant at the midclavicular line close to the costal margin. Our preferred trocar scheme is to have a 10-mm optical trocar in the umbilicus and a 10-mm optical trocar in the epigastrium which enters at the base of the falciform. A 12-mm trocar in the subxiphoid position is used for dissecting and stapling the gastric pouch and creation of the jejunojejunostomy. A second 12-mm trocar in the left upper quadrant is used for stapling the gastric pouch and is later expanded to introduce the EEA stapler to create the gastrojejunostomy. A 5-mm trocar in the left anterior axillary line is used by the second assistant and a 10-mm trocar in the right upper quadrant is used for a fan liver retractor and serves as an optical port during the creation of jejunojejunostomy. A fixed Nathanson or Genzyme liver retractor can be inserted through a separate 5-mm incision as an alternative.

  - Alternative techniques have been described and are valid and can be tailored to the surgeon's preference and patient habitus. We have found this to be the most reproducible across a wide range of patient sizes and the most ergonomic. The abdomen should be insufflated to 15 mm Hg. At times 20 mm Hg may be necessary to enhance visualization.

Two insufflators are useful in maintaining pneumoperitoneum, especially if suction is used. The surgeon and anesthesia team should be aware of hemodynamic and respiratory alterations during insufflations.

- **Abdominal survey:** Assess the abdomen for feasibility of gastric bypass. Any unexpected anatomy or adhesions should be evaluated. Most important to successful completion of gastric bypass is the ability to expose the diaphragm and angle of His. If the left lobe of the liver is too large to retract or fatty and friable, creation of the gastric pouch maybe too difficult or dangerous. In this case, the surgeon may decide to abort the case and subject the patient to a low-calorie diet, convert the procedure to sleeve gastrectomy or a two-staged gastric bypass.

- **Creation of the gastric pouch:** We prefer to start with the creation of the gastric pouch and creation of the gastrojejunostomy, as this is the most challenging part of the case. Others feel that creation of the Roux limb first is more appropriate.

- **Dissection of the angle of His:** The patient should be in maximal reverse Trendelenburg. The first assistant retracts the liver exposing the gastroesophageal (GE) junction, gastric fundus, and diaphragm. The second assistant retracts the fundus of the stomach caudally and to the patient's left with an atraumatic grasper. The surgeon retracts the fat pad overlying the GE junction to the patient's right with his or her left hand via the subxiphoid trocar. With a hook electrocautery or ultrasonic dissector, in the right hand via the left upper quadrant port, the angle of His is dissected free of the GE junction and off the left crus. Bulging of retroperitoneal fat through this space suggests adequate dissection. Care should be taken to avoid injury to the spleen. In case this dissection is difficult due to the size of the liver or patient habitus, it can be completed from behind the stomach after the first couple of staple firings. Freeing the angle of His marks the target of the staple line in creating the gastric pouch (Fig. 29.1).

- **Perigastric dissection:** In order to perform the first staple firing, the gastric wall along the lesser curvature should be freed from the fat containing its blood supply. A spot is chosen about 5 cm from the GE junction, which is generally between the second and third vessel on the lesser curvature. Some surgeons prefer longer pouches in order to decrease tension off the gastro-jejunal (G-J) anastomosis. The neurovascular fat bundle is freed with combination of blunt and sharp dissection using blunt graspers alternating with judicious use of the ultrasonic shears to seal individual vessels,

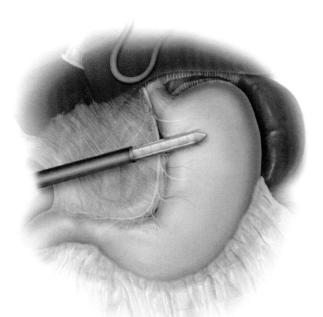

Figure 29.1 Angle of His has been dissected. Perigastric window approximately 5 cm below GE junction created for firing of first stapler.

taking care not to injure the gastric wall. The majority of the dissection is done with the surgeon's left hand via the subxiphoid trocar. The surgeon's right hand acts as a place holder and gently pushes the gastric wall away from the fat. The second assistant should retract the stomach at this point anteriorly to create adequate tension for dissection. Bleeding can make this dissection difficult and should be controlled quickly if occurs. Care must be made to not track superiorly or inferiorly in the perigastric fat which can devascularize a larger portion of the stomach than necessary (Fig. 29.1).

■ **Stapling the pouch:** Before beginning, it is important to confirm that the anesthesiologist has removed all tubes from the esophagus. The lesser sac is entered via the perigastric dissection. The surgeon's right hand holds the place open while a 45 mm × 3.5 mm stapler is inserted via the subxiphoid trocar. It is important that this first staple line is perpendicular to the lesser curvature. The subsequent staple firings are performed from the left upper quadrant 12-mm trocar aiming toward the left crus with the surgeon's left hand retracting the forming pouch to the patient's right. After the second staple firing, it may be necessary to free up posterior adhesions to the pancreas and dissect posterior gastric vessels. This can be done with the ultrasonic scalpel. The second assistant can grasp the posterior fundus and retract it to the patient's left. This results in a smaller pouch size. Generally, the pouch is created with one 45 mm × 3.5 mm and two to three 60 mm × 3.5 mm staplers. We prefer using stapling line buttressing material (Seamguard, Gore, Flagstaff AZ) for all except the first two staple lines in order to reduce bleeding. The resultant pouch is approximately 30 mL in volume. Once the pouch is created, the staple lines should be checked for completeness and hemostasis. The staple lines that do not have buttressing material on the remnant stomach can be over sewn to prevent bleeding from the excluded stomach (Figs. 29.1 and 29.2).

■ **Transoral Anvil:** A 25-mm EEA anvil can be sutured to an orogastric tube or the DST series EEA OrVil (CovidienCovidien, Mansfield, MA) can be passed through the mouth into the gastric pouch. The anesthesiologist should be instructed that the tube end should enter the mouth and pass with ease. The anvil should be guided into the mouth with the convex end up toward the hard palate. It does get hung up on the hard palate and behind the arytenoids. A jaw thrust can facilitate passage

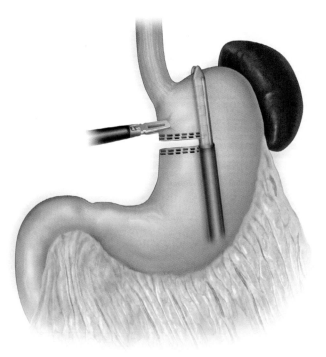

Figure 29.2 Stapling completed toward angle of His dissection.

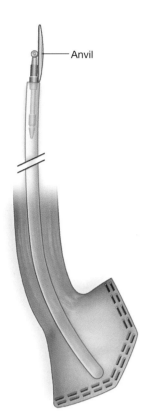

Figure 29.3 Transoral passage of anvil into gastric pouch.

Anvil

into the esophagus. The tip of the tube should be visible against the staple line. It can be guided into place by the surgeon's graspers. Ideally it should be on the patient's left side of the first staple line or the junction of the first and second staple line. A small gastrotomy is created with the ultrasonic shears just big enough to allow passage of the tube. The tube is gently withdrawn from the gastric pouch while the anesthesiologist assists in guiding the anvil into the mouth. No resistance should be felt while traction is applied to the tube. If resistance is encountered, it is generally in the places described above. If the anvil gets caught in the esophagus, an endoscope should be passed to evaluate the site of obstruction or to help push the anvil into position. The tube is withdrawn out of the body. It is not sterile at this time and should be manipulated with clamps or towels. Traction should be stopped when the white cuff of the anvil is seen. The sutures to the tube are cut and the tube is passed off the field. The anvil should fit snuggly in the gastrotomy. If it is gaping open, then a purse string suture around the device should be applied (Figs. 29.3 and 29.4).

■ **Alternative technique:** The anvil of an EEA can be placed into the stomach via a separate gastrotomy prior to complete transection of the gastric pouch from the remnant stomach. The gastrotomy is stapled closed and the anvil is pulled through a small hole in the pouch.

■ **Creation of Roux limb:** The camera is placed in the umbilical port and the patient is placed in a level position. The end of the omentum is identified and grasped by the surgeon's left hand and the second assistant. The omentum is then split in a line headed toward the left phrenic vessels (Fig. 29.5). Care must be taken to make note of the location of the transverse colon to avoid injury. Once two leaves of omentum are created, they can be tucked away on each side. The transverse colon is rolled cephalad and the ligament of Treitz is identified. The first assistant can aid in retracting the colon with the liver retractor. The surgeon runs the bowel for 75 to 100 cm from the ligament. The bowel can be tucked away in the left upper quadrant. The second assistant grasps the proximal end of the bowel and the surgeon's left hand is

Part IV: Bariatric

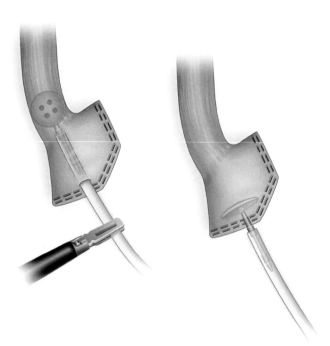

Figure 29.4 Transoral passage of anvil into gastric pouch.

on the distal end (the future site of gastrojejunostomy). The bowel is held tightly while a blunt dissector such as a 10-mm right angle is used to dissect a space between the bowel and mesentery. A 45 mm × 2.5 mm stapler with buttress material is used to transect the bowel. It is important to maintain orientation of which are the proximal and distal ends of the bowel (Fig. 29.6).

■ **Gastrojejunostomy with the EEA:** The staple line on the distal end (being held by the surgeon's left hand, on the patient's right) is opened using ultrasonic shears. Once open, the distal end is distinct from the proximal end, and the ends of the

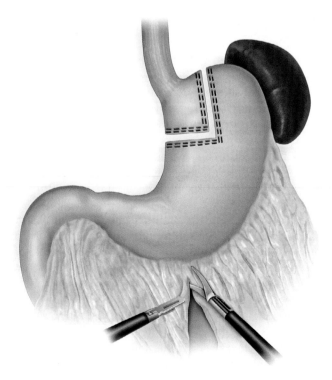

Figure 29.5 Division of greater omentum.

Figure 29.6 Creation of Roux limb.

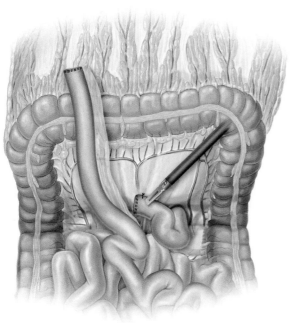

bowel can be let go. The left upper quadrant 12-mm port is enlarged to about
2.5 cm and the subcutaneous and muscle layers are spread using a large Kelly
clamp. The hole should allow passage of two fingers which can further spread the
opening. The EEA stapler should be wrapped in a disposable camera bag secured
to the shaft with a Steri-strip. This allows for subsequent removal of the stapler
without contaminating the abdominal wound. The stapler is placed through the
abdominal wall. This can be challenging, and it is helpful to use the curve of the
instrument. Once inside the abdomen, the surgeon grasps the open end of
the bowel at the 10 o'clock position while the second assistant holds open the
staple line. They work together to guide the stapler into the bowel. It is important
to allow the bowel to accommodate the stapler so it is does not tear. Here again,
the curve of the stapler can be used to facilitate this process. The stapler is placed
curve down, and once in the bowel, it can be flipped upward to keep the bowel
on the stapler and the graspers can be taken off. The patient is returned to the
reverse Trendelenburg position and the Roux limb is brought up to the gastric
pouch containing the anvil. The spike of the EEA is brought out to reveal the
orange stripe. The first assistant's liver retractor can help hold the bowel tightly
over the stapler. The liver is retracted to reveal the anvil and pouch. The anvil is
grasped with a 10-mm right angle clamp with the surgeon's left hand from the
subxiphoid position while the right hand drives the EEA and Roux limb toward
the anvil anterior to the transverse colon and remnant stomach (antecolic, antegastric). As the anvil and stapler are married, ensure that there is no kinking or fold-
ing of the bowel that can serve as an obstruction. Confirm there is no fat or remnant
stomach that is being caught in the stapler. The "green" line appearing on the
stapler signifies a complete union of the stapler. It should be fired, with an audible
"click" heard. The stapler is opened and removed from the small bowel. A gentle
rotation can aid in this. The stapler should be withdrawn from the body by undo-
ing the Steri-strip on the shaft and pulling the bag over the device and then out of
the body. The 12-mm trocar can be replaced with the addition of towel clamps to
maintain pneumoperitoneum. The corners of the anastomosis can be reinforced
with 2-0 Vicryl sutures. The anastomosis is inspected from inside the small bowel
for completion and bleeding. Bleeding sites should be sutured from the outside of
the anastomosis. Once satisfactory, the open end of the bowel is stapled closed

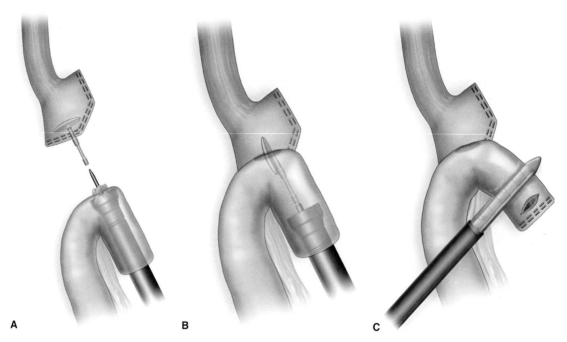

A   B   C

Figure 29.7 (A–C) Creation of gastrojejunostomy with EEA circular stapler.

with a 60 mm × 2.5 mm load with buttressing material. When doing this, it is critical to make sure the mesenteric end of the bowel is within the staple line. The end of the bowel should be removed from the body. The anastomosis can be tested by passage of an orogastric tube and instillation of methylene blue or with an endoscope and insufflations of air. If leak is encountered, sutures can be used to oversew the area in question (Figs. 29.7–29.9).

- **Jejunojejunostomy:** With the camera in the umbilical port, the surgeon runs the Roux limb from the anastomosis for 150 cm. The cut end of the biliopancreatic limb is identified and approximated to the site of anastomosis. Some surgeons suture the two together, but we find this unnecessary. An enterotomy is made on each side with the ultrasonic shears on the antimesenteric surface. The surgeon now moves to the patient's right side and the camera is placed in the right upper quadrant 10-mm trocar site. A 60 mm × 2.5 mm stapler is introduced via the 12-mm subxiphoid incision, and the surgeon manipulates the bowel on either end of the stapler. Once on the stapler, the bowel and the stapler are raised anteriorly to allow the mesenteries to align. The stapler is fired and withdrawn from the body. The staple line is examined for bleeding. The enterotomy is closed with two layers of permanent suture in a running fashion. Alternatively, the enterotomy can be stapled closed. It is important to

Figure 29.8 Creation of jejunojejunostomy.

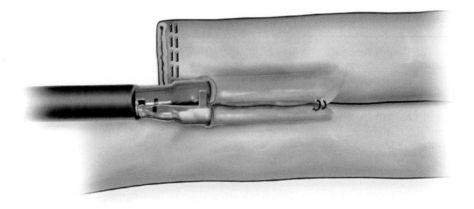

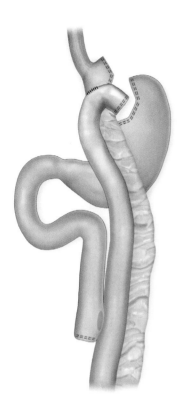

Figure 29.9 Completed antecolic-antegastric Roux-en-Y gastric bypass.

take note not to narrow the anastomosis during this step. A stitch is placed in the crotch of anastomosis (Fig. 29.8).

■ **Closure of mesenteric defects:** The jejunojejunostomy defect can be closed as a continuation of the outer layer of the enterotomy or with a separate permanent suture and is done from the patient's right side. It is important to include a bite of serosa to prevent the closure from opening once the patient loses weight. Closure of Peterson's defect (between the Roux limb and transverse colon mesentery) is performed from between the patient's legs. It may be necessary to place another 5-mm trocar in the patient's left lower quadrant to perform this closure ergonomically. The closure is performed with permanent suture from the base of the defect to the level of the transverse colon. Again, it is important to include bites of serosa in the closure. The Roux limb should be flipped to the patient's right side after closure of this defect. And proper orientation of the limbs is confirmed one last time. We do not feel it is necessary to routinely leave a drain (Fig. 29.9).

■ **Closure:** We close all 10- or 12-mm trocar sites with 0 Vicryl figure of eight transfascial sutures using a suture passer. The site of the EEA stapler may require more than one suture. The umbilical site can be closed this way or from the outside. We prefer prolene suture at the umbilicus. All wounds are irrigated and closed with running absorbable subcuticular suture.

Alternate Techniques

■ **Gastrojejunostomy:**

■ **Hand-sewn:** A two-layered anastomosis can be performed between the Roux limb and the gastric pouch with absorbable 2.0 or 3.0 sutures. This can be performed with a free needle or an Endostich (Covidien, Mansfield, MA) device. Advantages (compared to EEA) include decreased cost, lower rate of postoperative ulcers, strictures, and lower wound infection rate. Disadvantages include longer operative times, greater skill in suturing, and greater variability in size of anastomosis. No difference in long-term weight loss or leak rate is noted in the literature.

- **Linear stapler:** This is generally performed with an outer layer of hand-sutured anastomosis, followed by a linear stapler, and the enterotomy is either sutured or stapled closed. Advantages (compared to EEA) include decreased wound infection rate and decreased cost. Disadvantages: Requires suturing skills and variable size of anastomosis. No difference in leak has been shown.
- **Retrocolic versus antecolic Roux limb:** The Roux limb can be passed in front of or through the mesocolon. In addition, if retrocolic, it can be ante- or retrogastric. We prefer an antecolic approach, as described. Advantages of a retrocolic approach are as follows: potentially decreased tension on the gastrojejunal anastomosis and no division of the omentum is necessary. Disadvantages include potential difficulty in dissection through the mesocolon, bleeding in the mesocolon, need to close the defect in the mesocolon, and higher rate of internal hernia through this space.

 POSTOPERATIVE MANAGEMENT

After extubation, the patient should be transferred to a bed capable of withstanding the weight of bariatric patient. Hospital staff should be protected against injury when transferring patients with the assistance of hover technology air mattress transfer systems if possible. After discharge criteria from the post-anesthesia care unit are met, the patient should be transferred to a floor that is familiar with bariatric patients and surgery. Routine use of monitored settings is not necessary, unless the patient has significant obstructive sleep apnea or cardiovascular disease. The patient is maintained NPO for the first 24 hours, with IV fluid, urinary catheter in place with an IV dilaudid PCA supplemented by ketorolac. The patient should ambulate on the evening of surgery, have compression devices in place when in bed, and have 5000 units of subcutaneous heparin administered every 8 to 12 hours to prevent VTE. Incentive spirometry and chest therapy is also necessary to prevent atelectasis and pneumonia.

On post operative day 1, a contrast upper gastrointestinal series is obtained to evaluate for patency of anastomosis. Some centers forgo this study if there are no clinical signs of leak. Clear liquids are initiated, and the urinary catheter is removed. On postoperative day 2, if the patient continues to tolerate liquids, the IV is discontinued, oral medications are initiated and the diet is advanced to puree. Most patients can be discharged on the afternoon or evening of postoperative day 2.

Patients stay on a pureed diet for 2 weeks after surgery and slowly transition to more formed food over the next month. Patients should take a proton pump inhibitor, multivitamin fortified with iron, calcium, and vitamin D. Patients are also instructed to take about 70 grams of protein a day, generally in the form of shakes in the first few weeks following surgery. Interface with specialized dieticians are crucial in maintaining postoperative patient health and nutrition.

 COMPLICATIONS

Several early and late complications are possible after laparoscopic Roux-en-Y gastric bypass (LRYGB). The overall rates of serious complications is usually less than 5% in most series, and generally lower than that of open gastric bypass, particular in the area of wound and pulmonary complications.

- **Anastomotic leak:** Probably the most dreaded complication, it generally occurs less than 3% of the time in most large series by experienced surgeons and is rare after the surgeon's first hundred cases, stressing the significance of the learning curve. Tachycardia, fever, low urine output, and elevated WBC are all signs of a leak.

Stable patients should undergo imaging by contrast examination or CT scan. If patients are unstable or doubt exists as to the diagnosis, there should be no hesitation in proceeding to the operating room for diagnostic laparoscopy. Leaks are not limited to the gastrojejunal anastomosis but can occur in the pouch, the remnant stomach, and the jejunojejunostomy. A leak should be suspected if a patient deteriorates in the setting of a normal upper GI series that may not evaluate some of these other sites. Managing early leaks generally means reoperation and direct suture repair, drainage, and distal feeding tube. Delayed leaks may be managed by percutaneous drain placement and feeding tube placement. Oral feeds should be held for several weeks to allow the leak to heal, and an upper GI demonstrates patency without leak.

- **VTE:** Pulmonary embolus is a significant source of perioperative fatality in this population. As discussed earlier, all measures should be made to prevent DVT, including screening of high-risk individuals, early ambulation, and mechanical and chemical prophylaxis and IVC filter in the highest risk individuals. If suspected, patients should be anticoagulated, and a CT pulmonary angiogram should be obtained. PE and gastrointestinal leak can often have the same symptoms (tachycardia and hypoxia). If one is suspected, both should be ruled out.

- **Bleeding:** Can occur in up to 5% of cases and can be intra-abdominal or intraluminal. Staple lines are a frequent cause of bleeding and absorbable buttressing can reduce the incidence of bleeding. If bleeding occurs, it may be necessary to hold nonsteroidal anti-inflammatory drugs and VTE prophylaxis. Endoscopy and re-operation to oversew staple lines may be necessary to control bleeding.

- Later formation of marginal ulcers or formation of gastrogastric fistula can be a source of gastrointestinal bleeding. Smokers and those with untreated *H. pylori* are at higher risk of ulcer formation.

- **Stricture:** This can also occur in 3% to 5% of cases. Emesis and intolerance to oral intake in the first few months after surgery may suggest stricture formation at the GJ anastomosis. It can generally be managed with outpatient endoscopic dilation, unless the patient is severely dehydrated. Two to three balloon dilations are usually necessary. Patients with untreated *H. pylori* are at higher risk of stricture. There is also a slightly higher stricture rate using the EEA stapler to form the anastomosis, particularly the 21-mm EEA.

- **Internal hernia:** One of the few complications that occur more frequently after laparoscopic bypass as opposed to open surgery, probably due to less adhesion formation. Closure of the mesenteric defects and use of antecolic Roux limb has reduced the incidence of this complication. It can present with chronic or acute pain, vomiting or acutely with signs of ischemic bowel. The presentation may be insidious as the herniated bowel is usually the excluded segment so vomiting may not be present. If suspected and the patient is stable, a CT scan should be ordered. Dilated bowel, dilated gastric remnant, or "swirling" of the mesentery suggests internal hernia. If the CT is negative and symptoms persist, diagnostic laparoscopy should be undertaken.

- **Nutritional complications:** The majority of gastric bypass patients can have normal vitamin and micronutrient levels when adequate supplementation is administered. Patients are, however, at risk of iron, vitamin D, calcium, and vitamin B12 deficiency. Other deficiencies can occur but are rarer. Protein calorie malnutrition is generally not seen, unless there are very poor diet choices or a distal gastric bypass has been performed. Patient compliance with long-term follow-up is critical in preventing deficiencies.

RESULTS

- **Safety:** Despite the multiple potential complications that can exist in this relatively high-risk population, with this rather complex surgery, the overall major complication at high volume is generally less than 5% with a mortality less than 0.5%. Patients with a history of VTE, sleep apnea, and higher BMIs are at increased risk of complication and death.

■ **Weight loss:** In terms of weight loss, many large series of laparoscopic gastric bypass with about 2-year follow-up have demonstrated that the average percent excess weight loss (%EWL) ranges from 60% to 80%. Ten-year data available on gastric bypass from the Swedish obesity study suggests that weight loss is maintained over a long period of time and that gastric bypass is superior to other solely restrictive mechanisms of bariatric surgery.

■ **Comorbidities:** Resolution of comorbidities is frequent and dramatic after gastric bypass. Meta-analysis of all published series of laparoscopic gastric bypass (and other bariatric procedure) by Buchwald demonstrated that diabetes resolves or improved in 86% of subjects. Hypertension improves in 78.5% of patients. These patients can frequently be free of medications. Eighty-five percent of patients with obstructive sleep apnea had resolution and were able to come off CPAP. Lipid profile improvement is seen in 93% of patients. In addition, patients can also see improvement in GERD, asthma, infertility, stress urinary incontinence, osteoarthritis, normal pressure hydrocephalus, and mood.

■ **Overall survival:** Perhaps most significantly, gastric bypass is associated with an increase in overall survival of obese patients. In a study comparing patients having undergone gastric bypass with matched obese patients obtaining a drivers license, not undergoing surgery with 7 year follow-up, there was a 40% reduction in death noted. While not a randomized study, the findings highly suggest a survival benefit from having undergone surgery. The reduction in mortality was primarily due to decreased cardiovascular disease.

✧ CONCLUSIONS

■ Obesity is a prevalent and growing health problem with few adequate long-term solutions.

■ Surgical weight loss is currently the most effective means of weight loss for morbidly obese individuals. That is, those with a BMI > 40 kg/m^2 or BMI > 35 kg/m^2 and a comorbidity.

■ Patients should be appropriately educated prior to surgery, have demonstrated inability to lose weight by other means, and be of reasonable risk to undergo surgery.

■ Preoperative evaluation and preparation can be extensive and involve multiple specialists including nutritionists, psychiatrists, cardiologists, sleep specialists, gastroenterologists, and endocrinologists.

■ Laparoscopic Roux-en-Y gastric bypass is a complex and technically demanding procedure and surgeon and institution volume has been shown to reduce complications.

■ Operating room equipment and postoperative care units should be customized to address the need of bariatric patients.

■ Several variations of technique have been described in performing gastric bypass:
  ■ Position: French vs. American
  ■ Order of steps: Proximal first vs. distal first
  ■ Type of anastomosis: Circular stapled, linear stapled, or hand-sewn
  ■ Position of Roux limb: Ante-colic vs. retro-colic (can be retro or ante-gastric)

■ Common themes: Small restrictive gastric pouch (approximately 30 ml); approximately 2 cm anastomosis, bypassed bowel of varying lengths, closure of mesenteric defects.

■ Postoperative care aims to have patients ambulate early and prevent VTE, identify early leaks, and feed patients as early as possible and have them return to an ambulatory lifestyle.

■ Various complications are possible, but overall rate of major complications is low, with most complications being treatable.

■ Weight loss after LRYGB is significant and durable, is associated with profound and frequent resolution of comorbidities, and is associated with increased overall survival.

Recommended References and Readings

Adams TD, Gress RE, Smith DC, et al. Long-term mortality after gastric bypass surgery. *N Engl J Med.* 2007;357:753–761.

Apovian CM, Cummings S, Anderson W, et al. Best practice updates for multidisciplinary care in weight loss surgery. *Obesity (Silver Spring).* 2009;17(5):871–879. PMCID: 2859198.

Brethauer S. ASMBS position statement on preoperative supervised weight loss requirements. *Surg Obes Relat Dis.* 2011;7(3):257–260.

Buchwald H, Avidor Y, Braunwald E, et al. Bariatric surgery: A systematic review and meta-analysis. *JAMA.* 2004;292(14):1724–1737.

Flegal KM, Carroll MD, Ogden CL, et al. Prevalence and trends in obesity among US adults, 1999–2008. *JAMA.* 2010;303(3):235–241.

Flum DR, Belle SH, King WC, et al. Perioperative safety in the longitudinal assessment of bariatric surgery. *N Engl J Med.* 2009;361(5):445–454. PMCID: 2854565.

Greenberg I, Sogg S, Perna MF. Behavioral and psychological care in weight loss surgery: best practice update. *Obesity (Silver Spring).* 2009;17(5):880–884.

Mason EE, Ito C. Gastric bypass. *Ann Surg.* 1969;170(3):329–339.

National Institutes of Health UDoHaHS. Gastrointestinal surgery for severe obesity. Consensus statement of the NIH consensus development conference.; 1991 [updated 1991; cited]. Available from: http://consensus.nih.gov/1991/1991gisurgeryobesity084html.htm.

Podnos YD, Jimenez JC, Wilson SE, et al. Complications after laparoscopic gastric bypass: A review of 3464 cases. *Arch Surg.* 2003;138(9):957–961.

Poitou Bernert C, Ciangura C, Coupaye M, et al. Nutritional deficiency after gastric bypass: Diagnosis, prevention and treatment. *Diabetes Metab.* 2007;33(1):13–24.

Ren CJ, Cabrera I, Rajaram K, et al. Factors influencing patient choice for bariatric operation. *Obes Surg.* 2005;15(2):202–206.

Rubino F, Kaplan LM, Schauer PR, et al. The Diabetes Surgery Summit consensus conference: Recommendations for the evaluation and use of gastrointestinal surgery to treat type 2 diabetes mellitus. *Ann Surg.* 2010;251(3):399–405.

Schauer PR, Ikramuddin S, Hamad G, et al. Laparoscopic gastric bypass surgery: Current technique. *J Laparoendosc Adv Surg Tech A.* 2003;13(4):229–239.

Simpfendorfer CH, Szomstein S, Rosenthal R. Laparoscopic gastric bypass for refractory morbid obesity. *Surg Clin North Am.* 2005;85(1):119–127, x.

Sjostrom L Lindroos AK, Peltonen M, et al. Lifestyle, diabetes, and cardiovascular risk factors 10 years after bariatric surgery. *N Engl J Med.* 2004;351:2683–2693.

Winegar DA, Sherif B, Pate V, et al. Venous thromboembolism after bariatric surgery performed by Bariatric Surgery Center of Excellence Participants: Analysis of the Bariatric Outcomes Longitudinal Database. *Surg Obes Relat Dis.* 2011;7(2):181–188.

Wittgrove AC, Clark GW, Schubert KR. Laparoscopic gastric bypass, Roux-en-Y: Technique and results in 75 patients with 3–30 months follow-up. *Obes Surg.* 1996;6(6):500–504.

Part IV: Bariatric

30 Laparoscopic Sleeve Gastrectomy Technique

Raul J. Rosenthal and Wasef Abu-Jaish

 ## INDICATIONS AND CONTRAINDICATIONS

The morbid obesity epidemic continues to spread throughout industrialized nations. Bariatric surgery continues to be the only proven method to achieve sustained weight loss in the majority of patients. Currently, the four most common bariatric operations in the United States are Roux-en-Y gastric bypass (RYGB), adjustable gastric band (LAGB), laparoscopic sleeve gastrectomy (LSG), and biliopancreatic diversion with duodenal switch (BPD-DS). These operations are now performed laparoscopically at most bariatric centers. The adoption of laparoscopic techniques has led to a dramatic increase in the annual number of bariatric procedures performed.

Sleeve gastrectomy (SG), a relatively new surgical approach, was initially conceived as a restrictive component of the BPD-DS in the era of open bariatric surgery. With the advent of minimally invasive surgery in the late 1980s, LSG has been proposed as a step procedure in high-risk patients, followed by a second step RYGB or BPD-DS, and, recently, as a stand-alone bariatric approach.

When evaluating a potential patient for bariatric surgery, a multidisciplinary team should be used. This team includes a dietitian and a mental health professional who are familiar with bariatric surgery. Their purpose is to obtain past dietary and behavioral eating history, discuss postoperative dietary expectations, and decide whether the individual is an appropriate candidate for this type of operation. Support for the surgery from family members and friends is important. If the team believes that the patient is not appropriate for the procedure, then consideration should be given to nonoperative medical management with appropriate counseling.

Since the National Institutes of Health (NIH) Consensus Conference convened in 1991, surgical approaches have been identified as the best course of treatment for patients with clinically severe obesity, who have a body mass index (BMI) of at least 35 kg/m^2 and associated comorbid conditions.

In most institutions, LRYGB, LAGB, and LSG are offered to all patients. Following the NIH recommendations, most centers in the United States recommend LRYGB as the procedure of choice or gold standard in patients with a BMI over 40 kg/m^2 with or without comorbidity. As the experience with LSG increases, attempts are being made to define indications for LSG as a first or final step. Most centers agree that there is

TABLE 30.1	Indications
Indication/Procedure	**Characteristics**
Two-stage procedure	
First step in super-super morbidly obese patient	Followed by RNYGB or BPD
First step to a nonbariatric second procedure	Low BMI of 35–40
	Followed by hip replacement, recurrent incisional hernia, pull through procedure for ulcerative colitis, renal/liver transplantation
Single-stage procedure	
Final step in ASA IV morbidly obese patient	Low EF, heart/liver/kidney transplant recipient
Final step in poor candidate for LRYGB or BPD-DS	Smoker
	Warfarin
Final step in extremes of age	Adolescents
	Elderly age ≥70 yrs
Final step in a high-risk stomach	Chile, Colombia, Japan: high incidence of gastric cancer
Patient preference/refusal to undergo anatomic rearrangement of their intestinal anatomy or placement of an implanted device	
Low BMI of 35–40 with comorbidity	
Final step in Crohn's/Celiac disease or UC	
BMI 30–35 with the metabolic syndrome	Under protocol only
Other indications: liver cirrhosis. Dense adhesions of small bowel, expected complex colorectal surgery in patients with diverticular disease, huge abdominal hernia, necessity to continue specific medications (immunosuppressant, anti-inflammatory)	

BPD-DS, biliopancreatic diversion and duodenal switch; BMI, body mass index; BPD, biliopancreatic diversion; EF, ejection fraction; LRYGB, laparoscopic Roux-en-Y gastric bypass; RYGBP, Roux-en-Y gastric bypass; UC, ulcerative colitis.

enough evidence to recommend LSG in the presence of serious contraindications or for poor risk surgical candidates for LRYGB, BPD-DS, and LAGB. Owing to the two International Consensus Summits for SG, held in 2007 and 2009, this procedure has been recognized as an established bariatric procedure and is rapidly becoming accepted as an acceptable procedure for morbid obesity.

Additional indications include patients with liver cirrhosis (without severe portal hypertension), dense adhesions of small bowel (high risk for bowel obstruction after RYGB or BPD-DS), large recurrent abdominal wall hernias in the presence of obesity (lower incidence of recurrence after weight loss), and expected complex colorectal surgery in patients with diverticular or inflammatory bowel disease. More controversially, LSG may have a role in patients with a low BMI of 30 to 35 kg/m^2 with the metabolic syndrome. The latter should be conducted under Institutional Review Board protocol only (Table 30.1).

The potential benefits of performing SG (Table 30.2) include that, due to its "relative" technical simplicity, it can be performed laparoscopically in high BMI patients (super-super morbid obesity). Minimal follow-up is required when compared with other well-established procedures such as LAGB (no need for adjustments with LSG) and RYGB/BPD-DS (no marginal ulcerations and micronutrient malabsorption with LSG). It is an attractive option for patients with chronic conditions, such as Crohn's/celiac disease or ulcerative colitis, which preclude extensive intestinal surgery.

As mentioned before, LSG provides an effective decrease in operative risk and alleviates technical difficulties when implemented as a first-stage procedure for super-obese and high-risk patients. It can be converted to a malabsorptive procedure such as BPD-DS or to a LRYGB in case of failure of weight loss and/or severe GERD.

When contemplating bariatric surgery indications, factors that are taken into consideration by surgeons and patients are the following: insurance coverage, age, BMI, associated comorbid illnesses, efficacy, and morbidity. There is also the so-called patient preference when discussing surgical options. LSG is attractive to patients who do not want to undergo anatomic rearrangement of their intestinal anatomy (RYGBP or BPD-DS)

TABLE 30.2   **Advantages and Disadvantages**

Advantages
1. The stomach is reduced without major changes in either anatomy or continuity
2. The pyloric preservation prevents dumping syndrome and might add to the restrictive component
3. The patient can be discharged from hospital within 2 days postoperatively
4. It provides an effective first-stage procedure for super-obese patients
5. It is useful for patients with conditions such as Crohn's disease, celiac disease, or ulcerative colitis, which preclude intestinal bypass.
6. It can be performed laparoscopically, even in patients who weigh over 500 lbs
7. Minimal follow-up is required when compared with other well-established procedures such as laparoscopic adjustable gastric banding and Roux-en-Y gastric bypass
8. There are no problems with malabsorption and nutritional deficiencies as seen in biliopancreatic diversion with duodenal switch
9. It provides a good educational base for resident doctors lacking experience in the surgical treatment of gastric ulcers
10. It can be converted to a malabsorption procedure (biliopancreatic diversion with duodenal switch) in case of failure or to laparoscopic Roux-en-Y gastric bypass for severe gastroesophageal reflux disease

Disadvantages
1. The risk of stapling complications such as leaks, bleeding, and stenosis
2. The irreversibility of the procedure

or placement of an implanted device (LAGB). While all procedures are similar in their "final effect," by inducing rapid weight loss and resolution of comorbidities, there can be a significant difference in its efficacy and morbidity.

The disadvantages of LSG include the risk of stapling complications, such as leaks, bleeding, and stenosis, and the irreversibility of the procedure.

There are to our knowledge no studies that discuss in the detail the contraindications for LSG (Table 30.3). Three clinical scenarios can be considered as absolute contraindications:

1. Patients with severe and documented GERD. The performance of LSG in this clinical scenario could worsen the GERD by creating a high-pressure system in a patient who already has insufficient lower esophageal sphincter. Furthermore, LSG removes the gastric fundus, and as a result an antireflux procedure becomes impossible for those patients who are not candidates for RYGB or BPD-DS.
2. Patients with Barrett's esophagus. There is scientific evidence that for morbid obesity patients with severe GERD, gastric bypass is the procedure of choice. Additionally, by removing the greater curvature of the stomach with LSG, we eliminate the portion of the stomach that can potentially be used as a graft (interposition) in those cases when esophagectomy is indicated.
3. Patients with liver cirrhosis and severe portal hypertension (Childs B/C).

In this clinical scenario, LSG has a high risk for complications and mortality, as with any other surgical procedure. It would be of interest to evaluate LSG as a treatment

TABLE 30.3   **Contraindications**

Absolute
1. Severe and documented gastroesophageal reflux disease
2. Barrett's esophagus
3. Liver cirrhosis and severe portal hypertension

Relative
1. Perioperative risk of cardiac complications
2. Poor myocardial reserve
3. Significant chronic obstructive airways disease or respiratory dysfunction
4. Noncompliance of medical treatment
5. Psychological disorders of a significant degree
6. Significant eating disorders
7. Large hiatal hernias

Part IV: Bariatric

option for morbidly obese patients with liver cirrhosis and portal hypertension who would undergo a decompressive procedure, such as transjugular intrahepatic portosystemic shunt followed by a LSG.

There are several relative contraindications for LSG that are common in other surgical procedures, including the following: perioperative risk of cardiac complications, poor myocardial reserve, significant chronic obstructive airways disease or respiratory dysfunction, noncompliance of medical treatment, psychological disorders of a significant degree, and significant eating disorders (Table 30.3).

PREOPERATIVE PLANNING

All patients undergoing surgery should meet the NIH criteria for obesity surgery and have completed a comprehensive, multidisciplinary, preoperative program. The standardized comprehensive preoperative program includes an initial information session conducted by one of the bariatric surgeons.

After the initial information session, patients are preliminarily evaluated by a specialized bariatric nurse clinician, a psychologist, and the patient's own primary care physician. During these visits, the patients are provided with written materials, in addition to direct contact with care providers, with regard to weight loss and weight loss surgery. Patients are then evaluated by a bariatric surgeon, who conducts a preoperative quiz and full consultation. The consultation includes discussion of surgical options and expectations of postoperative life.

After the surgical consultation, the patients see a nutritionist, who provides further written information. Additionally, patients are required to adhere to a strict preoperative high-protein liquid diet 2 weeks before the date of surgery. This serves two functions: it minimizes liver size and prepares patients for the postoperative experience.

Preoperative evaluation should include a thorough history, a complete endocrinological workup, psychological testing, and counseling by a dietician, as with any other bariatric procedure. At our institutions (Cleveland Clinic Florida & University of Vermont/Fletcher Allen Health care) as well as most bariatric centers, patients undergo upper abdominal sonography to exclude gallstones and barium swallow/upper GI or an esophagogastroduodenoscopy (EGD) to exclude anatomic variations of the upper digestive tract, such as hiatus hernias. Hiatus hernias are repaired when present.

The planned procedure (LSG, possible open procedure, possible gastric bypass, intraoperative EGD/upper endoscopy), the risks, benefits, and alternatives of the procedure are explained to the patient and his/her family in detail. The risks include but are not limited to medical, surgical, intraoperative, postoperative, and early and late complications. Medical complications include but are not limited to death, anesthesia and medically adverse effects, deep vein thrombosis, pulmonary embolism, myocardial infarction, stroke, and respiratory and renal failure. Surgical complications include but are not limited to early and late complications, intra-abdominal bleeding, injury to nearby structures such as liver, spleen, esophagus, small and large bowel, infection with abscess formation, staple line leak, stenosis, stricture, reflux symptoms, and delayed gastric emptying. Other potential risks and complications include wound infection or bleeding at the trocar sites, incisional hernia, and failure to lose weight or regain weight. A consent form is obtained after all of the patient's and their family's questions are answered.

SURGICAL TECHNIQUE

Mechanism of Action

LSG involves removing most of the stomach (70% to 80%), including the fundus, and creating a gastric "tube" 100 to 130 mL in capacity. The efficacy of SG has been attributed to the reduction of gastric capacity (restrictive effect) and/or to the orexigenic and anorexigenic intestinal hormone modification (hormonal effect). Currently, both hormonal changes and a hindgut theory have been postulated to be involved. The mechanism of weight loss following LSG is mainly due to a restricted calorie intake, which results from the combination of the small capacity, low distensibility of the sleeve, and the resultant immediate high intraluminal pressure. Both might be responsible for the satiety effect of this procedure.

The role of the pylorus as another potential mechanism of increased intragastric pressure remains to be determined. There are, however, other mechanisms that must be considered, such as hormonal changes that result in alliesthesia and anorexia. Although resection of the fundus may lower ghrelin levels by reducing the volume of ghrelin-producing cells, it has been suggested that the low levels of this hormone after surgery are in fact attributable to the paracrine effect exerted by endogenous gastrointestinal hormones, such as glucagon-like peptide-1 (GLP-1), GLP, ghrelin, and other hormones. However, it is doubtful that decreased levels of ghrelin are the sole reason for the weight loss achieved by LSG. The insulin, GLP-1, and peptide YY levels increase similarly after LRYGB and LSG with marked improvement in glucose homeostasis, as well as appetite suppression and excess weight loss (EWL). Adequate weight loss plays a key role in alleviating comorbidities and can be achieved by complete removal of the gastric fundus, which is not only important for eliminating ghrelin production but also for making the inlet of the stomach small enough so that the patient will feel full quickly.

The incorporation of laparoscopy in bariatric surgery has increased the demand and application of minimally invasive techniques in the treatment of morbid obesity. The adoption of these techniques has led to a dramatic increase in the annual number of bariatric procedures performed. SG can be performed by open or conventional multiport laparoscopy. More recently, some surgeons have performed the procedure using a single-incision or hybrid NOTES transvaginal approach.

On the morning of surgery, the patient is injected subcutaneously with 5,000 units of unfractionated heparin to prevent venous thromboembolic complications. Then low-molecular-weight heparin is continued during hospitalization, whereas the higher risk venous thromboembolism patient may be treated beyond this period up to an entire post-operative month. A peripheral intravenous (IV) line is placed and a second-generation cephalosporin is administered intravenously and continued for the first 24 hours postsurgery. The patient is placed on the operating room table in the supine position with a footboard. Sequential compression devices are placed on the lower extremities. General anesthesia is administered and a urinary catheter is inserted. The anesthetist inserts, applies suction to, and then immediately removes the orogastric tube before starting the operation. The esophageal temperature probe is removed to prevent migration into the stomach during stapling. The operating surgeon stands at the patient's right side together with the second assistant (camera operator) and the first assistant at the left with the scrub nurse. We have found that the safest way to enter the abdomen in morbidly obese patients is under direct vision using a device that allows visualization of the abdominal wall layers sequentially with a zero-degree laparoscope. When performing LSG, there is so far no general agreement or standard technique regarding the number of trocars used, bougie size, staple line reinforcement, complete or partial removal of the gastric antrum, intraoperative testing, EGD, drain placement, and postoperative upper gastrointestinal study among most bariatric surgeons. The entire abdomen is prepped and draped in usual sterile surgical fashion. A seven-trocar technique is used (Fig. 30.1). The aim of the operation is to create restriction and reduce the size of the stomach to a 100-cc tube by resecting the greater curvature (Fig. 30.2).

The main steps of this operation are as follows:

1. Access to the abdominal cavity
2. Trocars placement (Fig. 30.1)
3. Creation of pneumoperitoneum
4. Liver retraction (Fig. 30.3)
5. Inspection of the gastroesophageal (GE) junction for possible hiatus hernia
6. Identification of the pylorus (Fig. 30.4)
7. Dissection of the stomach from the greater omentum up to the GE junction (Figs. 30.5 and 30.6)
8. Identification the left crus of the diaphragm at the esophagogastric junction to ensure complete mobilization of the gastric fundus (Figs. 30.7 and 30.8)

Figure 30.1 Trocar placement.

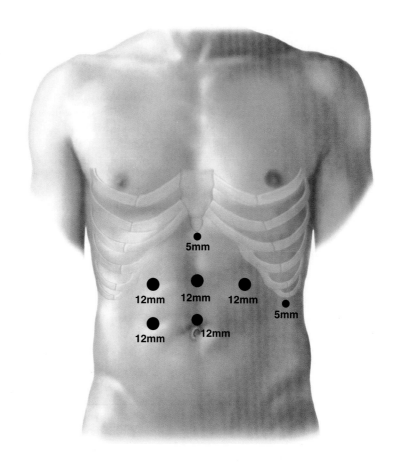

5mm

12mm   12mm   12mm

5mm

12mm   12mm

Figure 30.2 Illustration showing sleeve gastrectomy.

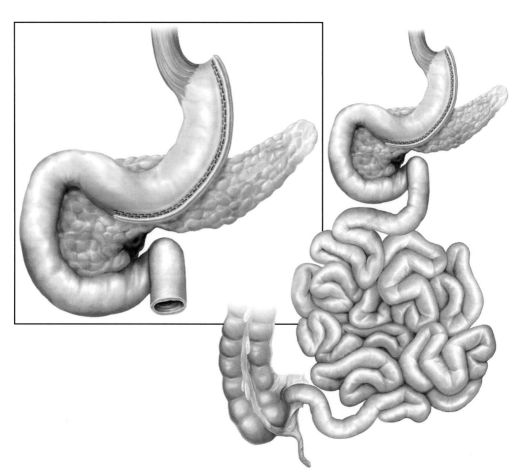

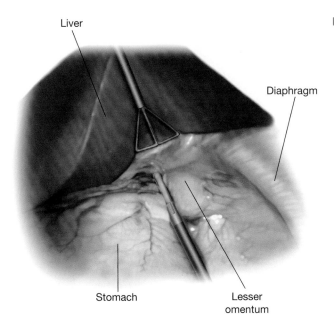

Liver

Diaphragm

Stomach

Lesser
omentum

Figure 30.3 Liver retraction.

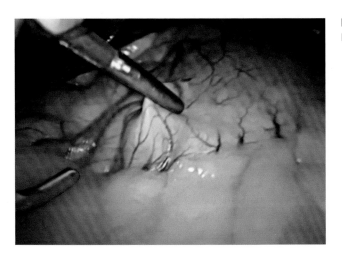

Figure 30.4 Identification of the
pylorus.

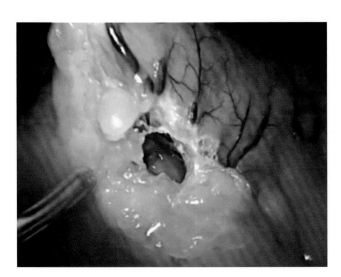

Figure 30.5 Dissection of the short
gastric vessel along the greater
curvature starts about 5 cm from the
pyloric channel.

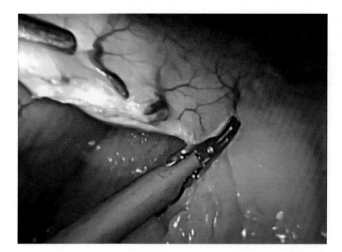

Figure 30.6 Dissection of the short gastric vessel along the greater curvature starts about 5 cm from the pyloric channel.

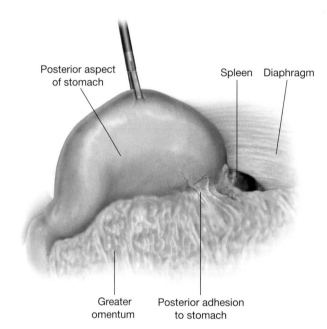

Figure 30.7 Posterior dissection of the stomach.

Posterior aspect of stomach

Spleen   Diaphragm

Greater omentum

Posterior adhesion to stomach

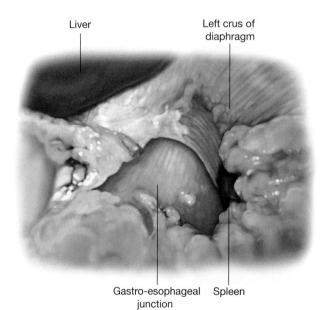

Figure 30.8 Identification the left crus of the diaphragm at the esophago-gastric junction to ensure complete mobilization of the gastric fundus.

Liver

Left crus of diaphragm

Gastro-esophageal junction   Spleen

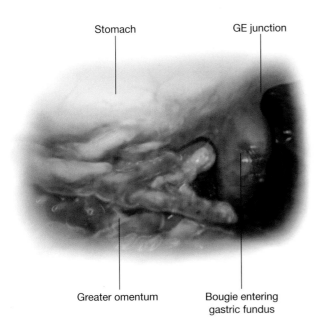

Stomach   GE junction

Greater omentum   Bougie entering
                   gastric fundus

Figure 30.9 Transoral insertion of
the bougie.

 9. Transoral insertion of the bougie (Fig. 30.9)
10. Vertical transaction of the stomach to creation the gastric sleeve (Fig. 30.10)
11. Imbrication of the staple line (Fig. 30.11)
12. Removal of the bougie (Fig. 30.12)
13. (+/−) intraoperative testing: air insufflation, methylene blue and EGD
14. Drain placement (Fig. 30.13)
15. Placement of the specimen in the endobag and retrieval (Figs. 30.14 and 30.15)
16. Fascial closure of the 15-mm trocar site and skin closure

For all laparoscopic SG patients at our institution, we adopted the following technique:

Access to the abdominal cavity is gained through a 1-cm supraumbilical incision using the Xcel trocar® (Ethicon Endo-Surgery, Cincinnati, OH, USA) in the middle of the left rectus sheath above the umbilicus. To create the pneumoperitoneum, warm CO_2 is insufflated to achieve an intra-abdominal pressure of approximately 15 mm Hg. The patient is placed in a slightly reverse Trendelenburg position with left side up to facilitate additional trocar placement and exposure. Four additional 12-mm and two 5-mm bladeless trocars are inserted under direct visualization. The liver retractor is placed through the 5-mm subxiphoid trocar (Fig. 30.3). The lateral segment of the left lobe of the liver is then elevated out of the way to expose the GE junction and the gastric fundus. The retractor is then fastened to the table.

With the trocars in proper position, the fundus of the stomach is grasped and then retracted caudally, exposing the gastrophrenic ligament to assess for the presence of a

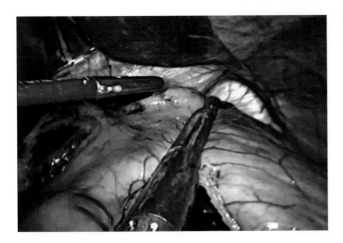

Figure 30.10 Vertical transaction of
the stomach to create the gastric
sleeve.

Liver   GE junction   Diaphragm

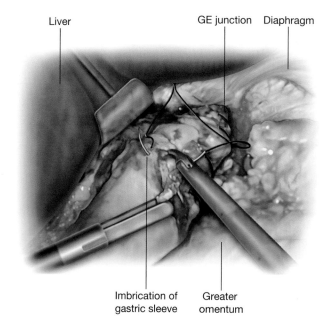

Figure 30.11 Imbrication of the staple line.

Imbrication of   Greater
gastric sleeve   omentum

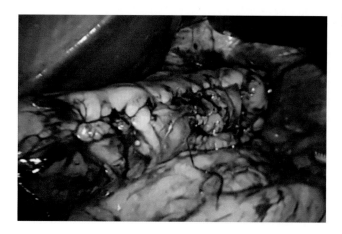

Figure 30.12 Sleeve completed.

Liver   Blake drain
               (placement)

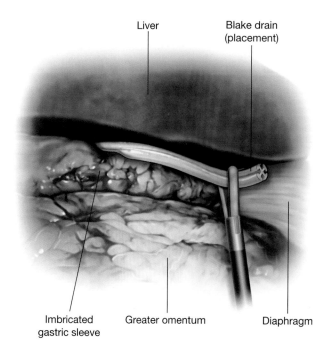

Figure 30.13 Drain placement.

Imbricated   Greater omentum   Diaphragm
gastric sleeve

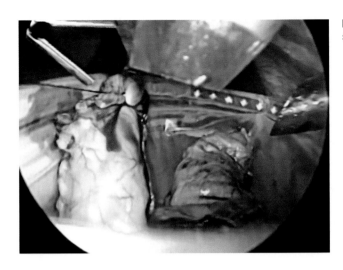

Figure 30.14 Placement of the specimen in the endobag.

hiatus hernia. The pyloric channel is identified, beginning opposite the crow's foot, approximately 5 to 7 cm proximal to the pylorus, and the stomach is separated from the greater omentum using the Harmonic scalpel™ (Ethicon Endo-Surgery) ultrasonic shear device by taking down the greater omentum and the short gastric vessels of the greater curvature all the way up to the GE junction (Fig. 30.4).

The peritoneal covering over the left crus of the diaphragm is taken down to identify the esophagogastric junction and to ensure complete mobilization of the gastric fundus.

It is important to identify and mobilize the angle of His with exposure of the left crus of the diaphragm to delineate the GE junction and to facilitate complete resection of the gastric fundus (Fig. 30.8). Retrogastric adhesions are taken down with the Harmonic scalpel™ (Ethicon Endo-Surgery) device to allow for complete mobilization of the stomach, to eliminate any redundant posterior wall of the sleeve, and to exclude the fundus from the gastric sleeve (Fig. 30.7).

The area is irrigated with warm normal saline until hemostasis has been assured.

The cardia of the stomach, the distal esophagus, and the esophagogastric junction are supplied in the right and anterior side by branches of the left gastric artery and left inferior phrenic artery. The posterior and left sides are vascularized mainly by fundic branches of the splenic artery and, if present, by the posterior gastric artery. The arterial supply of the esophagus is segmental. Complete dissection of the fundus requires

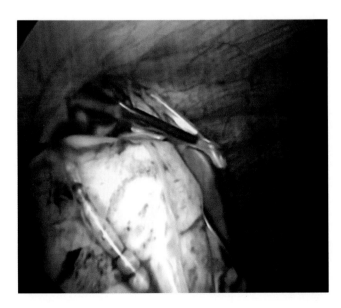

Figure 30.15 Retrieval of the specimen through the right lower quadrant trocar site.

necessarily division of the short gastric vessels, posterior gastric artery, and phrenic branches when present. A "critical area" of vascularization may occur laterally, just at the esophagogastric junction at the angle of His. A resection line avoiding the "critical area" may partly solve the problem by leaving 1 to 2 cm of gastric remnant just at the GE junction.

In our experience, this technique was adopted in all cases (greater than 400) with one leak occurrence, and the residual capacity of the gastric sleeve remained unchanged.

Other factors considered for the development of gastric leak in this area are the increased intraluminal pressure and the diminished thickness of the gastric wall at the fundus.

After complete mobilization of the stomach, a 38 to 42F bougie is inserted transorally into the stomach and through the pylorus under direct vision and is placed against the lesser curvature (Fig. 30.10). This helps to calibrate the size of the gastric sleeve, prevents any constriction at the GE junction, and provides a uniform shape to the remaining stomach.

After securing the bougie against the lesser curvature of the stomach, the main part of the corpus and the gastric fundus are transected in vertical fashion up to the angle of His.

The gastric sleeve is created using a linear stapler (EndoGIA, US Surgical, Norwalk, CT, USA), with two sequential 4.8/45-mm green load firings for the antrum, followed by two or three sequential 3.8 to 3.5/45-mm purple/blue loads for the remaining gastric corpus and fundus or Echelon™ Endopath (Ethicon Endo-Surgery; Johnson & Johnson, Cincinnati, OH, USA) with gold cartridge (Fig. 30.10).

A long laparoscopic reticulating 45-mm EndoGIA linear cutting stapler (Covidien, Norwalk, CT, USA) loaded with a green (4.8 mm) cartridge is inserted through the 15-mm trocar in a cephalad direction to transect the thick antrum of the stomach. Then, a sequential application of the purple/blue (3.8 mm and 3.5 mm) load cartridge is utilized, creating a gastric sleeve with an estimated capacity of less than 150 mL. Care must be taken not to narrow the stomach at the incisura angularis. It is important to inspect the stomach anteriorly and posteriorly to ensure no redundant posterior stomach is present (Fig. 30.10).

In all cases, the staple line is reinforced/imbricated with a running 2-0 Vicryl suture on an SH needle over the bougie from each direction to ensure hemostasis along the staple line and for possible leakage prevention. One suture is used from the superior staple line. A second suture is used from the inferior portion. The sutures are tied together at the staple line midportion (Fig. 30.11). The left upper quadrant is irrigated with warm normal saline above the spleen and once hemostasis has been assured, the bougie is removed (Fig. 30.12). Throughout the years, technical modifications have been introduced. Reinforcement by oversewing the staple line was adopted to reduce bleeding and leaks.

With LSG we do not routinely test the integrity of the staple line unless clinically indicated or after revisional procedures. If the decision is made to perform intraoperative testing, we proceed as follows: The patient is placed flat, and an atraumatic clamp is placed near the pylorus. The integrity of the staple line is tested by either insufflating air after immersing the sleeve under saline, infusing 60 cm^3 of methylene blue, or intraoperative EGD.

A large bore 19Fr Blake drain is placed in the subhepatic area near the staple line at the conclusion of the procedure to identify any potential postoperative bleeding and/or leak. The drain is exteriorized through the right upper quadrant trocar site and secured with 2-0 nylon and put to self-suction (Fig. 30.13). The use of drains after gastrointestinal surgery has long been debated. Most bariatric surgeons use drains for the early detection of the presence of bleeding or leaks and to try to obviate the need for emergent repeat operation in the case of a leak, allowing a nonoperative treatment option. It is our routine to use a large bore drain after all bariatric procedures. From the beginning, we have left this drain in place until the seventh postoperative day (POD). This is a practice we imported from our general surgery experience, and in some cases from our initial series of bariatric surgery, we detected some leaks after the seventh POD. The duration of cavity drainage is also controversial; however, the tendency has been to maintain the drain until the third or fourth POD or before the patient's discharge.

Using the same working trocars, other associated surgical pathologies, such as paraesophageal hernia, umbilical hernia, cholecystectomy, and diagnostic liver biopsy, are addressed at the same time.

The resected stomach is extracted in a retrieval bag (15-mm Endo Catch II. Specimen Retrieval Pouch. Covidien-Mansfield, MA,USA), or is grasped at the antral tip by a laparoscopic grasper and retrieved through one of the enlarged trocar site (15 mm) (Figs. 30.14 and 30.15). The trocars should be removed under direct vision to identify any bleeding points. The 15-mm trocar-site-enlarged fascia is closed with absorbable, figure-of-eight Vicryl #1 suture. Fascial defects on the other trocar site are not routinely closed but the skin is approximated with absorbable subcuticular Monocryl 4-0.

The mean operative time is 60 minutes (range 58 to 190) with a mean blood loss of 20 mL (range 0 to 300). There have been no perioperative deaths in our series.

 POSTOPERATIVE MANAGEMENT

All bariatric patients are transferred to the intermediate care unit after routine monitoring in the recovery room. Moderate-to-severe obstructive sleep apnea patients are prescribed continuous positive airway pressure while they are sleeping. Occasionally, we admit patients to the intensive care unit if their respiratory demands exceed the capability of the floor staff. IV antibiotics are continued for 24 hours in most cases. Ambulation is started as soon as possible. Low-molecular-weight heparin is continued during hospitalization for most patients, whereas the higher risk venous thromboembolism patients may be treated up to an entire postoperative month.

Early postoperative ambulation and generous use of incentive spirometry is encouraged. Adequate postoperative analgesia is essential to improve mobility and decrease pulmonary-related complications. We initially use a patient-controlled analgesia pump and then convert to an oral morphine elixir after the first POD. On the first POD, a water-soluble contrast as well as a thin barium swallow is performed to exclude leakage and to serve as a baseline study for future follow-up (Fig. 30.16).

Figure 30.16 Postoperative upper GI contrast study.

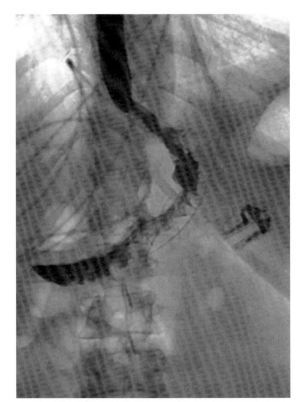

Part IV: Bariatric

Lower extremity duplex is performed to rule out deep venous thrombosis. The patients are discharged on POD 2 or 3 when they meet our discharge criteria: stable vital signs, negative upper GI study, negative lower extremity duplex study, ambulation, well-hydrated, and able to tolerate liquid diet.

We discharge the patients on a liquid diet and they are continued on a semisolid/liquid diet for another 2 weeks with instructions to start multivitamin substitution daily thereafter. Proton pump inhibitor in the form of solutabe is prescribed for 3 months to control any reflux symptoms.

Postoperative management involves scheduled visits for education and counseling with physicians, nurse practitioners, nutritionists, and nurse clinicians.

The patients are strongly encouraged to attend a monthly support group meeting and see the dietitian on a routine basis, as well as a mental health professional if one is needed or requested.

Patients are seen 2 weeks postoperatively, and then follow-up is conducted at 3, 6, and 12 months, and annually thereafter, as it is routine in all centers of excellence in the United States. At each postoperative visit, a nonfasting blood sample is drawn. The measurements include total/corrected calcium, albumin, vitamin D, iron, ferritin, folic acid, zinc, magnesium, vitamin B1, B6, and B12 concentrations, and complete blood count. Owing to the drastic change in diet (quality and quantity), we prescribe oral multivitamin supplementation postoperatively at least temporarily for these patients.

 COMPLICATIONS

Major complication rates reported in these studies are relatively low. For all studies, the complication rates range up to 24% and, for the larger studies ($n > 100$), up to 15%. The reported leak, bleeding, and stricture rates are 2.2, 1.2, and 0.63%, respectively, for all studies reporting detailed complication data ($n = 2367$).

Overall, the complication rate of LSG is equivalent to RYGB, BPD-DS, and LAGB with less or absent nutritional complications, dumping syndrome, internal hernia, marginal ulcers, foreign body, and port access problems that plague more traditional bariatric operations.

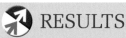 RESULTS

The American Society for Metabolic and Bariatric Surgery, in its position statement, analyzed the published reports in the literature and concluded that LSG is a promising procedure for the surgical management of morbid obesity. More recently, a systematic review of the current literature reporting either complications or weight loss outcomes after LSG in adult human subjects has been completed. This review includes 36 studies, two randomized controlled trials, one nonrandomized matched cohort analysis, and 33 uncontrolled case series. Three were multicenter trials while the remaining studies were from single institutions. These 36 studies report on a total of 2,570 patients. Intermediate-term follow-up is now reported in the literature with 3-, 4- and 5-year follow-up periods. The postoperative 30-day mortality rate is 0.19% in the published literature. The mean percentage EWL after SG was reported in 24 studies ($n = 1662$) and was 33% to 85%, with an overall mean EWL of 55.4%. The follow-up period for the weight loss data was 3 to 60 months.

During the consensus section of the second annual International Consensus Summit for LSG (ICSSG) in 2009, the audience responded as follows:

1. There was enough evidence published to support the use of LSG as a primary procedure to treat morbid obesity and indicated that it is on par with LAGB and RYGB, with a yes vote at 77%.
2. There is a perception among most bariatric surgeons that in order to achieve acceptable long-term weight loss, the bougie size should not be larger than 40Fr; however,

it has also been a concern that the lower the bougie size, the higher the incidence of staple line disruption.

3. The responders reported postoperative occurrence of a high gastric leak in 1.5% and a lower gastric leak in 0.5%.

4. A total of 81.9% of the surgeons reported no conversions from a laparoscopic to an open SG.

5. A total of 65.1% of the surgeons reported that they reinforced the staple-line of the gastric tube; of these, 50.9% over-sew the staple line, 42.1% use a buttress on the staple line, and 7.0% do both, depending on the circumstances (e.g., a figure-of-eight stitch where each buttress meets).

6. Nearly two thirds (64.1%) leave a drain, with 93.2% of these using a closed-suction (Blake/Jackson–Pratt) and 6.8% using a Penrose drain.

 CONCLUSIONS

LSG is rapidly gaining popularity as a primary, staged, and revisional operation for its proven safety, as well as short-term and midterm efficacy. It is a safe procedure with less short- and long-term morbidity, as well as negligible mortality when compared with other well-established operations. It is technically a simple operation, and it causes satisfactory weight loss along with resolution and/or improvement of comorbidities.

There are still important questions that remain unanswered. What will the future of LSG look like? Will LSG replace any of the current procedures such as LAGB? Will the long-term results be superior or equivalent to the current procedures endorsed by CMS and American Society for Metabolic and Bariatric Surgery?

LSG has clearly been demonstrated to be a safe and efficacious procedure in the treatment of morbid obesity. The most compelling argument that is positioning this procedure as superior to the current options is the lack of long-term complications. The difference in morbidity is significant when comparing the long-term follow-up of LSG to RYGB and LAGB. Currently, several new laparoscopic and endoscopic approaches, such as gastric imbrication, gastroplasties, balloons, and removable devices, are being tested under US FDA supervision. We hope that they may provide a better and less invasive option for weight loss and resolution of comorbidities than the current surgical approaches. However, it is too early to predict the efficacy and safety of these new procedures when implemented in clinical practice.

Recommended References and Readings

Abu-Jaish W, Rosenthal RJ. Sleeve gastrectomy: A new surgical approach for morbid obesity. *Expert Rev Gastroenterol Hepatol.* 2010;4(1):101–119.

Akkary E, Duffy A, Bell R. Deciphering the sleeve: Technique, indications, efficacy, and safety of sleeve gastrectomy. *Obes Surg.* 2008;18(10):1323–1329.

Brethauer SA, Hammel J, Schauer PR. Systematic review of sleeve gastrectomy as a staging and primary bariatric operation. *Surg Obes Relat Dis.* 2009;5:469–475.

Broglio F, Koetsveld PV, Benso A, et al. Ghrelin secretion is inhibited by either somatostatin or cortistatin in humans. *J Clin Endocrinol Metab.* 2002;87:4829–4832.

Chousleb E, Szomstein S, Podkameni D, et al. Routine abdominal drains after laparoscopic Roux-en-Y gastric bypass: A retrospective review of 593 patients. *Obes Surg.* 2004;14:1203–1207.

Clinical Issues Committee of the ASMBS. Updated position statement on sleeve gastrectomy as a bariatric procedure. *Surg Obes Relat Dis.* 2010;6:1–5.

Consten EC, Gagner M, Pomp A, et al. Decreased bleeding after laparoscopic sleeve gastrectomy with or without duodena switch for morbid obesity using a stapled buttressed absorbable polymer membrane. *Obes Surg.* 2004;14(10):1360–1366.

Croce E, Olmi S. Chirurgia del reflusso gastroesofageo UTET, Torino, 2006, p. 18.

Dallal RM, Mattar SG, Lord JL, et al. Results of laparoscopic gastric bypass in patients with cirrhosis. *Obes Surg.* 2004;14(1):47–53.

Dapri G, Cadie`re GB, Himpens J. Reinforcing the staple line during laparoscopic sleeve gastrectomy: Prospective randomized clinical study comparing three different techniques. *Obes Surg.* 2010;20(4):462–467

Deitel M, Crosby RD, Gagner M. The First International Consensus Summit for Sleeve Gastrectomy (SG), New York City, October 25–27, 2007. *Obes Surg.* 2008;18:487–96.

Frezza EE. Are we closer in finding the treatment for Type II diabetes mellitus in morbid obesity – are the incretins the key to success? *Obes Surg.* 2004;14(7):999–1005.

Frezza EE. Laparoscopic vertical sleeve gastrectomy for morbid obesity. The future procedure of choice? *Surg Today.* 2007;37:275–281.

Frezza EE, Wachtel MS, Chiriva-Internati M. The multiple faces of glucagon-like peptide 1-obesity, appetite, and stress: What is next? A Review. *Dig Dis Sci.* 2007;52(3):643–649.

Fris RJ. Preoperative low energy diet diminishes liver size. *Obes Surg.* 2004;114:1165–1170.

Gagner M, Deitel M, Kalberer TL, et al. The Second International Consensus Summit for sleeve gastrectomy, March 19 21, 2009. *Surg Obes Relat Dis.* 2009;5:476–85.

Karamanakos SN, Vagenas K, Kalfarentzos F, et al. Weight loss, appetite suppression, and changes in fasting and postprandial ghrelin and peptide-YY levels after Roux-en-Y gastric bypass and sleeve gastrectomy: A prospective, double blind study. *Ann Surg.* 2008;247(3):408–410.

Livingston EH, Huerta S, Arthur D, et al. Male gender is a predictor of morbidity and age a predictor of mortality for patients undergoing gastric bypass surgery. *Ann Surg.* 2002;236:576–582.

Meier JJ, Gallwitz B, Schmidt WE, et al. Glucagon-like peptide 1 as a regulator of food intake and body weight: Therapeutic perspectives. *Eur J Pharmacol.* 2002;440:269–279.

National Institutes of Health. Gastrointestinal surgery for severe obesity. *NIH Consens Statement.* 1991;9(1):1–20.

Norrelund H, Hansen TK, Orskov H, et al. Ghrelin immunoreactivity in human plasma is suppressed by somatostatin. *Clin Endocrinol.* 2002;57:539–546.

Peterli R, Wölnerhanssen B, Peters T, et al. Improvement in glucose metabolism after bariatric surgery: comparison of laparoscopic Roux-en-Y gastric bypass and laparoscopic sleeve gastrectomy: A prospective randomized trial. *Ann Surg.* 2009;250(2):234–241.

Ramos AC, Zundel N, Neto MG, et al. Human hybrid NOTES transvaginal sleeve gastrectomy: Initial experience. *Surg Obes Relat Dis.* 2008;4:660–663.

Saber AA, El-Ghazaly TH, Dewoolkar AV, et al. Single-incision laparoscopic sleeve gastrectomy versus conventional multiport laparoscopic sleeve gastrectomy: Technical considerations and strategic modifications. *Surg Obes Relat Dis.* 2010;6: 658–664.

Schauer PR, Ikramuddin S, Gourash W, et al. Outcomes after laparoscopic Roux-en-Y gastric bypass for morbid obesity. *Ann Surg.* 2000;232(4):515–529.

Suzuki K, Prates JC, DiDio LJ. Incidence and surgical importance of the posterior gastric artery. *Ann Surg.* 1978;187(2):134–136.

Szomstein S, Arias F, Rosenthal RJ. How we do laparoscopic sleeve gastrectomy. *Contemp Surg.* 2008;64(3):126–130.

Tucker O, Szomstein S, Rosenthal R. Indications for sleeve gastrectomy as a primary procedure for weight loss in the morbidly obese. *J Gastrointest Surg.* 2008;12:662–667.

Yehoshua RT, Eidelman LA, Stein M, et al. Laparoscopic sleeve gastrectomy-volume and pressure assessment. *Obes Surg.* 2008; 18(9):1083–1088.

31 Laparoscopic Adjustable Gastric Banding

Ninh T. Nguyen and Brian R. Smith

 ## INDICATIONS AND CONTRAINDICATIONS

In 1991, the National Institutes of Health Consensus Development Conference established the current indications for bariatric surgery which have remained in effect since that time. These guidelines recommend bariatric surgery for the following patients:

- Acceptable operative risks, well-informed and motivated
- Evaluated by a multidisciplinary team
- Failure of established weight control programs
- Body mass index (BMI) ≥ 40 or ≥ 35 with at least one high-risk, obesity-related comorbid condition

The prominent obesity-related comorbid conditions include hypertension, type 2 diabetes, dyslipidemia, obstructive sleep apnea, cardiomyopathy, and pseudotumor cerebri. Other common obesity-related comorbidities include gastroesophageal reflux, osteoarthritis, infertility, cholelithiasis, venous stasis, and urinary stress incontinence. With a large body of evidence supporting the efficacy of bariatric surgery in ameliorating the above comorbidities, debate over the role of bariatric surgery specifically to treat these conditions, more than the obesity, has begun. In February 2011, the FDA approved the expanded use of the Lap-Band (Allergan Inc., Irvine, CA, USA) for adults with obesity who have failed more conservative weight reduction alternatives and have a BMI of 30 to 40 with at least one obesity-related comorbid condition.

Relative contraindications to bariatric surgery include the following:

- Alcohol or drug dependence
- Ongoing smoking
- Uncontrolled psychiatric disorders such as depression or schizophrenia
- Untreated, severe underlying psychiatric disorders, specifically depression and schizophrenia.
- Inability to comprehend the requirements for postoperative nutritional and behavioral changes
- Unacceptable cardiorespiratory risk (American Society of Anesthesiologists class IV)
- End-stage hepatic disease

The patients best suited for gastric band placement are those who have less weight to lose (BMI < 40), are willing to exercise regularly, and those willing to significantly change their eating habits. Patients who tend to take-in high-calorie foods or those who graze continuously throughout the day are less well suited to gastric banding, as are those unable to perform regular exercise to augment the dietary restriction or those who live far enough from their surgeon to preclude regular band adjustments.

PREOPERATIVE PLANNING

Patients preparing for laparoscopic adjustable gastric banding (LAGB) require both pre-operative medical evaluation as well as optimization prior to surgery. Medical clearance requires a comprehensive and thorough review of the patient's medical history, specifically looking for factors which can predict an adverse outcome. Independent predictors of surgical morbidity and mortality include age ≥45 years, male gender, BMI ≥50 kg/m^2, risk for pulmonary embolism, and hypertension. Collectively, these clinical findings can be used to calculate Obesity Surgery Mortality Risk Score which has been validated at multiple institutions. Patients with 0 or 1 comorbidity are considered low risk or class A with a 0.2% risk of mortality. Those in class B have two or three comorbidities and are at intermediate risk of 1.2%. Class C patients are highest risk and have four or five comorbidities with a corresponding mortality of 2.4%. BMI ≥ 50 kg/m^2 and cigarette smoking have also been shown to be associated with higher postoperative surgical morbidities. Basic preoperative work-up should include the following:

- Comprehensive history and physical
- 12-lead EKG
- Basic blood chemistries, lipid profile, and nutritional panel
- Chest radiograph

The choice of operation for a particular patient must take into account several issues including patient's preference, surgeon's expertise, BMI, patient's metabolic conditions, and other associated comorbidities. While gastric bypass is largely considered the most effective procedure at achieving long-term weight loss, it is also the most effective at reducing the metabolic derangements of obesity, including diabetes, hypertension, and dyslipidemia. However, these benefits come with a slightly higher overall mortality rate. For gastric bypass, average 30-day mortality is 0.16%, compared with that of LAGB placement at 0.06%. For this reason, high-risk patients, including older patients with more comorbidities, should be counseled with regards to the perioperative risks between gastric bypass and LAGB.

The benefit of preoperative weight loss prior to bariatric surgery has been debated. A recent randomized trial demonstrated that patients who achieve ≥5% excess body weight loss (EBWL) prior to surgery had significantly lower weight and BMI and a higher EBWL at 1 year. The success of preoperative weight loss is felt to predict patients with the discipline and willingness to follow a healthy lifestyle that will ultimately translate to sustained long-term weight loss. As a result, many surgeons will place patients on one of many available forms of preoperative weight loss diet for 2 to 4 weeks prior to surgery, with a goal of 5% to 10% EBWL. Many forms of commercial dietary programs are available for these purposes, often consisting of a high-protein, low-fat, low-carbohydrate, predominately liquid diet. An additional benefit of this preoperative liquid diet is decreased liver size and density which makes manipulation of the left lobe of the liver easier during surgery.

SURGICAL PROCEDURE

All patients should receive routine deep venous thrombosis (DVT) chemoprophylaxis immediately prior to arrival in the operating room, as initial development of DVT is felt to occur intraoperatively in this high-risk population. In addition, sequential compression device is placed prior to anesthetic induction. Routine preoperative antibiotic prophylaxis is also indicated. A second-generation cephalosporin is adequate but typically requires increased dosing in morbidly obese patients. There are two adjustable gastric bands currently on the market, including the Lap-Band™ (Allergan Inc., Irvine, CA, USA) and the Realize® Band (Ethicon Endo-Surgery, Cincinnati, OH, USA). Regardless of which band is implanted, it is advisable to have a second band available for backup at the time of surgery in the event that one is contaminated or damaged at the time of implantation. Each band also has a separately packaged replacement port available as a stand-alone when necessary.

Patient Positioning

Patient positioning is often dictated by surgeon's preference. Some surgeons prefer the French or lithotomy position. The main advantage of this position is access in between the patient's legs and inline trajectory of one's laparoscopic instruments. This centers the surgeon over the operative field and improves posture while minimizing shoulder fatigue. However, this position can be difficult and time consuming and places patients at risk for nerve injury if not positioned properly. Most surgeons have evolved to a completely supine position with arms outstretched on and secured to arm boards. For LAGB placement, supine positioning is recommended. A footboard is also recommended to minimize patient slippage inferiorly during reverse Trendelenburg positioning, as is an upper thigh strap to minimize lateral slippage during rotation of the patient. All bolsters placed behind the patient's neck and/or shoulders by anesthesia to facilitate endotracheal intubation should be removed prior to initiation of surgery. A Foley catheter is optional. Routine cardiac noninvasive monitoring is essential. Invasive monitoring, including arterial and central venous catheters, is not routinely indicated and is only utilized in selected cases where such additional monitoring is necessary.

Technique

Standard technique includes a five-trocar configuration (Fig. 31.1). Initial cannulation of the abdominal cavity with Veress needle is typically through the camera port, located

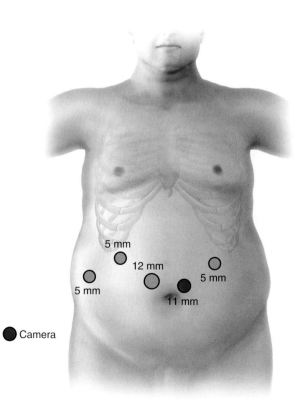

Figure 31.1 Port placement for laparoscopic adjustable gastric banding.

5 mm

12 mm

5 mm

5 mm

11 mm

● Camera

in the left supraumbilical region. Upon insufflation to 15 mm Hg, the Veress is removed and a 15-mm trocar is inserted followed by camera confirmation of no visceral injury from entry. Subsequent 5-mm trocars are placed in the far left and right subcostal margins just above the viscera, along with right epigastric (12 mm) and right upper quadrant (5 mm) trocars. The far right subcostal trocar secures a serpentine liver retractor for anterior retraction of the left lobe of the liver. Alternatively, the subxiphoid 5-mm trocar site can be used to accommodate a Nathanson liver retractor. The operating surgeon utilizes the epigastric and right upper quadrant trocars while the assistant utilizes the left subcostal trocar and the laparoscope.

The band is inserted through the 15-mm trocar, either utilizing a blunt grasper or specific band introducers are commercially available for intra-abdominal placement. Once the band is in the abdominal cavity, it can be placed in the left upper quadrant in preparation for placement. A small peritoneal window between the stomach and the diaphragm is dissected at the angle of His for eventual band passage. The gastrohepatic ligament is then incised with thermal energy and the right crus of the diaphragm exposed. The *pars flaccid* dissection begins immediately anterior to the base of the right crus and is initiated with thermal energy. Blunt dissection is then continued along the anterior decussation of both diaphragmatic crura which is avascular. A tunnel is created between the crura and the retroesophageal fat pad. One of several commercially available 10-mm articulating band graspers is then passed through this tunnel and articulated and brought through the previously created window at the angle of His. The band is then secured to the band grasper, which is un-articulated and withdrawn through the tunnel, drawing the band around the gastric cardia. The band is then disconnected from the band grasper and the tubing may need to be drawn through the buckle prior to closure, depending on the brand (Fig. 31.2). The band is then closed over the cardia using the buckle attached to the band (Fig. 31.3). Gastric plication of the body to the cardia to cover the band anteriorly is then performed with several interrupted sutures (Fig. 31.4). This plication, along with the pars flaccida approach posteriorly, serves to discourage band slippage. Another plication suture is also placed on the medial aspect of the gastric cardia, immediately below the band to minimize the risk for slippage.

The band tubing is then grasped and brought out to the 15-mm port site, taking great care to avoid abrupt angles upon exit through the fascia. The 15-mm port site is then closed utilizing a suture passing device, and a pocket in the subcutaneous tissue is created to accommodate the port. The suture tails of the fascia closure can be saved to secure the port to the fascia. Band tubing is then shortened to appropriate length and connected to the saline-flushed port, again taking great care to avoid abrupt angles or redundancy in the tubing. The port is then secured to the fascia with the previous suture tails or with a commercially available securing device, which comes with the

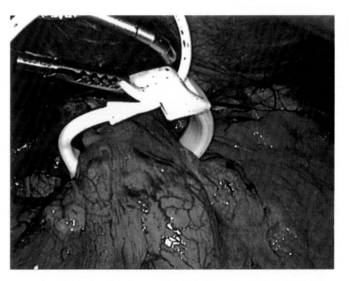

Figure 31.2 Placement of adjustable gastric band using the pars flaccid approach.

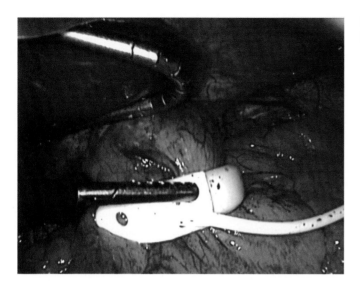

Figure 31.3 Closure of the adjustable gastric band.

Realize band. Soft tissue is closed over the port, followed by skin closure. All instruments and trocars are then removed and closure of the 12-mm port site is optional at the surgeon's discretion. Port sites are then closed at the skin level.

 POSTOPERATIVE MANAGEMENT

Patients without significant cardiac issues can be transferred to a ward bed. Cases where continuous monitoring may be indicated postoperatively include a significant cardiac history, any intraoperative cardiorespiratory issues, or severe obstructive sleep apnea. Higher-risk patients are admitted for overnight observation while lower-risk patients can be discharged on an ambulatory basis. Patients begin a diet of sugar-free clear liquids on the evening of the surgery. Ambulation also begins on the evening of surgery. Medication adjustments are vital, particularly in diabetic patients, and must take place immediately postoperatively. While each patient must be individualized, often utilizing half of the patient's preoperative dose of diabetic medications serves as an appropriate starting point after surgery.

Diet is advanced to sugar-free full liquids upon discharge for the first 2 weeks postoperatively. Patients are then transitioned to pureed diet, soft foods, and finally a modified regular diet over the ensuing 6 weeks. Postoperatively, patients are counseled

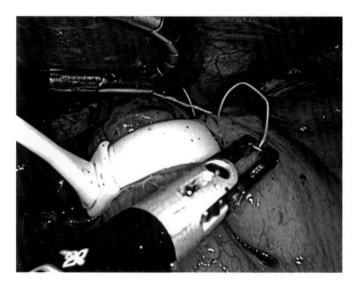

Figure 31.4 Placement of anterior gastrogastric sutures to minimize postoperative slippage.

regarding appropriate behavioral and dietary changes. Overall dietary guidelines include routine low-calorie, low-fat, and low-sugar food intake. Patients are encouraged to take in three small meals per day with healthy snacks in between and to eat slowly, stopping at the first sign of feeling full. Specific efforts at protein intake at each meal are encouraged. Patients are counseled to take eight 8-ounce cups of water daily and should avoid taking beverages concurrently with meals. Carbonated beverages result in gas expansion of the small gastric pouch that lead to significant discomfort and hence should be avoided. Vitamin and mineral supplementation is essential to avoid deficiencies in vitamins A, D, B1, B6, B12, calcium, and folate. As banding is not a malabsorptive procedure, these deficiencies are less pronounced yet not entirely absent, predominately due to dietary restrictions encouraged after surgery. As such, a daily multivitamin is usually adequate for most LAGB patients. Routine daily physical activity is encouraged, and participation in monthly bariatric support groups has been shown to result in significantly improved and sustained weight loss. Postoperative follow-up typically occurs at 1 week, 1, 3, 6, 9, and 12 months, and then every 4 months thereafter. Evaluation for late complications, behavioral counseling, and monitoring for nutritional deficiencies are the main goals of these routine visits.

Band adjustments are the hallmark of progressive weight loss. The first band adjustment typically takes place beyond 4 weeks postoperatively, as the majority of wound healing has taken place by that time. In addition, the band usually provides adequate restriction upon placement, and only after several weeks of weight loss does the band become sufficiently loose to require adjustment to augment restriction. Adjustments are office-based procedures and can be done with or without fluoroscopic guidance. A long Huber needle is used to access the subcutaneous port with the port pinned between the fingers of the opposite hand. Local anesthetic is not indicated. It is recommended that all fluid in the band be completely aspirated with each adjustment prior to infusion in order to ensure accuracy of the adjustment. Addition of fluid typically ranges between 0.5 and 1 mL of saline per adjustment, depending on the brand of band. Older bands had smaller reservoirs, requiring adjustments ranging from 0.1 to 0.5 mL. Alternatively, adjustments can be performed under direct fluoroscopic imaging to visualize the amount of desired restriction based on contrast retention and passage through the adjusted band. The authors find this unnecessary and cumbersome, but the practice is common in certain practices.

 COMPLICATIONS

Complications after LAGB placement range from those that are perioperative, to late complications, to eventual band explantation. Relatively low perioperative complications rates range from 2.3% to 2.8% and largely account for the good safety profile of LABG. These complications tend to include those issues related more to obesity and major surgery than to the band itself. They include pulmonary complications, wound infections, venous thromboembolism (VTE), postoperative hemorrhage, and band failure/leak, each with a rate less than 1%. The most common late complication after LAGB remains prolapse/slippage (Fig. 31.5), occurring in approximately 3% of patients. This rate has decreased in recent years with adoption of the pars flaccida technique and gastric plication over the band anteriorly, decreasing the posterior and anterior prolapsed rates, respectively. Band erosion occurs in 1% to 2% of patients and rarely causes significant morbidity. This process occurs slowly over time and often presents with a port infection as the herald sign. As the band erodes through the wall of the stomach, the serosa typically heals over the band, preventing leakage of gastric contents but permitting luminal infection to ascend along the tubing and eventually infect the port. Band removal is indicated once erosion is discovered. Port and tubing problems, including port inversion or kinking of the tube, can be as high as 4% at 5 years. Correction of these problems is often a local procedure.

The most common indications for band explantation include band slippage, pouch dilation, gastric inlet obstruction (Fig. 31.6), band erosion, and inadequate weight loss. In a prospective multicenter trial, band removal rates due to slippage and pouch dilation

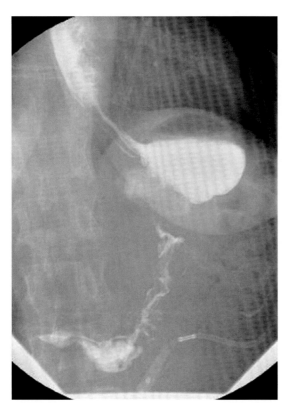

Figure 31.5 Upper gastrointestinal contrast study demonstrating band slippage. Note the horizontal plane of the band. A normal band should reside at a 30° angle from the horizontal plane on an AP film.

(5.3%), obstruction (4.6%), inadequate weight loss (3.5%), and erosion (1%) as well as other conditions (3.5%) totaled 18% of the patients within 5 years. Rates of band removal in other studies have been similar, ranging from 1.4% to 5.8%. Most complications from LAGB are not life-threatening, making this the operation of choice when patient comorbidities serve as a deterrent to the more risky gastric sleeve or bypass. Mortality rates have been consistently low at 0.01%.

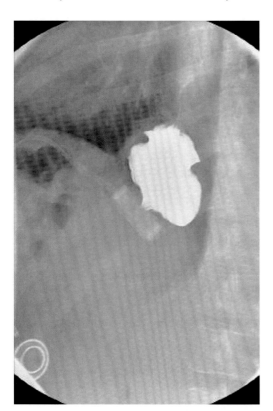

Figure 31.6 Band obstruction despite complete evacuation of all fluid from the band.

Weight Loss Outcomes

Bariatric surgery has been shown repeatedly to be the most definitive and successful treatment for severe obesity compared to conventional medical therapy. Lifetime risk of death from extreme obesity is decreased by 35% in individuals who undergo bariatric surgery compared to control individuals. However, the safety of bariatric surgery has come under increasing scrutiny since the early part of this century. Bariatric Centers of Excellence were developed by the American College of Surgeons and the American Society of Metabolic and Bariatric Surgery, and many insurance carriers have followed by only covering bariatric surgery performed at these centers. The Leapfrog Group has added bariatric surgery to the growing list of procedures with improved mortality when performed at high-volume centers (>125 annual cases).

LAGB has consistently yielded the lowest EBWL percentages of all bariatric operative procedures. A recent randomized controlled trial comparing gastric bypass to LAGB revealed a 41.8% EBWL at 2 years and 45.4% at 4 years. The same trial also revealed statistically better EBWL in those patients with BMI less than 50 kg/m^2 compared to those whose preoperative BMI was above 50 kg/m^2, suggesting LAGB is not ideal for the larger super morbidly obese. These results were consistent with another prospective randomized trial between the two different band devices available. In this trial, those patients with preoperative EBW < 50 kg had a better postoperative weight loss at 2 years (55% EBWL) compared to larger patients with EBW > 50 kg (44%; $P = .004$). These two studies provide evidence to help counsel super obese and larger patients away from LAGB and toward a more invasive procedure such as sleeve gastrectomy and gastric bypass. Other studies have demonstrated EBWL closer to 50% at 1 year.

Improvement in obesity-related medical comorbidities has been shown to be similar to other weight loss procedures. However, results tend to be more time (and hence weight loss) dependent than with gastric bypass. Predictors of poor weight loss and/or failure, defined by either conversion to another procedure or < 20% EBWL at 4 years postoperatively, included male sex for those undergoing LABG. Overall failure rate in the randomized trial was 16.7% at 4 years for LAGB. The FDA) recently approved the Lap Band for use in patients with BMI ≥ 30 and at least one obesity-related medical comorbidity. This approval represents the first formal US government movement toward expansion of surgery to patients with a lower BMI for the treatment of both obesity and the concomitant comorbidities.

CONCLUSIONS

Of the standard bariatric operations currently available and widely covered by insurance, gastric banding remains the safest and second most commonly performed operation. However, such safety is traded for the lower long-term weight loss outcomes of the standard operations currently being performed. Morbidity of gastric banding has been largely overcome with improved techniques of surgery and adjusting the band. It appears that males are more likely to fail with LAGB as are the super obese. However, with the FDA lowering the BMI threshold recently for band placement to 30, bands will likely continue to play an integral role in the bariatric surgery lineup as the entry-level operation for the foreseeable future.

Recommended References and Readings

Buchwald H, Avidor Y, Braunwald E, et al. Bariatric surgery: A systematic review and meta-analysis. *JAMA.* 2004;292:1724–1737.

Buchwald H, Estok R, Fahrbach K, et al. Trends in mortality in bariatric surgery: A systematic review and meta-analysis. *Surgery.* 2007;142:621–632.

Buchwald H, Estok R, Fahrbach K, et al. Weight and type 2 diabetes after bariatric surgery: Systematic review and meta-analysis. *Am J Med.* 2009;122:248–256.

Gravante G, Araco A, Araco F, et al. Laparoscopic adjustable gastric bandings: A prospective randomized study of 400 operations performed with 2 different devices. *Arch Surg.* 2007;142:958–961.

Hinojosa MW, Varela JE, Parikh D, et al. National trends in use and outcome of laparoscopic adjustable gastric banding. *Surg Obes Relat Dis.* 2009;5:150–155.

Livingston EH, Langert J. The impact of age and Medicare status on bariatric surgical outcomes. *Arch Surg.* 2006;141:1115–1120.

Martin LF, Smits GJ, Greenstein RJ. Treating morbid obesity with laparoscopic adjustable gastric banding. *Am J Surg.* 2007;194:333–343.

Mechanick JI, Kushner RF, Sugerman JH, et al. American Association of Clinical Endocrinologists, the Obesity Society, and American Society for Metabolic & Bariatric Surgery medical guidelines for clinical practice for the perioperative nutritional, metabolic, and nonsurgical support of the bariatric surgery patient. *Endocr Pract.* 2008;14(S1):1–83.

Nguyen NT, Slone JA, Nguyen XT, et al. A prospective randomized trial of laparoscopic gastric bypass versus laparoscopic adjustable gastric banding for the treatment of morbid obesity; Outcomes, quality of life, and costs. *Ann Surg.* 2009; 250:631–641.

Pories WJ, Swanson MS, MacDonald KG, et al. Who would have thought it? An operation proves to be the most effective therapy for adult-onset diabetes mellitus. *Ann Surg.* 1995;222:339–352.

Rubino F, Kaplan LM, Schauer PR, et al. The diabetes surgery summit consensus conference. Recommendations for the evaluation and use of gastrointestinal surgery to treat type 2 diabetes mellitus. *Ann Surg.* 2010;251:399–405

Sjostrom L, Lindroos AK, Peltonen M, et al. Lifestyle, diabetes, and cardiovascular risk factors 10 years after bariatric surgery. *N Engl J Med.* 2004;351:2683–2693.

Part IV: Bariatric

32 Robot-assisted Laparoscopic Biliopancreatic Diversion with Duodenal Switch

Ranjan Sudan

 ## INDICATIONS/CONTRAINDICATIONS

The biliopancreatic diversion with duodenal switch (BPD/DS) has more weight loss, but it is technically complex and has more malabsorptive side effects than the other bariatric operations. The first BPD/DS was performed by Hess in 1988 and is a modification of the original biliopancreatic diversion (BPD) described by Scopinaro. In the BPD/DS, a sleeve gastrectomy is performed and the pylorus is preserved. This modification is associated with reduced dumping, marginal ulcerations, diarrhea, and protein malnutrition compared to the Scopinaro operation. The first laparoscopic BPD/DS in humans was described in 2000, and the same year the first robot-assisted procedure was performed. While any patient with morbid obesity with a body mass index (BMI) of more than 40 kg/m^2 or more than 35 kg/m^2 with comorbid medical conditions may be a candidate for a BPD/DS, those with severe diabetes, severe hypercholesterolemia, or higher BMI may benefit more with the BPD/DS than other bariatric operations. It is also a good option for revisions from a previous failed restrictive operation such as a laparoscopic adjustable gastric band, a sleeve gastrectomy, or a vertical banded gastroplasty. Compliance with diet and micronutrient intake as well as lifestyle modification, and regular follow-up to monitor for vitamin deficiencies, will give the best results. Contraindications for a BPD/DS are those for any bariatric operation such as unacceptable anesthetic risk or unresolved psychological issues, but more specifically those medical conditions in which a malabsorptive procedure is contraindicated such as Crohn's disease or end-stage liver disease.

 ## PREOPERATIVE PLANNING

Detailed clinical history and physical examination helps detect co-existing medical problems and guides further investigations such as cardiac echography, sleep apnea studies, and pulmonary evaluations. Suitable medical consultations are obtained on the basis of individual assessment of the patient to optimize their health prior to surgery. Routine laboratory investigations include a comprehensive metabolic panel, hemogram, thyroid tests, HbA1c, lipid profile, and vitamin levels. Electrocardiograms and chest radiographs are also obtained. Nutritional deficiencies are easier to correct in patients prior to their undergoing a malabsorptive operation. Patients are also asked to update their screening mammograms, Papanicolaou's smears, and colonoscopy, as indicated for cancer screening.

In addition, all patients undergo psychological and nutritional evaluations to assess their understanding of the lifestyle changes that are necessary for the success of a bariatric operation, ability to comply with medical instructions, rule out untreated psychiatric disorders or addictions and maladaptive eating behaviors.

 ## SURGICAL TECHNIQUE

Pertinent Anatomy

In order to perform the sleeve gastrectomy and the duodenal switch, it is necessary to recognize the location of the pylorus and the gastroduodenal artery. The pylorus is thicker, has a slightly more pale appearance and is identified by the overlying vein of Mayo. The gastroduodenal artery lies posterior to the first part of the duodenum and provides a useful landmark where the first part of the duodenum is transected.

Identifying the incisure is important to avoid narrowing the stomach tube when performing the sleeve gastrectomy. The lesser sac is entered across from the incisure near the greater curvature of the stomach. By keeping the dissection close to the stomach, the gastroepiploic vessels are preserved, avoiding excessive bleeding. The gastrosplenic ligament is also thin in this location, facilitating division with an ultrasonic dissector. To prevent a delayed perforation of the stomach, transmission of thermal energy near the gastroesophageal junction is avoided when dividing the proximal short gastric vessels.

The ileocecal valve is an important landmark because the bowel is measured and marked from it in order to create the distal anastomosis.

Positioning

The patient is placed supine with the right arm by the patient's side. The left arm is placed on an arm board and can be extended to provide the operating surgeon with standing room by the patient's side, and the anesthesiologist sufficient access for intravenous lines and other monitoring devices, as needed. The extremities are suitably padded and protected to prevent pressure sores or a neuropathy. A Foley catheter is placed, but it is not necessary to place routine arterial catheters. The endotracheal tube is positioned with a low profile, ensuring an adequate distance between the operating table and the anesthetic cart, to allow the robot to be brought in over the patient's right shoulder. A thermal blanket is used on the lower body so that it does not interfere with the operation.

There are three phases of the operation, and the operating team changes its position in relationship to the patient in each phase. At the beginning of the operation, the team stands near the head of the patient and face toward the patient's feet. The surgeon is to the patient's left, the camera operator is in the middle, and the assistant is to the right. During this phase, the distal ileoileal anastomosis is performed, and an appendectomy is optional.

In the second phase of the operation, the team moves to the patient's side and face toward the patient's head. The camera operator and surgeon are on the patient's left while the assistant is on the patient's right. During this phase of the operation, the sleeve gastrectomy, division of the duodenum, and placement of the alimentary limb in a retrocolic position is completed. Many surgeons will also elect to perform a cholecystectomy in this phase.

In the last phase, the operating surgeon moves to the robotic console from where the robotic arms and the camera are controlled, and the assistant moves to the patient's left side.

Technique

Pneumoperitoneum is obtained using a left upper quadrant Veress needle and the abdomen is entered in the midline, about 15 cm inferior to the xiphoid, using a 12 mm optical trocar, and a zero-degree scope. Additional clear non-cutting trocars are positioned in the anterior and midclavicular lines as shown in Figure 32.1. All port sites are pre-injected with a local anesthetic.

The operation is divided into three major phases as outlined above:

Phase 1

With the patient in Trendelenburg position and tilted to the left, the team stands near the patient's head and identifies the ileocecal valve to perform the ileoileal anastomosis, and an optional appendectomy.

If the surgeon decides to perform an appendectomy, a 2.5 mm leg-length stapler load is used to divide the base of the appendix, and its mesentery is divided close to the appendix to facilitate its removal from one of the ports.

In order to perform the ileoileal anastomosis, marking sutures are placed at 100 cm and 250 cm from the ileocecal valve (Fig. 32.2). The bowel is divided 250 cm proximal to the ileocecal valve with a 2.5 mm leg-length stapler and the mesentery is divided using the ultrasonic dissector. A two-inch piece of blue drain (non-latex sterile tourniquet) is attached to the stapled edge of the alimentary limb to facilitate its subsequent passage through the retrocolic tunnel.

The distal ileoileal anastomosis is performed by making small enterotomies at the 100 cm mark on the common channel and near the stapled edge of the biliary limb (Fig. 32.3). A 60 mm long staple load with 2.5 mm leg-length is used to create the side-to-side anastomosis. The enterotomy is closed with intra-corporeal suturing to prevent narrowing of bowel.

Figure 32.1 Trocar placement.

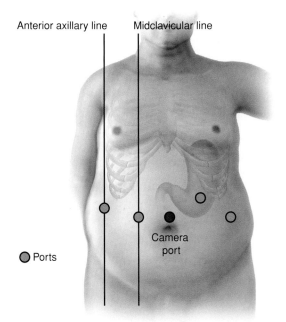

Anterior axillary line   Midclavicular line

Camera port

⬤ Ports

Figure 32.2 Marking sutures are placed at 100 cm and 250 cm from the ileocecal valve.

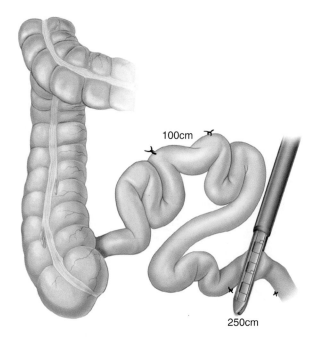

The mesenteric defect between the biliary limb and the common channel is closed with a running permanent 2-0 suture.

Phase 2

With the patient placed in steep reverse-Trendelenburg position, the Nathanson liver retractor is inserted just to the left of the xiphoid and is used to elevate the liver. The falciform ligament may need to be divided or sutured to the anterior abdominal wall if it obscures visualization.

This phase begins with a cholecystectomy. The cystic duct and artery are dissected, double clipped proximally, and single clipped distally before dividing. The gallbladder is taken off the liver bed by using cautery or ultrasonic dissectors and placed in an

Figure 32.3 The distal ileoileal anastomosis is performed by making small enterotomies at the 100 cm mark on the common channel and near the stapled edge of the biliary limb.

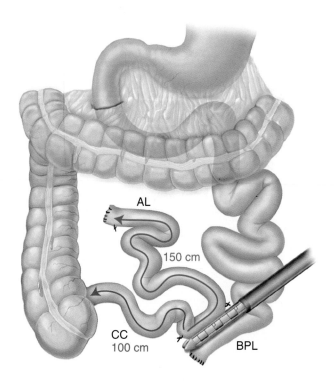

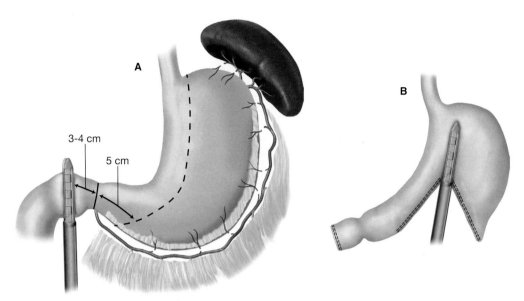

A

3-4 cm

5 cm

B

Figure 32.4 The greater curvature of the stomach is mobilized to about 4 cm distal to the pylorus, and the duodenum is divided using 3.5 mm leg-length stapler load. The sleeve gastrectomy starts 5 cm proximal to the pylorus.

endobag for retrieval later. The gallbladder may also be left in place for later removal with the help of the robot in phase three.

Next, the lesser sac is entered across from the incisure, near the greater curvature of the stomach. The greater curvature of the stomach is then mobilized to about 4 cm distal to the pylorus, and the duodenum is divided using a 3.5 mm leg-length stapler load (Fig. 32.4). In order to position the stapler in this location, a window is created on the superior aspect of the duodenum, using a right angle clamp. The areolar tissue overlying the second part of the duodenum, where it turns to become the third part, is cleared to facilitate the retrocolic passage of the alimentary limb.

The rest of the greater curvature of the stomach is then mobilized to the angle of His using the ultrasonic dissector. After completing the division of all of the short gastric vessels, the sleeve gastrectomy is performed by dividing the stomach about 5 cm proximal to the pylorus. This part of the stomach is thick and at least 4.5 mm leg-length staples are used for the Initial two firings. Using a 45 mm long stapler cartridges makes it is easier to create a smooth curve so that there is no encroachment of the stomach lumen toward the incisure. After the first two cartridges are fired, the rest of the stomach is divided using 3.5 mm leg-length, 60 mm long stapler cartridges with the intent to create a 150 to 250 mL stomach tube. An Allergan® sizing tube is used as a guide to size the stomach pouch and can be used to insufflate the stomach with methylene blue to check for leaks. After the stomach is resected, a long suture is secured to one of the ends on the specimen to facilitate its removal at the end of the operation. The staple lines may be reinforced with buttress material or suture, particularly if the stomach is thick or the integrity of the staple line is in question. Bleeding along the staple line can easily be controlled with hemoclips. The patient is next taken out of the steep reverse Trendelenburg position, and the omentum is elevated to create a window in the transverse mesocolon. A blunt grasper or the ultrasonic dissector can be used to open the transverse mesocolon. Using the blue tubing as a handle, the alimentary limb is delivered through a retrocolic tunnel to the first portion of the duodenum where it is anchored to the proximal duodenum with a stay suture. The robot is then engaged in position to perform the duodenoileostomy.

Phase 3

The robot is brought over the patient's right shoulder and the robotic camera is inserted through the umbilical port. The robotic instrument ports are inserted using a cannula-in-cannula technique in the right anterior axillary, right midclavicular, and left midclavicular ports. A grasper in the right anterior axillary line port is used to retract the stay

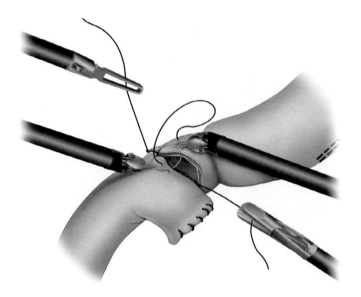

suture and help align the bowel for suturing. Two robotic needle drivers are then brought in from the remaining robotic ports and used to perform a two-layer robot-sewn anastomosis (Fig. 32.5). First, the posterior seromuscular row is completed using running 2-0 braided nylon suture. Next, the bowel is opened using the robotic ultrasonic dissectors and a running full-thickness posterior row of 2-0 absorbable suture is placed and then continued anteriorly to close the bowel. The placement of seromuscular anterior layer of sutures completes the formation of the two-layer anastomosis. Methylene blue is insufflated to check for leaks. The omentum is again lifted to identify the mesentery of the alimentary limb and close the defect between the alimentary limb mesentery and the retroperitoneum. A 2-0 permanent braided nylon is used to close this defect robotically completing the rearrangement of the bowel (Fig. 32.6). The robot is then disengaged and the gallbladder and stomach specimens are removed. Grasping the long suture attached to the stomach specimen helps retrieve it though the midline port-site. Usually, the port-site does not need to be dilated to retrieve the stomach specimen. Following the irrigation and suctioning of the right upper quadrant of the abdominal cavity, the absence of leaks is confirmed and ports are removed. The skin incisions are closed with subcuticular absorbable suture. A drain is not placed routinely.

 POSTOPERATIVE MANAGEMENT

Patients are encouraged to ambulate early and the liberal use of incentive spirometry. Prophylactic doses of low-molecular weight heparin are used for the duration of the patient's hospital admission. A patient-controlled analgesic pump is used for pain control, and patients are given acetaminophen orally, as a scheduled dose, to reduce the need for narcotic medication. Due to the probability of gastroparesis, a liquid diet is initiated only after the patient passes flatus. Over the ensuing weeks, the diet is gradually advanced to solid foods, and supplemented with vitamins and minerals. It is important to include the water-soluble analogues of fat-soluble vitamins for BPD/DS patients.

 COMPLICATIONS

A leak may present with tachycardia, fever, and significant abdominal pain. It should be investigated radiographically or even surgically, if needed. A pulmonary embolism may develop despite prophylactic anticoagulation and is often suspected in a dyspneic

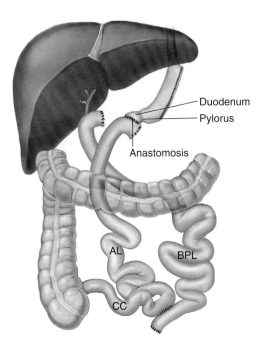

Figure 32.6 The robot is used to create the duodenoileal anastomosis and close the defect between the alimentary limb mesentery and the retroperitoneum. The orientation of the rearranged bowel is shown.

Duodenum
Pylorus
Anastomosis
AL
BPL
CC

patient. Results of blood gas results and computerized tomographic angiogram confirm the diagnosis. Superficial or deep wound infections are infrequent and may need treatment with antibiotics or drainage. Bowel obstructions or vitamin deficiencies (particularly vitamin D) can develop long term.

RESULTS

Patients lose more than 70% of their excess body weight long term, and the cure rate for diabetes type 2 is as high as 98% to 99%. Rates of resolution of other medical condition including hypertension, hypercholesterolemia, and sleep apnea are also high. Results of initial robotic BPD/DS series are available.

CONCLUSIONS

The BPD/DS is a less commonly performed but very effective bariatric operation. By using the robot, a complex bariatric procedure can be performed safely with fewer ports and easier intracorporeal suturing.

Recommended References and Readings

Aills L, Blankenship J, Buffington C, et al. ASMBS Allied Health Nutritional Guidelines for the Surgical Weight Loss Patient. *Surg Obes Relat Dis.* 2008;4(5 Suppl):S73–S108.

Hess DS, Hess DW, Oakley RS. The biliopancreatic diversion with the duodenal switch: Results beyond 10 years. *Obes Surg.* 2005; 15(3):408–416.

Marceau P, Biron S, Hould FS, et al. Duodenal switch: Long-term results. *Obes Surg.* 2007;17(11):1421–1430.

Ren CJ, Patterson E, Gagner M. Early results of laparoscopic biliopancreatic diversion with duodenal switch: A case series of 40 consecutive patients. *Obes Surg.* 2000;10(6):514–523; discussion 524.

Scopinaro N, Gianetta E, Civalleri D, et al. Bilio-pancreatic bypass for obesity: II. Initial experience in man. *Br J Surg.* 1979;66(9): 618–620.

Sudan R, Puri V, Sudan D. Robotically assisted biliary pancreatic diversion with a duodenal switch: A new technique. *Surg Endosc.* 2007;21(5):729–733.

Part IV: Bariatric

33 Single-Incision Laparoscopic Bariatric Surgery

Sunil Sharma and Alan A. Saber

 ## INDICATIONS AND CONTRAINDICATIONS

There is a growing trend toward surgical techniques that facilitate less abdominal trauma. This has the potential to complement and expand the benefits of traditional laparoscopic surgery that stems from less abdominal trauma, less postoperative pain, analgesia requirement, hospital stay, less scarring, and better cosmetic outcome.

With the emergence of natural orifice translumenal endoscopic surgery, more attention has been directed toward the single-incision transumbilical laparoscopic approach for minimally invasive surgery. Single-incision surgery brings together the cosmetic advantages of natural orifice translumenal endoscopic surgery and the familiarity of conventional laparoscopic surgery. As instruments become more flexible, along with availability of multichannel ports, the single-incision approach could represent the future direction of minimally invasive surgery.

The predetermined exclusion criteria for the single-incision bariatric approach includes patients who have undergone previous bariatric surgery, upper abdominal open surgery, or upper abdominal ventral hernia mesh repair and super-morbid obesity.

 ## PREOPERATIVE PREPARATIONS

As with any form of bariatric surgery the essential prerequisites before surgery are to attend a weight loss surgery information seminar, psychological evaluation and clearance, nutrition evaluation, medical evaluation, workup and clearance. We have found that by instructing all of our bariatric patients to consume a high-protein low-calorie liquid diet for 2 to 4 weeks before their scheduled surgery enables the liver to shrink, making its retraction more feasible. All patients should be involved in the decision-making process. They should receive a detailed description of the risks and benefits of all bariatric procedures.

Deep vein thrombosis prophylaxis is achieved using anticoagulation, compression stockings, and lower extremity sequential compression devices. Preoperative intravenous antibiotic prophylaxis is administrated before making the skin incision.

Operative Strategy and Technical Considerations

The feasibility of the single-incision approach is enhanced when tailored according to each patient's body habitus. In patients with a relatively low BMI, peripheral obesity, a small liver, and a short umbilicus–xiphoid distance, we proceed with transumbilical single incision. In addition to the cosmetic advantages of a hidden intraumbilical single incision, the umbilicus provides a safe zone for abdominal access while minimizing the torque effect of an obese patient's thick abdominal wall. In contrast, for patients with a much greater BMI, central obesity, a large liver, and a long umbilicus–subxiphoid distance, we advance the single incision toward the epigastric area.

TAP Block

The single-incision approach involves a single incision as opposed to multiple tiny incisions, scattered all over the abdomen in a standard laparoscopic operation. We take advantage of this situation by selectively blocking the nerves supplying the periumbilical area. This is achieved by ultrasound-guided transversus abdominis plane (TAP) block. When the block is performed correctly, the single incision stays relatively pain-free, thereby reducing the requirement for narcotic analgesics and enabling for a faster recovery and earlier discharge from the hospital.

Anatomy

The anterior abdominal wall (skin, muscles, parietal peritoneum) is innervated by the anterior rami of the lower six thoracic nerves (T7 to T12) and the first lumbar nerve (L1). Terminal branches of these somatic nerves course through the lateral abdominal wall within a plane between the internal oblique and transversus abdominis muscles. This intermuscular plane is called the TAP. Injection of local anesthetic within the TAP can therefore potentially provide unilateral analgesia to the skin, muscles, and parietal peritoneum of the anterior abdominal wall (Fig. 33.1).

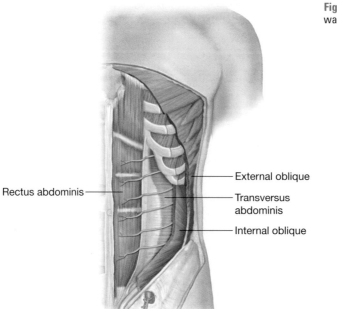

Figure 33.1 Anatomy of the abdominal wall.

Rectus abdominis

External oblique

Transversus abdominis

Internal oblique

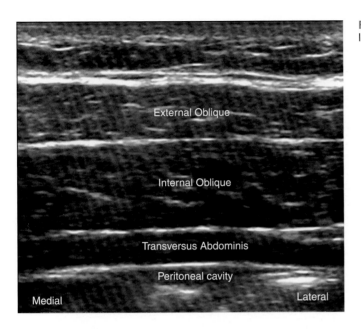

Figure 33.2 Ultrasound showing layers of the abdominal wall.

Block Technique

Scanning Technique

Ultrasound-guided TAP block:

■ Using ultrasound guidance, it is easy to identify the fascial plane between the internal oblique and the transversus abdominis muscles.
■ The patient is placed in a supine position exposing the costal margin and the iliac crest.
■ A linear, high-frequency transducer is recommended for this block.
■ After preparing the skin and transducer in sterile fashion, the transducer is placed in an axial (transverse) plane, above the iliac crest, and at the anterior axillary line.
■ The three muscular layers of the abdominal wall are identified as follows: the external oblique (most superficial), the internal oblique (most prominent), and the transversus abdominis muscles below it (Fig. 33.2). The terminal branches of the anterior rami are expected to lie within the TAP between internal oblique and the transverse abdominis muscles above the iliac crest. The peritoneal cavity lies deep to the transversus abdominis muscle layer and may be identified by the peristaltic movements of bowel loops.

Needle Insertion

■ A 120- to 150-mm 22G short beveled block needle is inserted in-plane with the transducer, in an anterior-posterior direction Alternatively, a spinal needle may be used and connected to the syringe via short extension tubing.
■ The needle is inserted some distance away from the transducer. This permits a shallower needle trajectory and improves needle shaft and tip visualization.
■ In obese patients with protuberant abdomen, manual retraction of the abdominal wall by an assistant is a useful maneuver to facilitate needle insertion.
■ Accurate placement of the needle tip may be facilitated by **"hydrodissection"** of the appropriate plane. This is achieved by injection of a small amount of fluid (1 to 2 mL of saline or local anesthetic).
■ It is important to deposit local anesthetic deep to the fascial layer that separates the internal oblique and the transversus abdominis muscles.

Local Anesthetic Injection

■ A total of 20 to 30 mL of local anesthetic (e.g., ropivacaine 0.5% to 0.75%) is injected into this plane on each side (Fig. 33.3).

Figure 33.3 Ultrasound-guided
TAP Block.

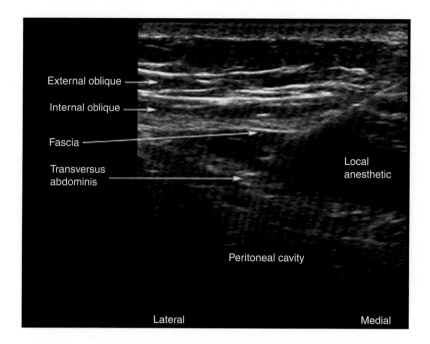

- Correct needle tip position and deposition of local anesthetic is indicated by the appearance of a hypoechoic fluid pocket immediately deep to the hyperechoic fascial plane below the internal oblique and above the transversus abdominis. If the needle tip is intramuscular, a pattern of fluid spread consistent with intramuscular fluid injection will be seen.
- During local anesthetic injection, it is advisable to scan the abdomen cephalad and caudad to determine the extent of longitudinal spread. Medial and lateral scanning will determine the extent of horizontal spread.

Technical and Physical Challenges in Single-Incision Approach

Lost Triangulation and Trocar Placement Strategy

Achieving adequate triangulation is a basic principle of traditional laparoscopic surgery.

Trocars could be directed from multiple points of entry, guiding instruments toward the target organ, where adequate manipulation could be achieved. (Fig. 33.4A)

Operating through a single incision with only rigid instruments would be challenging, because the surgeon would either implement a coaxial positioning of instruments (Fig. 33.4B) or a "crossing" arrangement (Fig. 33.4C). In the coaxial technique, both instruments emerge through the umbilicus and are parallel to one another; thus, controlling both instruments outside the abdomen would pose a challenge, because the surgeon's hands would be at such close proximity. On the other hand, when rigid instruments are crossing, there would be a considerably more comfortable range of movement on the outside; however, on the inside, the left hand controls the right instrument, and vice versa, posing a challenge for first-time single-incision adopters. As the overall flexibility of the instruments increases, triangulation issues can be overcome without sacrificing external maneuverability.

Flexible instruments have articulating shafts, steering the tip of the instrument toward the target organ and restoring lost triangulation. Thus, combining flexible and rigid instruments has resulted in a more comfortable configuration (Fig. 33.4D,E), increasing maneuverability and the feasibility of advanced surgical procedures using a single incision.

Conflict of Instruments

Multiple instruments inserted at close proximity through a common port of entry produce an undesirable limitation of movement both inside and outside. Many advanced

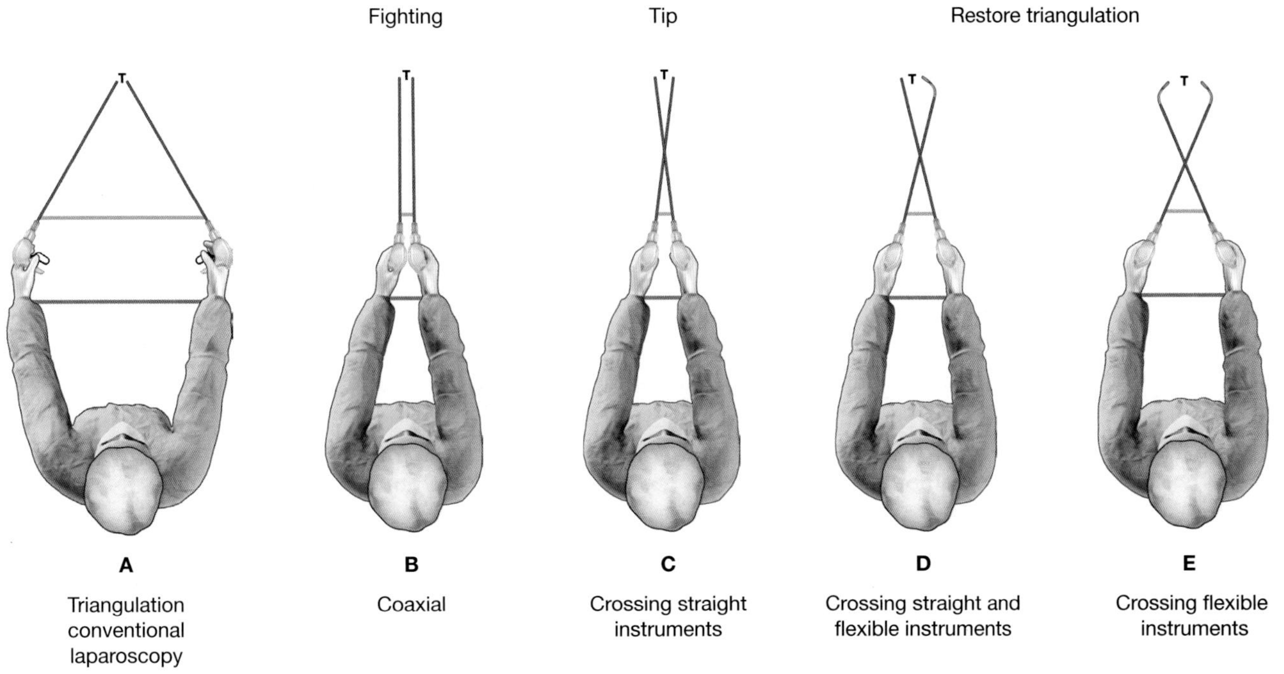

Fighting	Tip	Restore triangulation

A	B	C	D	E
Triangulation conventional laparoscopy	Coaxial	Crossing straight instruments	Crossing straight and flexible instruments	Crossing flexible instruments

Figure 33.4 Conflict of instrumentation and triangulation in single-incision laparoscopic surgery and trocar reduction. Reproduced with permission from Saber AA. Single incision laparoscopic surgery (SILS) and trocar reduction strategies for bariatric procedures. Adapted from: Dietel M, Gagner M, Dixon JB, Himpens J, Madan AK, eds. Handbook of Obesity Surgery. Toronto: FD Communications Inc. 2010:190–197.

procedures involve switching instruments and trocars more often, which could compromise the pneumoperitoneum. These challenges have led to the development of multichannel ports to avoid the clinching of laparoscopic instruments diverting from a common point.

If multichannel ports are not available, it is necessary to insert three trocars through the same umbilical skin incision but with different fascial incisions at different levels in a triangular fashion. Using a flexible tip laparoscope minimizes the external conflict of instruments, because its cable exits through the instrument's back end, keeping it away from the operative field.

Abdominal Wall "Torque Effect"
Utilizing the umbilicus (the thinnest part of abdominal wall) minimizes the torque effect on trocars inserted at such close proximity, providing a wider range of motion for the instruments and trocars in different directions. However, in incisions away from the umbilicus, the "torque effect" on trocars increases with the increasing thickness of the point of abdominal access, counteracting the movement of trocars and decreasing maneuverability.

Umbilical Recession
In super-obese patients a receded umbilicus can reduce the feasibility of the transumbilical approach, favoring the epigastric placement of trocars to ensure that the gastroesophageal junction is within the comfortable reach of the laparoscopic instruments.

Retraction of Large Liver
Bariatric patients have a higher incidence of fatty liver, potentially obscuring the operative field and presenting a challenge for the single-incision approach. Liver retraction can be achieved by internal retraction (i.e. sutures), external retraction (i.e. subxiphoid, transumbilical liver retractor), or using the mobilized portion of the stomach.

Part IV: Bariatric

Operative Technique for Single-Incision Sleeve Gastrectomy

The patient is placed in a supine or split leg position. The surgeon stands either on the right side or between the legs of the patient with the assistant on the left. Both the location of the single incision and the method of liver retraction are tailored according to the operative strategy discussed in the previous sections. For the transumbilical approach, the deepest point in the umbilical scar is pulled up using Kocher graspers while applying subtle pressure on the abdominal wall to tent up the umbilical scar. A 2.5-cm intraumbilical skin incision is created and deepened to the linea alba. A fascial opening up to a length of 2 cm is established. Larger incisions can result in a loose port, promoting gas leakage and an inadequate pneumoperitoneum. The SILS™ Port (Covidien, Norwalk, CT) is folded at its lower edge (opposite to the insufflator) and advanced under direct vision into the abdomen using a clamp. Once the bottom half of the port is introduced into the abdomen, the port is released. Two 5-mm trocars and one 15-mm trocar are introduced through the access channels. The pneumoperitoneum is initiated to a pressure of 15 mm Hg. A 5-mm flexible tip laparoscope is inserted.

Using a 5-mm LigaSure™ and 5-mm flexible grasper, the greater curvature of the stomach is mobilized, beginning from a point 6 cm proximal to the pylorus, staying close to the wall of the stomach, all the way up the greater curvature to the angle of His, dividing both gastrocolic and gastrosplenic ligaments. This is followed by liver retraction, as detailed, according to each patient's body habitus and liver size (Fig. 33.5).

It is important to identify and mobilize the angle of His, with exposure of the left crus of the diaphragm, to facilitate complete resection of the fundus. Retrogastric adhesions are taken down with the LigaSure™. This allows complete mobilization of the stomach, eliminates any redundant posterior wall of the sleeve, and excludes the fundus from the gastric sleeve.

Once the stomach is completely mobilized, a 34F orogastric tube is inserted orally, placed against the lesser curvature and through the pylorus. This calibrated size of the gastric sleeve prevents constriction at the gastroesophageal junction and incisura angularis and provides a uniform shape to the entire stomach.

The gastric transection is started at a point 6 cm proximal to the pylorus, leaving the antrum and preserving gastric emptying. A long laparoscopic roticulating 60-mm XL endo-GIA stapler with green cartridge 4.8-mm staples and a synthetic absorbable buttressing material is inserted through the 15-mm trocar in a cephalad direction. The stapler is fired consecutively along the length of the orogastric tube until the

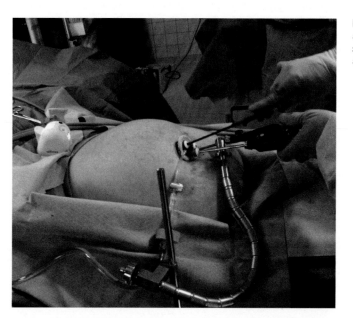

Figure 33.5 Umbilical port, trocars, and liver retractor placement during single-incision sleeve gastrectomy and adjustable gastric band.

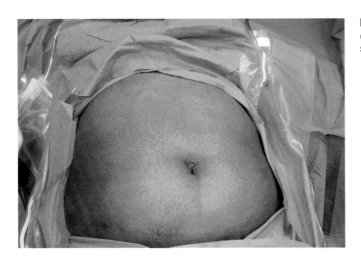

Figure 33.6 Operative picture after completion of single-incision sleeve gastrectomy.

angle of His is reached. Care must be taken not to narrow the stomach at the incisura angularis. It is important to inspect the stomach anteriorly and posteriorly to ensure that there is no redundant posterior stomach. Approximately 80% of the stomach is separated. The entire staple line is inspected for bleeding and tested for leakage. Insufflating air under saline and infusing methylene blue into the remaining stomach tests the integrity of the staple line. The resected stomach is extracted along with the SILS™ Port without the need for an Endobag. The fascial defect of the port site is closed with a figure-of-eight 2-0 nonabsorbable suture to prevent port site hernia formation. The skin incision is closed with 4-0 absorbable suture in a subcuticular fashion (Fig. 33.6).

Technique for Single-Incision Adjustable Gastric Band

The patient is placed in a supine position with the surgeon standing on the right side and the assistant standing on the left side of the patient. A 2.5-cm skin incision is placed intraumbilically. The incision should be large enough to accommodate the multichannel port and ultimately the subcutaneous access port for the adjustment of the gastric band. A safe entry to the abdomen with a 2-cm fascial incision is achieved using the open Hassan technique. The adjustable gastric band is inserted through the skin and the fascial defect into the abdominal cavity in an atraumatic fashion. A SILS™ port is placed and three 5-mm very low-profile trocars are placed at different levels. Pneumoperitoneum is established. A 5-mm flexible-tip laparoscope is used for visualization. The liver retractor is inserted either through the umbilical port or a 5-mm subxiphoid skin puncture with no port placement, in a fashion similar to that of single-incision sleeve gastrectomy (Fig. 33.5).

Using the endofinger device, the phrenoesophageal ligament is bluntly dissected at the angle of His exposing the apex of the left crus of the diaphragm; this represents the first landmark for the operation. Extensive dissection should be avoided to minimize the risk of slippage.

A flexible grasper is used to elevate the lesser curve of the stomach. L-hook electrocautery is used to open the pars flaccida of the gastrohepatic ligament exposing the right crus of the diaphragm. The peritoneum overlying the base of the right crus is incised using L-hook electrocautery.

Next, an articulating 5-mm blunt grasper is used to develop the retrogastric tunnel. The instrument is passed gently without resistance from the base of the right crus to the apex of the left crus at the 0 of His (Fig. 33.7). This will achieve a 45-degree angulation of the band. The distal end of the band tubing is held securely by the grasper and is passed through the retrogastric tunnel by an articulating grasper allowing the band to be placed within the retrogastric tunnel. The band is wrapped around the proximal stomach creating a small gastric pouch and the buckle is locked.

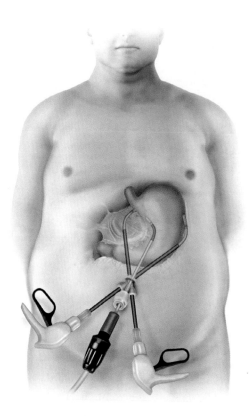

Figure 33.7 Operative strategy during single-incision laparoscopic adjustable gastric band placement. Note that the use of flexible blunt grasper facilitates retrogastric dissection.

The flappy part of the fundus below the band is then sutured to the pouch to imbricate the band. This is done using an endostitch device (Covidien) with a 2-0 nonabsorbable extra corporeal suture technique. The automated features of the endostitch device facilitate extra corporeal knot tying and overcome the challenges associated with the limited range of motion in the single-incision approach. It is important to make sure that the stomach is taken in each bite using seromuscular to seromuscular gastrogastric sutures. A total of four interrupted anterior gastrogastric sutures are placed to create the gastric plication necessary to reduce the risk of anterior slippage. Upon completion of the laparoscopic part, the band should be seen assuming a 45-degree tilt, with its buckle outside the anterior gastric wrap to minimize the risk of erosion.

The single-incision port is removed, and the tubing is exteriorized through the single umbilical incision and attached to the subcutaneous access port. The fascial defect is closed to avoid postoperative herniation. Four 2-0 nonabsorbable sutures are used to secure the access port to the anterior rectus fascia; this is done to avoid the rotation and subsequent inaccessibility to the port. The skin incision is closed with 4-0 absorbable suture in a subcuticular fashion.

Operative Technique for Single-Incision Roux-en-Y Gastric Bypass

Patient Position

The patient is placed in the supine position. The patient is properly strapped to the bed with a foot strap and appropriately cushioned on all the pressure points. After endotracheal intubation, a Foley catheter is inserted.

- TAP block: The TAP block is then performed in a sterile fashion as described.
- Creating pneumoperitoneum: The surgeon stands on the right side with the assistant on the left. Pneumoperitoneum is created by inserting a 150-mm Veress needle through umbilicus or left subcostal area. We have experienced that this step is very helpful in planning skin incision, undercutting the fascia and entering the peritoneal cavity.

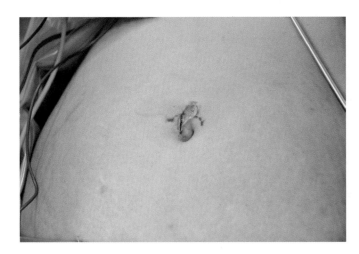

Figure 33.8 Umbilical incision.

- Incision: Both the location of the single incision and the method of liver retraction are tailored according to the operative strategy discussed in the previous sections. Our preferred incision is a 3-cm periumblical with small vertical extension as shown in Figure 33.8. About 10 mL of xylocaine is infiltrated at the umbilical site to evert the umbilicus. Skin incision is placed using a no. 15 blade, and then the subcutaneous fat is cut using electrocautery. The bulging peritoneum is opened by blunt dissection. Undercutting of fascia is performed to admit at least three fingers.
- Insertion of port: We prefer using GelPOINT™ port (Applied Medical) for single-incision gastric bypass. The inner ring of the wound protector is first inserted into the abdominal cavity. It is then rolled in until it becomes snug to the skin (Fig. 33.9). The GelPOINT port is then prepared by inserting three 5-mm ports and one 12-mm port as shown in the figure. The port is then mounted over the wound protector and the pneumoperitoneum is created (Fig. 33.10).
- Diagnostic laparoscopy: A 5-mm 45-degree angle scope is used to visualize the peritoneal cavity (Fig. 33.11). Alternatively a 5-mm flexible scope can also be used. If adhesions are seen, then lysis of adhesions is performed using the ultrasonic shears and also the liver size is assessed at this point. A snake retractor is used through a 5-mm port to retract the lateral segment of the left lobe of liver. Occasionally, a Nathanson retractor may be placed through a subxiphoid incision without a port if the liver is massively enlarged.
- Creation of gastric pouch: The pars flaccida overlying the caudate lobe of the liver is entered by blunt dissection. The lesser sac tunnel is visualized under the left gastric vessel. Three firings of articulating GIA 60-mm blue cartridges are used to create the gastric pouch. The first stapler is fired almost horizontal, the second one

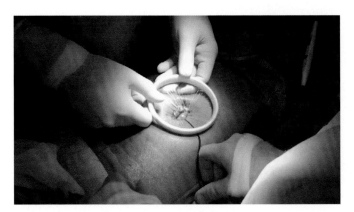

Figure 33.9 Wound protector.

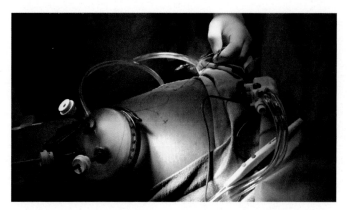

Figure 33.10 Gelpoint port.

is vertical, and the last one is through the angle of His (Fig. 33.12) creating a 10- to 20-mL gastric pouch. An Orovil™ (Covidien) tube is then passed by the anesthesiologist via the oral route. Using a point cautery the tube is delivered out through the posterior wall of the pouch about 1 cm away from the staple line. The tube is then gently pulled until the anvil is seen projecting out through the gastric pouch. The tube is then detached from the anvil and pulled out.

■ Creation of jejunojejunal anastomosis: We prefer doing an extra corporeal small bowel anastomosis as it significantly reduces the operating time. After identifying the ligament of Treitz, the jejunum is measured and transected at about 50 cm distal from the ligament of Treitz using an endoscopic linear cutter stapler 60-mm white cartridge. The tip of the Roux limb is then undermined for 3 cm using a harmonic scalpel. The Roux limb is then measured for about 100 to 150 cm. A stay suture is placed between the measured Roux limb and the tip of the biliopancreatic limb. The suture is cut long. The gelpoint port is then detached from the ring, desufflating the peritoneal cavity. By pulling the stay suture the two jejunal limbs are delivered out. Enterotomies are made at the appropriate antimesenteric sites, and using a linear cutter 60-mm white cartridge a jejunojejunal anastomosis is created (Fig. 33.13). The enterotomy site is then closed by firing another 60-mm white cartridge (Fig. 33.14). Silk suture is used to close the mesenteric defect, and Brolin stitch is placed to prevent the kinking of Roux limb. The anastomosis is then placed back into the abdominal cavity.

■ Creation of gastrojejunal anastomosis: The tip of the Roux limb is identified. Without twisting the mesentery the tip is delivered out. The staple line is excised

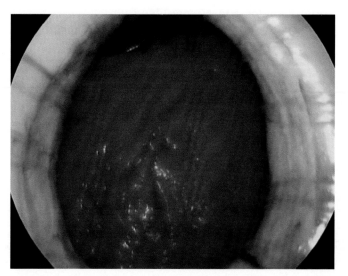

Figure 33.11 Diagnostic laparoscopy.

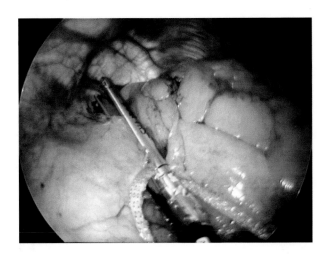

Figure 33.12 Creation of gastric pouch.

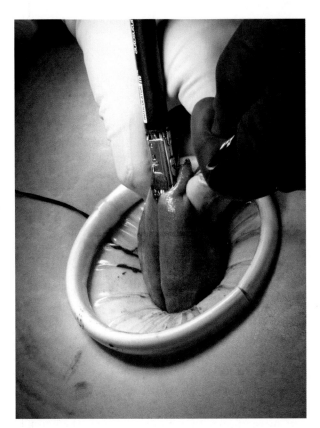

Figure 33.13 Extracorporeal jejunojejunal anastomosis.

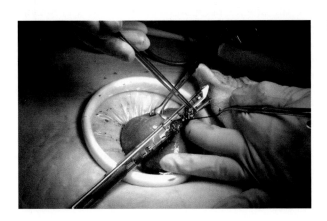

Figure 33.14 Closure of enterotomy.

Part IV: Bariatric

extracorporeally using electrocautery. A 25-mm EEA stapler is then passed through the gelpoint port and then introduced into the tip of the Roux limb. The spike of the stapler is then advanced to pierce the Roux limb at about 5 to 6 cm from the tip. Under direct vision the Roux limb with the tip of the spike is placed into the peritoneal cavity and gelpoint port is mounted back. Pneumoperitoneum is re-established and the 45-degree angle scope is again introduced. A flexible grasper is introduced to hold the anvil. The spike is then aligned to the anvil under direct vision and locked. After ensuring that there is no tension or twisting of mesentery, the stapler is fired and the GJ anastomosis is created. The nonviable open portion of the tip of the Roux limb is excised using a linear cutter 60-mm stapler. The specimen is removed after placing it in a specimen retrieval bag.

■ Testing the anastomosis: EGD is performed to do the air leak test and check for any internal bleeding.

Closure
The fascial closure is done by no. 1 PDS suture. Dead space is obliterated by subcutaneous vicryl sutures and the skin is approximated by subcuticular stitches.

Postoperative care
Postoperative gastrografin swallow is obtained on the first postoperative day to rule out leaks and obstruction in case of sleeve gastrectomy or gastric bypass and in case of gastric band to confirm the appropriate position of the band with no obstruction or extravasation. Deep vein thrombosis prophylaxis is achieved using anticoagulation, compression stockings, and a sequential compression device. The patient is discharged once they are tolerating a full liquid diet, are hemodynamically stable, afebrile, ambulating, able to maintain hydration, and pain is managed appropriately with oral analgesics.

 COMPLICATIONS

There have been very few minor early complications described; however, long-term data are required to rule out port site hernias, and weight regain.

 RESULTS

The scarce data documenting the early intraoperative and postoperative experience with single-incision bariatric surgery have shown that single-incision sleeve gastrectomy, adjustable gastric banding, and gastric bypass procedures are feasible and associated with a reasonable degree of safety. Postoperative weight loss is similar to those occurring after conventional multiport laparoscopic procedures, for both sleeve gastrectomy (1) and adjustable gastric banding (2). More importantly, no major operative or perioperative complications have been reported. Regarding the benefits of the single-incision approach, in addition to the cosmetic advantage, the potential advantages might include a shorter hospital stay or a reduced need for analgesia.

However, prospective randomized studies comparing multiport laparoscopic adjustable gastric banding, gastric bypass, and sleeve gastrectomy with their single-incision counterparts in large volumes with long-term follow-up are needed to confirm these initial results, identify the direct benefits, and assess the cost-effectiveness of the single-incision approach in broad detail.

✦ CONCLUSIONS

- The single-incision approach is a new emerging approach for bariatric surgery.
- The approach is particularly attractive for procedures that require a 2- to 3-cm incision to insert the adjustable band and the port as in adjustable gastric banding or to retrieve a large specimen as in sleeve gastrectomy.
- The single-incision approach has many potential advantages over the conventional laparoscopic approach, including less postoperative pain, less need for analgesia, and hospital stay. In addition it improves cosmesis and body images.
- However, some technical challenges are encountered during single-incision bariatric procedures including lost triangulation, conflict of instruments, umbilical recession, and large fatty liver.
- These could be overcome by using long flexible instrument, flexible tip scope, multichannel access ports, and liver retractor.

Recommended References and Readings

Saber AA, El-Ghazaly TH. Early experience with single-access transumbilical laparoscopic adjustable gastric banding. *Obes Surg.* 2009;19(10):1442–1446.

Saber AA, El-Ghazaly TH, Elian A. Single-incision transumbilical laparoscopic sleeve gastrectomy. *J Laparoendosc Adv Surg Tech A.* 2009;19(6):755–758.

Saber AA, El-Ghazaly TH, Elian A, et al. Single-incision laparoscopic sleeve gastrectomy versus conventional multiport laparoscopic sleeve gastrectomy: Technical considerations and strategic modifications. *Surg Obes Relat Dis.* 2010;6(6):658–664.

Saber AA, El-Ghazaly TH, Elian A, et al. Single-incision laparoscopic placement of adjustable gastric band versus conventional multiport laparoscopic gastric banding: A comparative study. *Am Surg.* 2010;76(12):1328–1332.

Tacchino RM, Greco F, Matera D, et al. Single-incision laparoscopic gastric bypass for morbid obesity. *Obes Surg.* 2010;20(8):1154–1160.

34 Open and Laparoscopic Procedures for SMA Syndrome

Markus W. Büchler and Thilo Welsch

 ## INDICATIONS/CONTRAINDICATIONS

The superior mesenteric artery syndrome (SMA syndrome or Wilkie's syndrome) is caused by the compression of the third part of the duodenum in the angle between the aorta and the SMA (Figs. 34.1 and 34.2). The entity was first described by the Austrian professor Carl von Rokitansky in his anatomy textbook in 1842. Subsequently, Wilkie published the first comprehensive series of 75 patients in 1927 and his name has become a common eponym for the SMA syndrome. Symptoms arise from the duodenal compression and comprise chronic or acute postprandial epigastric pain, nausea, vomiting, anorexia, and weight loss. Frequently, predisposing medical conditions associated with catabolic states or rapid weight loss result in a decrease of the aortomesenteric angle and subsequent duodenal obstruction. External cast compression, anatomic variants, and surgical alteration of the anatomy following spine or gastrointestinal surgery (e.g., ileoanal pouch anastomosis) can also precipitate the syndrome (Table 34.1).

Once radiologic studies have established SMA syndrome, first-line treatment is usually conservative with jejunal or parenteral nutrition for restoration of the aortomesenteric fat tissue. Nasogastric tube placement for duodenal and gastric decompression and mobilization into the prone or left lateral decubitus position often is effective in the acute setting. If conservative management fails, surgical procedures are indicated and include open or laparoscopic duodenojejunostomy or duodenal mobilization and diversion of the ligament of Treitz (Strong's procedure). Surgical exploration is further indicated if the SMA syndrome is expected to be caused by vascular pathology or by local tumor growth that require surgical intervention.

Indications for surgical treatment are as follows:

- Failure of conservative treatment
- Longstanding disease with progressive weight loss and duodenal dilatation with stasis
- The need for surgery for the causative pathology
- Complicated peptic ulcer disease secondary to biliary stasis and reflux

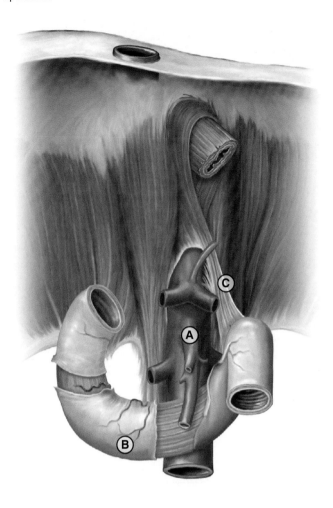

Figure 34.1 The SMA crosses the third part of the duodenum in the mesenteric root. A high insertion of the ligament of Treitz at the duodenojejunal juncture can displace the duodenum cranially into the vascular angle formed by the SMA and the aorta. *A,* SMA; *B,* third part of the duodenum; *C,* ligament of Treitz. Adapted from Welsch T, Buchler MW, Kienle P. (2007). Recalling superior mesenteric artery syndrome. *Dig Surg.* 24: 149–156.

⏩ PREOPERATIVE PLANNING

A detailed history (predisposing medical or surgical conditions, weight loss, epigastric pain, and conservative treatment strategies) and physical examination of the patient is mandatory in the preoperative setting. Patients who present with a history of characteristic symptoms suggesting SMA syndrome should undergo further radiographic studies

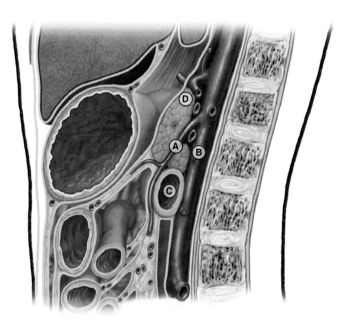

Figure 34.2 The SMA leaves the aorta at an acute angle that is sustained by the left renal vein and the uncinate process of the pancreas embedded in retroperitoneal fat and lymph tissue. A low aortomesenteric angle can lead to vascular compression of the duodenum. *A,* SMA; *B,* aorta; *C,* third part of the duodenum; *D,* pancreas. Adapted from Welsch T, Buchler MW, Kienle P. (2007). Recalling superior mesenteric artery syndrome. *Dig Surg.* 24: 149–156.

TABLE 34.1	Predisposing Conditions for Development of SMAS	

Chronic Wasting Disease	Postoperative States
Cancer	Bariatric surgery
Cerebral palsy	Proctocolectomy and ileoanal pouch anastomosis
Paraplegia	Nissen fundoplication
Juvenile rheumatoid arthritis	Aortic aneurysm repair
Cardiac cachexia	Spinal instrumentation, scoliosis surgery, or body casting
Drug abuse	
Trauma	**Anatomy and Congenital Anomalies**
Burn injury	High insertion of the ligament of Treitz
Brain injury	Intestinal malrotation, peritoneal adhesions
Multiple injuries	Low origin of the SMA
	Increased lumbar lordosis
	Intestinal malrotation
Dietary Disorders	**Local Pathology**
Anorexia nervosa	Neoplastic growth in the mesenteric root
Malabsorption	Dissecting aortic aneurysm

to establish the diagnosis. Upper gastrointestinal series, computed tomography (CT) scan or CT angiography, magnetic resonance (MR) angiography, conventional angiography, ultrasonography, and endoscopy have all been used for diagnosis. The following strict radiographic criteria have been established for diagnosis of the SMA syndrome by upper gastrointestinal series with contrast dye: (i) dilatation of the first and second parts of the duodenum, with or without gastric dilatation, (ii) abrupt vertical and oblique compression of the mucosal folds, (iii) antiperistaltic flow of contrast medium proximal to the obstruction, (iv) delay in transit of 4 to 6 hours through the gastroduodenal region, and (v) relief of obstruction in a prone, knee-chest or left lateral decubitus position.

Contrast-enhanced CT scan additionally demonstrates the aortomesenteric angle, distance and fat tissue, obstruction of the duodenum and a potential culprit for compression, for example, local neoplasia or an aneurysm. Contrast-enhanced CT scan and MR imaging seem to be equivalent in evaluating the exact angle and distance and are recommended by the authors (Fig. 34.3). Criteria for diagnosis mainly result from angiography studies (the former "gold standard"). An aortomesenteric angle of less than 22 to 25 degrees and a distance of less than 8 mm correlated well with the symptoms of the SMA syndrome.

Because of the superior information content and noninvasiveness, contrast-enhanced CT or MR angiography is more valuable if the cause for the SMA syndrome is unclear. In addition, upper gastrointestinal endoscopy should be performed to rule out intestinal intraluminal obstruction and gastric or duodenal ulcer disease that might be secondary to reflux or that might constitute a primary pathology mimicking SMA syndrome.

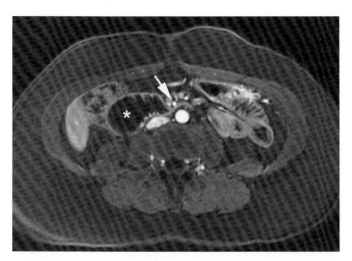

Figure 34.3 SMA syndrome in a 28-year-old female after gastrointestinal surgery. MR image demonstrating a moderately dilated second part of the duodenum (*) and compression by the SMA (*arrow*). The aortomesenteric distance was measured at 7 mm. Adapted from Welsch T, Buchler MW, Kienle P. (2007). Recalling superior mesenteric artery syndrome. *Dig Surg.* 24:149–156.

Preoperative assessment:

- Attempts of medical treatment failed or are contraindicated
- Proper imaging with contrast-enhanced CT scan or MR angiography of the abdomen and endoscopy (to rule out intrinsic abnormality) for surgical planning
- Optimize the patient's medical and nutritional status and nasogastric decompression

 # SURGERY

Several surgical approaches to resolve or bypass the SMA syndrome have been described:

- gastrojejunostomy
- open or laparoscopic duodenojejunostomy
- open or laparoscopic duodenal mobilization by division of the ligament of Treitz (Strong's procedure)

The first duodenojejunostomy for the SMA syndrome was done by Stavely in 1908 and has become the most frequent surgical procedure with a success rate of about 80%. Data reporting the outcome after different surgical procedures are historical. Lee et al. concluded after reviewing 146 cases operated after 1963 that duodenojejunostomy revealed the best results in severe cases and was significantly better compared to gastrojejunostomy and Strong's procedure. Today, laparoscopic procedures are increasingly performed, but studies comparing the outcome of laparoscopic duodenojejunostomy or duodenal mobilization are missing.

In this chapter, the authors describe the open Strong's procedure and the laparoscopic duodenojejunostomy for SMA syndrome. For either approach, the patient should undergo preoperative gastric decompression through a nasogastric tube.

Positioning

For the open Strong's procedure, the patient should be placed in a decubitus position. For the laparoscopic approach, the patient is placed in the lithotomy position with the legs extended in stirrups. The right arm is tucked at the patient's side. The operating surgeon stands between the legs, and the assistant stands to the patient's left side. Preoperative antibiotics are given 30 minutes prior to incision.

Laparoscopic Duodenojejunostomy

Recent reports have demonstrated that laparoscopic duodenojejunostomy can be safely and successfully performed without duodenal mobilization (Kocher maneuver). In the presented laparoscopic approach, a duodenojejunal bypass is created anastomosing the dilated third part of the duodenum with a proximal jejunal loop.

- A pneumoperitoneum is established and a 30-degree laparoscope is inserted through a 12-mm port near the umbilicus. The patient is placed in a 20-degree reverse Trendelenburg position. The surgeon operates through one right-handed 12-mm working trochar on the left side of the abdomen and one left-handed 5-mm port on the right abdomen. A third port (5-mm) is inserted in the left subcostal region and allows the assistant to retract the transverse colon cephalad.
- Once the transverse colon is elevated the dilated third part of the duodenum is seen below the transverse mesocolon and the ligament of Treitz can be identified. Dissection of the visceral peritoneum and base of the transverse mesocolon over the distal second part of duodenum and third part proximal to the superior mesenteric vessels is performed with laparoscopic scissors. This exposes the duodenum just proximal to the site of obstruction.
- A proximal jejunal loop 15 to 20 cm from the ligament of Treitz is mobilized to the exposed duodenal segment and the most caudal part of the duodenum is identified for the creation of the side-to-side anastomosis. The two limbs were secured with two stay sutures of 2-0 Vicryl.

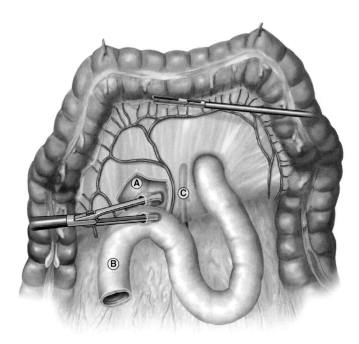

Figure 34.4 Laparoscopic duodenojejunostomy. The transverse colon is elevated with the assistant laparoscopic grasper. After incision of the mesocolon, the dilated third part of the duodenum (*A*) is clearly exposed. A proximal jejunal loop (*B*) is mobilized to the duodenum and the two limbs are side-to-side anastomosed using an endoscopic stapler device. Compression of the duodenum is caused by the superior mesenteric artery (*C*).

Part V: Other Gastric Operations

- Two small antimesenteric enterotomies are made with the hook cautery and gently dilated with an atraumatic grasper. The duodenojejunostomy is then performed using a 45-mm endoscopic gastrointestinal anastomotic (GIA) stapler (Fig. 34.4), and the remaining enterotomy is closed using a running 2-0 slowly absorbable suture. Finally, the abdomen is irrigated, a drain is positioned, and the trocars are removed.

Open Duodenal Mobilization by Division of the Ligament of Treitz (Stong's Procedure)

Strong first described the diversion of the ligament of Treitz with mobilization of the transverse and ascending duodenum for caudal displacement of the duodenum. The advantages of this procedure are that it does not violate the bowel and thus is the less invasive, quicker, and safer procedure. It has been correlated with an earlier postoperative recovery. The disadvantages are that the procedure can be aggravated or impossible due to adhesions and that caudal displacement of the duodenum cannot always be achieved because of interference with short vessels from the inferior pancreaticoduodenal artery to the duodenum. In recent years, Strong's procedure has also been performed laparoscopically.

- An epigastric midline incision is made and the abdominal cavity is explored.
- The ligament of Treitz is identified and divided with the electrocautery.
- Then the third part of the duodenum is completely mobilized from the mesenteric root. This results in a caudolateral shift of the duodenum resolving the duodenal compression in the aortomesenteric angle.
- No drain is placed and the abdomen is closed.

 POSTOPERATIVE MANAGEMENT

After duodenojejunostomy, the nasogastric tube is left in situ initially. A swallow study with oral contrast dye is performed on the first postoperative day. In the absence of a leak or a delay of the contrast dye passage through the anastomosis, a liquid diet is started. If liquid diet is well-tolerated, the nasogastric tube is removed. Patients are slowly advanced to pureed and solid diet as tolerated. Abdominal drains are generally removed on the second postoperative day.

Postoperative hospital stay after laparoscopic procedures is usually short lasting about 4 to 5 days. Patients should be followed regularly in the outpatient clinic for 3 months to check relief of symptoms and weight gain.

 COMPLICATIONS

Postoperative complications are rare. In a systematic review, the morbidity rate was calculated to 7% with no mortality. Patients can present with delayed gastric emptying requiring prolonged decompression with a nasogastric tube. Further, leakage of the duodenojejunostomy is a critical complication, and early diagnosis of this complication through the swallow study should prompt surgical re-exploration.

 RESULTS

Symptom relief is usually achieved early after the surgical procedure and the surgical results are excellent. From 1978 to 2010, duodenojejunostomy is reported to be successful in almost 100% of the patients, although there are only small series or case reports published in the literature owing to the paucity of the entity. A contemporary comparison of the different surgical procedures is not available, but in the past, duodenojejunostomy was considered to be superior to Strong's procedure. However, Strong's procedure is indicated only in selected patients without long-lasting duodenal dilatation and is limited by the extent of duodenal mobilization.

CONCLUSIONS

- SMA syndrome is a rare condition and is caused by the compression of the third part of the duodenum in the angle between the aorta and the SMA.
- There are numerous conditions that can cause SMA syndrome including catabolic states, anatomic abnormalities, scoliosis, external cast compression, gastrointestinal operations.
- Diagnosis is optimally confirmed through contrast-enhanced CT scan or MR angiography.
- The first-line treatment approach of SMA syndrome is conservative aiming to restore the aortomesenteric angle for duodenal decompression through nutritional support.
- Surgery is indicated if medical treatment fails.
- Historically, two major surgical approaches have been described: duodenojejunostomy and duodenal mobilization (Strong's procedure).
- Today, both procedures are increasingly performed laparoscopically with excellent results. The indications for Strong's procedure are limited, but duodenojejunostomy is the more invasive procedure.
- Complications are rare, and the most critical complication following duodenojejunostomy is anastomotic leakage. Postoperative contrast study is therefore recommended early before advancing dietary intake.

Recommended References and Readings

Fraser JD, St Peter SD, Hughes JH, et al. Laparoscopic duodenojejunostomy for superior mesenteric artery syndrome. *JSLS.* 2009; 13:254–259.

Lee CS, Mangla JC. Superior mesenteric artery compression syndrome. *Am J Gastroenterol.* 1978;70:141–150.

Massoud WZ. Laparoscopic management of superior mesenteric artery syndrome. *Int Surg.* 1995;80:322–327.

Morris TC, Devitt PG, Thompson SK. Laparoscopic duodenojejunostomy for superior mesenteric artery syndrome—how I do it. *J Gastrointest Surg.* 2009;13:1870–1873.

Munene G, Knab M, Parag B. Laparoscopic duodenojejunostomy for superior mesenteric artery syndrome. *Am Surg.* 2010;76:321–324.

Neri S, Signorelli SS, Mondati E, et al. Ultrasound imaging in diagnosis of superior mesenteric artery syndrome. *J Intern Med.* 2005; 257:346–351.

Richardson WS, Surowiec WJ. Laparoscopic repair of superior mesenteric artery syndrome. *Am J Surg.* 2001;181:377–378.

Strong EK. Mechanics of arteriomesentric duodenal obstruction and direct surgical attack upon etiology. *Ann Surg.* 1958;148:725–730.

Unal B, Aktas A, Kemal G, et al. Superior mesenteric artery syndrome: CT and ultrasonography findings. *Diagn Interv Radiol.* 2005;11:90–95.

Welsch T, Buchler MW, Kienle P. Recalling superior mesenteric artery syndrome. *Dig Surg.* 2007;24:149–156.

Wilkie DPD. Chronic duodenal ileus. *Am J Med Sci.* 1927;173:643–649.

35 Gastrostomy: Endoscopic, Laparoscopic, and Open

Jeffrey L. Ponsky and Melissa S. Phillips

 ## INDICATIONS/CONTRAINDICATIONS

The importance of nutritional support has been shown to decrease infectious complications, lead to better wound healing, and improve overall surgical outcomes. The most common approach for enteral access is through placement of a gastrostomy tube which can be placed through a percutaneous, laparoscopic, or open approach. Dysphagia and aspiration are common indications for gastrostomy tube placement and can result from multiple pathologies. Despite the approach taken, gastrostomy tube placement for nutritional support requires a functional gastrointestinal tract.

- Neurologic disease: This is the most frequently encountered indication for gastrostomy placement. Underlying neurologic pathology may range from an acute onset cerebrovascular event to those with a more slowly progressive process such as multiple sclerosis or amyotrophic lateral sclerosis. Additional indications may include severe dementia, hypoxic encephalopathy, and meningitis.
- Trauma: In addition to direct facial trauma, many people who undergo multisystem trauma require placement of a temporary gastrostomy for support during the recovery process. Patients with a high percentage of total body surface area burns may require supplemental nutritional support secondary to the induced state of catabolism.
- Aerodigestive malignancies: The indication for gastrostomy may be a direct result of the patient's primary malignancy, as would be the case in a nearly obstructing esophageal cancer or in dysphagia induced by a squamous cell carcinoma of the tongue. It may be, however, independent of the primary malignancy, being placed as a method for maintaining supplemental nutritional support during chemotherapy or to assure adequate caloric intake following a planned surgical resection.
- Pediatric indications: Pediatric patients have additional indications, such as congenital malformations, enzymatic deficiencies, or congenital neurologic syndromes. Examples of these conditions include tracheoesophageal fistulas, cerebral palsy, and seizure disorders.
- Decompression: Patients with unresectable malignant obstructions with a life expectancy greater than 4 weeks may be candidates for gastrostomy placement for decompression.

Other indications include severe radiation enteritis, refractory gastroparesis, or for redirection of gastrointestinal flow, such as following a duodenal perforation.

- Other indications: Gastrostomies have been used for refeeding of bile in patients with malignant biliary obstruction or for administration of intolerable medications. In patients who are unable to meet their caloric needs, such as those with inflammatory bowel disease or cystic fibrosis, supplemental tube feed support may also be indicated.

There are very few contraindications to gastrostomy tube placement although the approach for placement must be tailored to meet the specific needs of the patient. With the exception of a decompressive gastrostomy, an absolute contraindication for placement is a nonfunctioning gastrointestinal tract. Another specific contraindication is a limited life expectancy, generally accepted as less than 4 weeks. Patients in this situation should have a nasoenteric tube placed for temporary need given the cost and risks of a more permanent procedure. Patients with psychologically based eating disorders should also have a full evaluation including ethics consult before an invasive procedure is undertaken. Any patient with clinical decompensation, including fever of unknown origin or generalized sepsis, should undergo work up of this condition and gastrostomy tube placement should be delayed. Generally speaking, the percutaneous approach for gastrostomy is preferred in all patients without a specific indication for laparoscopic or open placement.

- Percutaneous approach: Relative contraindications for the endoscopic approach include morbid obesity, massive ascites, portal hypertension, and a history of peritoneal dialysis. Anatomic variations, such as the presence of a hiatal hernia or previous operations, must be considered. These factors can be overcome in many circumstances by the use of a good technique and the skill level of the endoscopist. Any patient with peritonitis should not undergo a percutaneous approach to gastrostomy but should be treated with immediate surgical exploration.
- Surgical approach: Laparoscopic or open gastrostomy is often reserved for patients who are not candidates for a percutaneous approach. This includes patients who have upper aerodigestive obstruction, commonly from malignancy, that does not allow the endoscope to pass. It may also be required for patients in whom there is a concern for interposed viscera (colon, liver, small bowel) between the gastric wall and the abdominal wall during a percutaneous attempt. In patients who have undergone a previous surgical intervention, an open approach may be required if significant intra-abdominal adhesions or postsurgical anatomy modifications fail to provide safe access to the stomach for gastrostomy tube placement.

⟫ PREOPERATIVE PLANNING

As mentioned in the "Indications" section, each patient should undergo evaluation as to which type of gastrostomy tube will offer the best benefit. The level of invasiveness increases with the different approaches from percutaneous to laparoscopic to open. The most common approach taken is a percutaneous endoscopic gastrostomy (PEG) which can be performed under sedation in an endoscopy suite.

All patients undergoing gastrostomy placement should have coagulation values and platelet levels checked. Subcutaneous heparin administration for deep venous thrombosis (DVT) prophylaxis is not a contraindication; however, full anticoagulation may need to be held temporarily. Any patient requiring general anesthesia should have the risks of this evaluated and an appropriate evaluation, such as cardiac clearance or consultation for a difficult airway, performed.

Any patient who has undergone previous surgical intervention should have evaluation to detail the postsurgical anatomy before undertaking gastrostomy placement. Old operative notes should be obtained and will help with determining the best treatment approach. In patients who have undergone imaging of the abdomen for other reasons, these studies should be evaluated to assess for the feasibility of a percutaneous approach.

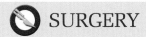

SURGERY

All patients undergoing gastrostomy placement should be prepared by fasting for 8 hours prior to the procedure. Intravenous access should be obtained in all patients. Patients should receive preprocedural antibiotics as this has been shown to decrease the risk for peristomal infection. Antibiotic coverage should be directed to skin flora and should be administered within 30 minutes of the procedure.

Operative Technique for Percutaneous Endoscopic Gastrostomy

Placement of a PEG was first described in 1980. Since its description, multiple modifications for placement have been developed. These can be broadly divided into procedures that introduce the gastrostomy orally, such as the "pull" or "push" techniques, and those that introduce the gastrostomy through the abdominal wall under endoscopic guidance, such as the introducer technique.

- Positioning and sedation: The patient is placed in the supine position and step-wise administration of intravenous medications, commonly a combination of narcotic and benzodiazepine, is given until adequate sedation has been obtained. Patient factors may necessitate the use of general anesthesia and should be evaluated before the procedure is undertaken.
- Upper endoscopy: Following the placement of a bite block, a standard gastroscope is passed through the mouth. The esophagus, stomach, and duodenum are then examined for any evidence of pathology. Specifically, one must take care to assure that there is no evidence of poor gastric emptying or of duodenal obstruction before PEG placement.
- Site selection: Finding the appropriate site for PEG placement is important as poor technique in this step can lead to inadvertent viscus injury. Attempts should be made to identify transillumination of the gastroscope when viewing the external abdominal wall. Next, the abdominal wall should be palpated under endoscopic visualization, watching for a one-to-one movement of the abdominal wall with finger indentation as seen by the gastroscope. Most important in the opinion of the authors is the use of the "safe tract" technique to confirm placement (Fig. 35.1A). A syringe is filled with local anesthesia, available in most kits, and the needle is introduced through the anterior abdominal wall while negative pressure is applied to the syringe. Endoscopically, the expected site is carefully monitored for the presence of the needle (Fig. 35.1B). If air is aspirated before the needle is seen in the gastric lumen, significant concern for interposed viscera is present. If this occurs, a new site should be selected. If the "safe tract" technique is unable to confirm a safe location, the percutaneous approach should be aborted and other techniques of gastrostomy considered.
- Obtaining access: After an appropriate location has been chosen, an introducer needle with a plastic catheter is introduced through the anterior abdominal wall (Fig. 35.2A). This catheter is grasped using an endoscopic snare while the needle is removed (Fig. 35.2B). A guidewire is then passed through the catheter and the endoscopic snare is relocated onto the guidewire. The guidewire is then advanced through the abdominal wall while the snare, other end of the guidewire, and endoscope are removed through the patient's mouth.
- "Pull" technique: The guidewire used in the "pull" PEG is soft and has a preformed loop at the mouth end. Once the guidewire has exited through the mouth, this loop is passed through the loop attached to the gastrostomy tube, forming a secure attachment. After application of a water-soluble lubricant, firm but gentle pressure is applied to the abdominal side of the guidewire as the gastrostomy tube is introduced through the mouth. The guidewire is used to advance the tube into the stomach and through the abdominal wall to the final position (Fig. 35.3). The guidewire is removed and the PEG is secured in place.

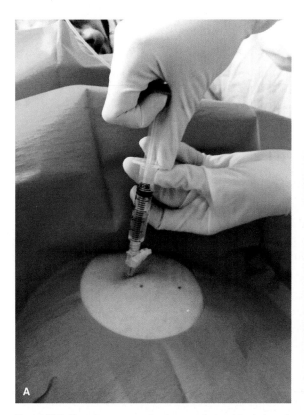

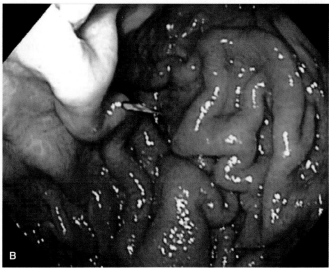

Figure 35.1 Percutaneous gastrostomy: safe-tract technique for selecting a safe location. The external view **(A)** shows transillumination and confirms lumen with visualization of air bubbles while the endoscopic view **(B)** confirms intragastric location of the needle simultaneous to air bubble appearance.

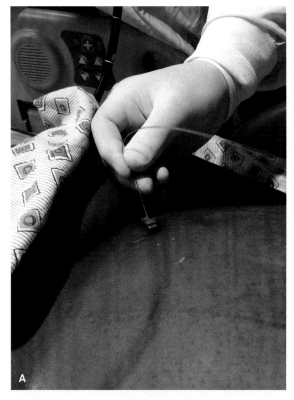

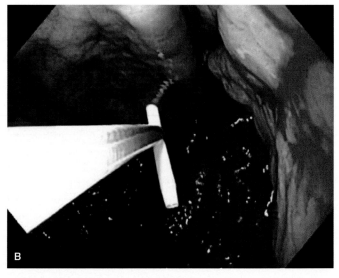

Figure 35.2 Percutaneous gastrostomy: access to the stomach. A catheter-covered needle is introduced, the needle removed, and guidewire inserted from the external view **(A)** and from an endoscopic view **(B)**.

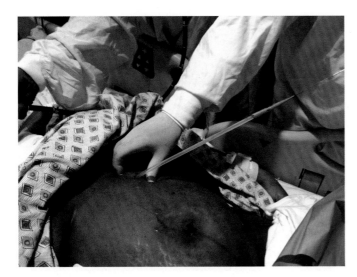

Figure 35.3 Percutaneous gastrostomy: introduction of the gastrostomy tube. The tube is inserted through the mouth, followed by the endoscope, and, in this case, the "pull" technique is used to pass the tube through the anterior abdominal wall.

- "Push" technique: The guidewire used for the "push" PEG is longer and more firm than that used for the "pull" approach and does not have an associated preformed loop. The associated gastrostomy tube is also longer and more tapered than that used for the "pull" approach. The gastrostomy tube is fed over the mouth side of the guidewire. While tension is held on both the mouth and the abdominal sides of the guidewire, the gastrostomy is advanced forward by applying gentle pressure to the bumper end. This allows the endoscopist to "push" the PEG through the abdominal wall from the mouth side. Once the bumper enters into the mouth, the endoscopist applies gentle traction to the abdominal side of the gastrostomy tube to align it into the final position. The guidewire is removed and the PEG is secured in place.

- "Introducer" technique: In this approach, endoscopic visualization is maintained throughout the entire procedure, which is performed from the abdominal wall side. The use of percutaneously placed t-tag anchors may be placed to provide fixation of the anterior gastric wall to the abdominal wall. Access to the gastric lumen is obtained with an 18G needle and a guidewire inserted. The needle is removed and an incision is then made where the wire pierces the skin. Using Seldinger technique, a dilator with break-away sheath is introduced using a twisting motion to facilitate introduction into the stomach. Care must be taken to assure that the dilator follows the path of the wire and does cause a kink. Again, endoscopic visualization is essential to the safety of this procedure. The guidewire and dilator are then removed, leaving the break-away sheath in place. Through this, a balloon tip gastrostomy, or alternatively a Foley catheter, can then be introduced. The sheath is then removed and the PEG is secured in place.

- Final touches: After the gastrostomy has been placed, the scope can be reintroduced to confirm positioning of the bumper (Fig. 35.4A). Literature has supported that this second pass may not be necessary, but the authors routinely confirm placement endoscopically at the completion of the procedure. When securing the gastrostomy tube at the completion of the procedure, care must be taken to avoid undue tension on the tube as this can lead to increased risks of wound complications (Fig. 35.4B).

Operative Technique for Surgical Gastrostomy: Open and Laparoscopic

Surgical gastrostomy is one of the earliest documented surgical procedures and was the gold standard for enteral access before the invention of the percutaneous approach. Operative gastrostomy still remains an important adjunct of care, as a significant number of patients are not candidates for PEG placement. Open and laparoscopic approaches are available and will be detailed here.

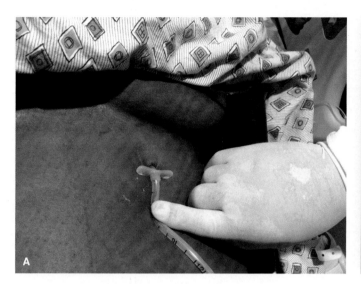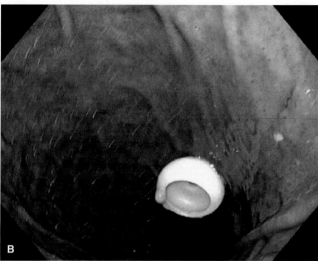

Figure 35.4 Percutaneous gastrostomy: final gastrostomy placement. Note the endoscopic view **(A)** shows good approximation of the internal bumper while the external view **(B)** allows for 2 to 3 mm of freedom to prevent local ischemia and erosion.

- Positioning and sedation/anesthesia: The patient is placed in the supine position. Open gastrostomy may be performed under local anesthesia with sedation or under general anesthesia. Laparoscopic approaches require general anesthesia for appropriate insufflation of the abdomen. The arms can be positioned perpendicularly to the torso on arm boards.

- Stamm gastrostomy: This technique for gastrostomy placement involves the development of a serosal-lined channel from the gastric wall to abdominal wall. This technique requires that an indwelling gastrostomy tube be present, otherwise the gastrocutaneous tract will close, losing access to the stomach. Through a small vertical midline incision, the anterior wall of the stomach is identified and a location is chosen that will reach the anterior abdominal wall without undue tension. Two purse-string sutures are then placed, one inside the other, to define the boundaries of the gastrostomy entry site (Fig. 35.5A). The gastrostomy is then placed in the center of these two sutures and a gastrostomy tube introduced through this incision (Fig. 35.5B). The authors prefer the use of a mushroom tip (dePezzar) catheter with a 20 to 24F diameter. The inner purse-string is tied, creating a secure closure around the gastrostomy tube, followed by the outer purse-string, which allows reinforcement of the gastrostomy tube by inverting it into the wall of the stomach (Fig. 35.5C). The external portion of the gastrostomy is then inserted (inside to outside) through the abdominal wall. The anterior gastric wall is secured to the abdominal wall using four absorbable sutures to encourage a mature gastrocutaneous tract. The catheter is secured to the abdominal wall at the level of the skin and the laparotomy site is closed.

- Janeway gastrostomy: This technique is based on the creation of a full thickness gastric tube to the anterior abdominal wall. The advantage of the Janeway approach is that a permanent, indwelling catheter is not required. The tract functions more as a small ostomy, allowing for intermittent access for feeding. The stomach is approached through a midline laparotomy. When compared to the Stamm approach, placement of a Janeway gastrostomy requires more extensive exposure of the stomach. The direction of the proposed gastric tube, either in the transverse or oblique direction, is chosen and the stomach is elevated in that direction. Creation of the full thickness gastric tube may be accomplished through firing of a commercially available stapling device with contained knife on an elevated piece from the anterior gastric wall (Fig. 35.6). This may also be performed as a hand-sewn approach if desired by the surgeon. This gastric tube must be of adequate length to reach through the abdominal wall intact without undue tension. The gastric tube is passed through the rectus sheath, similar to placement of an ostomy. The midline laparotomy is closed and covered to prevent contamination. The tip of the gastric tube is then removed. The

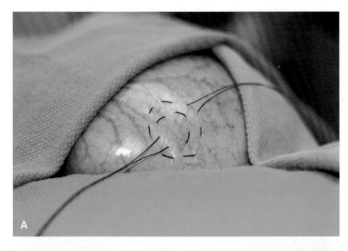

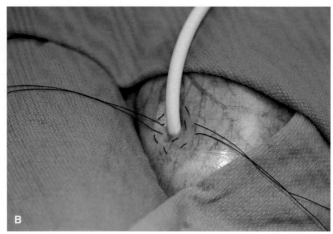

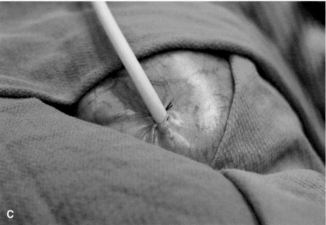

Figure 35.5 Open Stamm gastrostomy: note the double pursestring placement **(A)**, the gastrostomy tube insertion **(B)**, and the use of the sutures to invert the gastric wall **(C)**.

gastrostomy tube site is then matured, similar to an ostomy, using absorbable sutures. A straight tip gastrostomy or Foley catheter is placed for decompression until ileus improves. The catheter is then removed and inserted intermittently for feedings.

■ Laparoscopic Stamm gastrostomy: The most common laparoscopic approach is a modified Stamm gastrostomy. After general anesthesia, access to the abdominal cavity is obtained, usually with a trocar at the level of the umbilicus. One additional trocar, used as the working port for an atraumatic grasper, is placed in the right upper quadrant. The anterior gastric wall is grasped and, using the above criteria, a location is chosen for the gastrostomy. Using t-fasteners, the anterior gastric wall is then

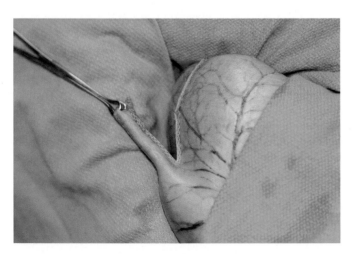

Figure 35.6 Open Janeway gastrostomy: note the use of staples to create a full thickness gastric tube, which will function as an intubatable connection through the abdominal wall.

secured to the abdominal wall. A 10-mm skin incision is then made and a needle introduced into the gastric lumen through the abdominal wall at this incision. A guidewire is passed into the stomach and the tract is serially dilated using Seldinger technique. The gastrostomy tube is then introduced, confirming appropriate placement using the laparoscope. The tube is secured in place. The abdomen is desufflated and the trocar sites closed.

■ Laparoscopic Janeway gastrostomy: Similar to the laparoscopic approach to Stamm gastrostomy, access to the abdomen is obtained with the camera port at the umbilicus and the working port in the right upper quadrant. One additional 12-mm port is placed in the left upper quadrant, allowing for the introduction of a commercially available stapling device. The anterior gastric wall is elevated and the directionality of the gastric tube is chosen. While this area is elevated, an articulating stapling device is used to create the full thickness gastric tube that will reach the abdominal wall without tension. Once created, an instrument through the left upper quadrant port is used to grasp the tip of the gastric tube, allowing it to exit through the abdominal wall without twisting. The abdomen is desufflated and the trocar sites are closed in standard fashion. The tip of the gastric tube is then amputated and it is matured in the manner described above in the open section. The catheter is introduced and left in place until ileus resolves.

POSTOPERATIVE MANAGEMENT

Gastrostomy tubes placed through a percutaneous approach may be used immediately for medications. Tube feeds can be initiated beginning 4 hours following the procedure. Surgically placed gastrostomy tubes, if straightforward, may be used according to these guidelines. For more difficult cases or those requiring extensive lysis of adhesions, the initiation of tube feeds should be delayed until the concern for postoperative ileus has passed.

All gastrostomy sites should be cleaned with soap and water and covered with dry gauze. Excessive tension on the gastrostomy tube should be avoided as this may increase wound complication rates or lead to conditions such as buried bumper syndrome, detailed below. These patients may have preexisting postoperative care needs related to the indication for gastrostomy tube placement, such as neurologic disease or trauma, which should continue to be addressed.

COMPLICATIONS

■ Wound complications: Wound problems are common following gastrostomy tube placement and most frequently consist of local skin irritation or small volume leakage around the tube. These can be treated conservatively, cleaning the site with soap and water daily and leaving open to air. True infectious complications, such as peritubal abscess, are rare and may require incision and drainage for resolution. The risk for infectious complications can be reduced by making the skin incision 1 to 2 mm larger than the gastrostomy tube to allow for egress of bacteria. Avoiding tension on the tube can also decrease the risk for tissue ischemia and reduce wound complications. Excessive tension on the gastrostomy can lead to buried bumper syndrome, a situation in which the bumper erodes through the gastric wall into the abdominal wall. Finally, administration of prophylactic antibiotics that cover skin flora has also been shown to decrease the risk for infectious complications related to gastrostomy placement. After surgical gastrostomy, patients are also at risk for developing standard postoperative wound infections at the site of incision(s).

■ Clogging of the gastrostomy: Intraluminal obstruction of a gastrostomy is more common with smaller diameter tubes. Prevention is the key. Routine tap water flushes, especially following medication administration, will help maintain patency. If clogging does develop, commercially available enzymatic products, hydrogen peroxide, or soda may help dissolve the obstruction. Clogged tubes that are not able to be opened may require removal and replacement.

■ Tube dislodgement: Early dislodgement is a complication that is more concerning after percutaneous approach, as surgical approaches provide direct fixation of the anterior stomach to the abdominal wall. Whether the gastrostomy was placed through surgical or percutaneous technique, an attempt may be made to replace the tube. This should be performed in an expedient manner as the tract may close spontaneously within a few hours. A water-soluble contrast study should be used to confirm intragastric placement before the replaced tube is used. If the tube is unable to be replaced, a stable patient with a benign abdominal examination can be treated with gastric decompression, bowel rest, and antibiotics until a repeat gastrostomy tube can be placed. Any patient who develops fevers, pain, feeding intolerance, or an acute abdomen should undergo emergent laparotomy or laparoscopy.

■ Perforation: Inadvertent visceral injury is rare. Following good operative judgment and using the above-mentioned techniques for percutaneous site selection, including the safe tract approach, reduces the risk for unintended injury to surrounding organs. The endoscopic approach also carries a small risk of esophageal or gastric perforation, most commonly occurring at the level of the cricopharyngeus.

■ Sedation/anesthesia-related complications: As many as 10% of patients undergoing conscious sedation experience hypoxemia with desaturation, but this is most commonly transient and without residual effect. Close monitoring with prompt intervention is required to maintain good outcomes. General anesthesia is relatively safe but does carry risks of cardiovascular collapse, myocardial infarction, stroke, allergic reaction, and DVT formation.

■ Rare complications: Rare cases of cancer seeding to the abdominal wall have been reported after endoscopic placement of gastrostomy in patients with aerodigestive malignancies. Use of a surgical approach or the percutaneous introducer technique can help eliminate this risk. Other complications include parotitis, abdominal cramping, osmolarity-related diarrhea, and nutritional deficiencies.

RESULTS

Results following gastrostomy placement are dependent on the original indication for enteral access, such as stroke, trauma, decompression for unresectable disease, or supplemental nutrition for catabolic states. The procedure and direct complications have only minor impact on overall outcome.

CONCLUSIONS

■ Gastrostomy tube placement is a safe and a reliable way to provide enteral access to the gastrointestinal tract for a variety of different indications. Common indications for gastrostomy include neurologic disease, trauma, and malignancies of the head, neck, or esophagus. Gastrostomy placement may also be necessary for decompression in patients with unresectable malignancy or for refractory gastroparesis.

■ Successful gastrostomy placement can be predicted in most patients and modifications in techniques can help overcome complicating factors, such as surgically altered anatomy, morbid obesity, ascites, or portal hypertension. Surgical indications for gastrostomy include the inability to pass a gastroscope secondary to obstruction, concern for inadvertent viscera interposition with failed "safe tract" technique, and postsurgical anatomy that precludes percutaneous gastrostomy.

■ Percutaneous approaches for gastrostomy include oral passage methods ("pull" and "push") and abdominal wall introducer methods. Patient-specific factors should be considered in the choice of the approach.

- The two main approaches to surgical gastrostomy include construction of a serosal-lined channel requiring indwelling catheter (the Stamm gastrostomy) or creation of a full thickness gastric tube that allows for intermitted catheterization for feeding (the Janeway gastrostomy). Either technique can be performed via an open or a laparoscopic approach.
- Complications from gastrostomy include wound complications, clogging, dislodgement, perforation, and those related to sedation. Good surgical technique, reducing tension on the gastrostomy, and routine catheter care will help decrease these risks. All patients should receive preprocedural antibiotics to decrease wound complications.
- Outcomes following gastrostomy are dependent on the indication for gastrostomy placement. The procedure and direct complications play only a minor role in overall recovery of the patient.

Recommended References and Readings

Cappell M. Risk factors and risk reduction of malignant seeding of the percutaneous endoscopic gastrostomy track from pharyngoesophageal malignancy: a review of all 44 known reported cases. *Am J Gastroenterol.* 2007;102(6):1307.

DeLegge M. Enteral access—the foundation of feeding. *JPEN J Parenter Enteral Nutr.* 2001;25:58.

Eisen GM, Baron TH, Dominitz JA, et al. American Society for Gastrointestinal Endoscopy: Role of endoscopy in enteral feeding. *Gastrointest Endosc.* 2002;55(7):794.

Eisen GM, Baron TH, Dominitz JA, et al. American Society for Gastrointestinal Endoscopy: Complications in upper GI endoscopy. *Gastrointest Endosc.* 2002;55(7):784.

Foutch P, Talbert G, Waring J, et al. Percutaneous endoscopic gastrostomy in patients with prior abdominal surgery: Virtues of the safe tract. *Am J Gastroenterol.* 1988;83:147.

Gauderer MWL, Ponsky JL, Izant R. Gastrostomy without laparotomy: A percutaneous endoscopic technique. *J Pediatr Surg.* 1980;15:872.

Holzman R, Cullen D, Eichhorn J, et al. Guidelines for sedation by nonanesthesiologists during diagnostic and therapeutic procedures. *J Clin Anesth.* 1994;6:265.

Lipp A, Lusardi G. Systemic antimicrobial prophylaxis for percutaneous endoscopic gastrostomy. *Cochrane Database Syst Rev.* 2006;18:CD005571.

Ljungdahl M, Sundbom M. Complication rate lower after percutaneous endoscopic gastrostomy than after surgical gastrostomy: A prospective, randomized trial. *Surg Endosc.* 2006;20:1248.

Mazaki T, Ebisawa K. Enteral versus parenteral nutrition after gastrointestinal surgery: A systematic review and meta-analysis of randomized controlled trials in the English literature. *J Gastrointest Surg.* 2008;12(4):739.

Moore FA, Feliciano DV, Andrassy RJ, et al. Early enteral feeding, compared with parenteral, reduces postoperative septic complications. The results of a meta-analysis. *Ann Surg.* 1992;216(2):172.

Pofahl W, Ringold F. Management of early dislodgment of percutaneous endoscopic gastrostomy tubes. *Surg Laparosc Endosc Percutan Tech.* 1999;9(4):253.

Ponsky JL, Gauderer MWL. Percutaneous endoscopic gastrostomy: a nonoperative technique for feeding gastrostomy. *Gastrointest Endosc.* 1981;27:9.

Russell T, Brotman M, Norris F. Percutaneous endoscopic gastrostomy: A new simplified and cost effective technique. *Amer J Surg.* 1984;148:132.

36 Gastric Electrical Stimulation for Chronic Gastroparesis

Jameson Forster

 ## INDICATIONS/CONTRAINDICATIONS

As a transplant surgeon who 13 years ago happened to become involved in placing gastric electrical stimulators for the treatment of gastroparesis, I have been impressed that the patients who suffer from this disease are as much psychologically impaired as they are nutritionally impaired. They are afraid of eating and scared to be anywhere but in a hospital bed; to later see these patients walking down the hospital hallway, well dressed, smiling, and engaged in life, all because they can now eat is astounding and gratifying. I have learned that being able to eat is an important part of being human. Gastroparetics suffers from nausea, vomiting, bloating, abdominal pain, weight loss, and early satiety. The disease is defined as having >10% of a standard meal remaining in the stomach after 4 hours. There needs to be an anatomically normal stomach, normal thyroid function, and no small bowel obstruction. The condition is frequently associated with diabetes mellitus of 20 years or more duration but may develop from unknown causes (idiopathically) or following abdominal surgery.

Since the gastric electrical stimulator does not cause gastric contractions, I have felt that we should not use the term "pacemaker," even though the device resembles a cardiac pacemaker. To actually pace the stomach, one needs to use a pulse lasting 1,000-fold longer, which can only be accomplished with an external power source.

A surgeon should not venture out alone in this endeavor but be an integral part of a multidisciplinary team that cares for these complicated patients. The other members should include gastroenterologists, with an interest in motility disorders, dietitians, psychologists, psychiatrists, pain specialists, and nurse practitioners. Conditions that often mimic gastroparesis but require a significantly different approach include rumination syndrome, conditioned vomiting, regurgitation, gallbladder dyskinesia, gastric outlet obstruction, and severe constipation. Medical treatment includes Erythromycin, Reglan, Domperidone, Tegaserod, Bethanechol, phenothiazines, ondansetron, tricyclic antidepressants, and antihistamines.

Surgeons have previously played only a minor role, since any resections short of total gastrectomy have proven ineffective in promoting gastric emptying or reducing nausea and vomiting. Pyloroplasties, gastrostomies, and/or subtotal gastric resections do not help. A jejunostomy feeding tube may allow a malnourished patient to be safely fed without the expense and risk associated with total parenteral nutrition (TPN).

PREOPERATIVE PLANNING

Patients should have recently documented normal esophagogastroduodenoscopy (EGD) and colonoscopy. An abdominal ultrasound should be obtained to rule out gallstones and a biliary scan with measurement of the gallbladder ejection fraction is appropriate, if there is a suggestion of biliary colic. Thyroid function studies are also required. Since postoperative infections are difficult to treat, prevention is the key. For patients with a history of infections, I suggest nasal swabs to make certain MRSA is not present and treatment with Bactroban if positive. Showers with chlorhexidine soap for a week prior to surgery are recommended. Ioban skin drapes are used during the operation so that neither the stimulator nor the electrodes come in contact with the skin; cefazolin as the preoperative intravenous antibiotic and for 24 hours postoperative is essential; a subcuticular closure with a running absorbable suture, dressed with dermabond, which seals and protects the skin from postsurgical infection, ends the case. Some patients may benefit from pyloroplasty, in an effort to improve gastric emptying which is not improved by the stimulator; others who come to surgery severely malnourished are often supplemented by placement of a feeding jejunostomy.

We have seen two early postoperative deaths in our series, for a mortality of about 1%, one elderly woman died from a pulmonary embolism and the other, also an elderly woman, died from a cardiovascular event. Morbidity includes no improvement in symptoms, migration of the device requiring reoperation, 10% incidence of infection, and a limited (7 to 8 years) battery life requiring replacement.

SURGERY

The patient is placed supine. After sufficient endotracheal anesthesia is established, nasogastric (NG) tube and Foley catheter are placed. Preoperative antibiotics are given and the lower chest and abdomen are prepped with chlorhexidine. The patient is draped using an Ioban Incise Drape. A small upper midline incision is made, approximately 5 cm in length. Once in the abdomen, exploration is done. The stomach is identified and the pylorus is located. If there was a prior cholecystectomy, the pylorus is usually adherent to the gallbladder bed and needs to be mobilized. Only when the pylorus is freed, can one properly measure along the greater curvature. Using a plastic ruler, we measure along the greater curvature and mark the stomach at 9.5 and 10.5 cm proximal to the pylorus, stretching the stomach as much as possible (Fig. 36.1). The

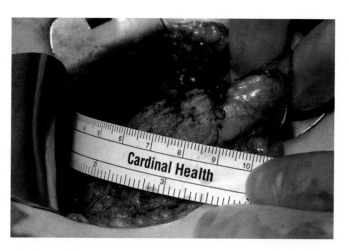

Figure 36.1 A plastic ruler is used to measure 9.5 and 10.5 cm proximal to the pylorus.

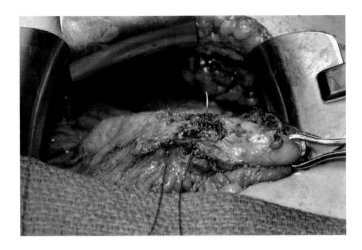

Figure 36.2 The needles are inserted tangentially through the gastric wall.

needles of each electrode are inserted tangentially through the gastric wall, radially inward, deep enough so that the needle is in the gastric muscle and not visible through the serosa. The two needles are placed a centimeter apart and coursing for at least a distance of 1 cm within the muscle (Fig. 36.2). With an endoscope, the gastroenterologist verifies that the needles have not traversed the mucosa and are not visible within the gastric lumen. During the endoscopy, the NG is clamped to allow the stomach to be insufflated. With the ceiling lights off but the operating room lights on, the surgeon gently pushes against the needles to clearly locate them, identifies that they are close to the incisura, and makes certain the needles are not visible to the endoscopist. If the needles are far from the incisura or if the needles are visible from the lumen, they are removed, cleaned with Betadine, and reinserted. Once proper position of the needles is ascertained, the needles are pulled through the stomach wall and left dangling until the endoscopy is completed. The endoscope is passed into the duodenum and retroflexed in the stomach to complete the examination. While the endoscope is being pulled out, care is taken to not also pull out the NG tube, which tends to stick to the sides of the endoscope. Once the endoscope is out, the stomach is decompressed using the NG tube. Both of the gastric electrodes are pulled into the gastric muscle wall by pulling on the monofilament, which is swedged onto the end of the electrode; this is safely done while the surgeon gently holds the stomach around the electrode (Fig. 36.3). Due to the slight difference in the diameter of the electrode and the monofilament, more force is needed to pull the electrodes into position than one would have thought; one feels a slight pop when the electrode gets into place. Once the electrode is in position, each anchor is sutured to the serosa with two interrupted stitches of 5-0 silk. Each monofilament is threaded through a plastic disk and two medium clips are placed to hold the monofilament to the disk. Each disk is stitched to the serosa with two sutures

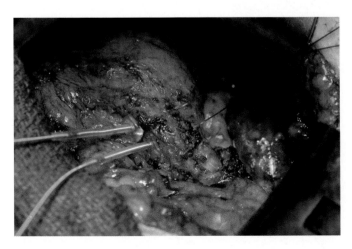

Figure 36.3 Each electrode is pulled into position.

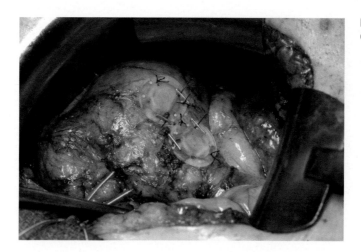

Figure 36.4 The final appearance of the electrodes.

of 5-0 silk (Fig. 36.4). An adequate-sized pocket is created on the right side of the incision, anterior to the rectus fascia, using electrocautery. The stimulator needs to be at a sufficient distance from the costal margin; so the pocket is often made lateral to the umbilicus while the incision is above the umbilicus. The electrodes are pulled into the pocket via a stab wound through the abdominal wall created with a tonsil clamp. The two electrodes are screwed into place on the stimulator. Either electrode can go into either track. The stimulator is interrogated and the load impedance is measured. The stimulator is sutured to the abdominal wall with three stitches of a 2-0 Ethibond suture. Two stitches are placed through the anterior rectus fascia and one of the plastic tracts and one stitch is placed through one tract and the abdominal wall and then through the abdominal wall and the second tract, being tied on top. The stimulator has to be positioned so that the writing is toward the skin, because only in that position can the interrogator change the settings of the stimulator. The pocket is closed with a running 3-0 PDS suture, bringing the edge of the subcutaneous fat to the top of the fascia. This suture separates the pocket from the skin and hopefully prevents a wound infection from getting

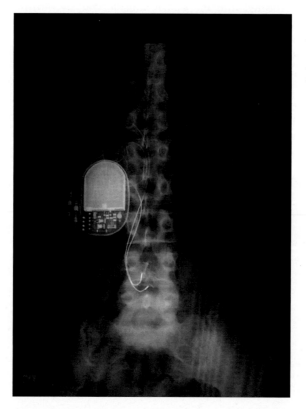

Figure 36.5 This is the x-ray of one patient's abdomen after placement of the stimulator. The important issue is to note the distance between the end of an electrode and the first clip. In follow-up for worsening symptoms, one needs to re-examine that distance and if greatly increased, the electrode may have pulled out of the stomach.

into the pocket. The stimulator is interrogated a second time and the load impedance rechecked. The fascia is closed with a running 0 PDS suture. The subcutaneous tissue is closed in two layers with interrupted 3-0 chromic sutures, and skin is closed with a running subcuticular 4-0 absorbable suture. The wound is dressed with dermabond.

 ## POSTOPERATIVE MANAGEMENT

The stimulator is usually not activated until after the operation is completed and the electrocautery is no longer in use. The settings used initially are those that the device selects. Postoperatively, we advance the diet slowly. With placement of the stimulator and electrodes alone, the patients are kept NPO for the first 24 hours. Then they are advanced to clear sips the second day, clear liquids the third day, full liquids the fourth day, a soft mechanical diet the fifth day, and discharged on the sixth day. If the patient had a pyloroplasty, the NG is left in for the first day, and then the same schedule is followed, with discharge being on the seventh day. Once the patients are taking liquids, their preoperative medications are resumed. The day after surgery the patients should get a flat and upright of the abdomen to establish the initial position of the electrodes relative to the medium clips, in order to allow for a check later on whether the electrodes had moved (Fig. 36.5). If a jejunostomy feeding tube had been placed, the tube is put to gravity for the first 24 hours. The next day feedings are started at 10 mL/hour of a 1 Kcal/mL formulation and are slowly advanced by 10 mL/hour every 6 hours until goal is reached. If the patient is severely malnourished, the rate may need to be advanced more slowly. Once the patient is eating sufficiently by mouth, the tube feedings are stopped. The tube placed at surgery can be exchanged for a low-profile Mickey tube at 2 weeks, if the patient needs to have small bowel access for the long term. Most patients will not need long-term access and the tube can be simply removed when both the patient and the gastroenterologist are comfortable doing so.

 ## COMPLICATIONS

The majority of patients do very well and are seen by the surgeon only once postoperatively until 7 to 8 years later when their battery is running out and they need a new stimulator. Unfortunately, some patients have an inordinate number of problems. After placement of the stimulator and its activation, some patients feel better almost immediately; we feel we need to wait 3 months to see the maximum effect of the stimulator. When a patient's symptoms abruptly worsen, a flat and upright x-ray of the abdomen should be done to make certain the electrodes have not pulled out of the stomach (Fig. 36.5) and the stimulator should be interrogated to make certain that the load impedance has not changed. An upper endoscopy should also be considered to verify that the electrodes have not eroded through the gastric wall and thus are visible from within the lumen.

If a patient is found to have the electrodes visible in the stomach's lumen, we assume that the entire system is contaminated and the electrodes, the stimulator, and the plastic disks all have to be removed, cultures have to be taken, and the patient should be appropriately treated with antibiotics.

Fluid collections around the stimulator need to be carefully aspirated and the fluid cultured. Not all such collections are infected; even if the cultures are negative, such patients need extended antibiotic therapy. Clearly, if there is infection in the pocket and around the stimulator, the stimulator, the electrodes, and the plastic disks are all removed. The pocket is left open and a wound vacuum assisted closure (VAC) device is used to help the healing process. Infections that do not clearly involve the system, even intra-abdominal abscesses, have been successfully treated without removing the device.

When patients develop pain associated with the stimulator, the stimulator may be moving. Unfortunately, the stimulators have become detached from the rectus fascia due to trauma and abdominal wall movement; this has been seen in patients who lean over a tub in their job washing clothes and or in patients whose stimulator is too close to the right costal margin. The patients will complain that such stimulators flip or stand upright. If the stimulator has completely loosened, it can coil up the electrodes and pull out the electrodes from the stomach wall.

RESULTS

About 90% of the patients achieve more than a 50% reduction in Total Symptom Score. Patients with diabetic and postoperative gastroparesis seem to do better than those with idiopathic gastroparesis. Gastric emptying time was reduced at 6 months but not at a year. About 89% of jejunostomies were removed at 1 year. After placement of the stimulator, diabetic patients have improved HgbA1c.

CONCLUSIONS

1. Gastroparesis is characterized by a dysfunctional stomach that no longer pushes food into the duodenum.
2. Treatment requires a team approach and relies on prokinetic medications.
3. The best surgical procedure is placement of a gastric electrical stimulator.

Recommended References and Readings

Buckles DC, McCallum RW. Treatment of gastroparesis. *Curr Treat Options Gastroenterol.* 2004;7:139–147.

Forster J, Sarosiek I, Delcore R, et al. Gastric pacing is a new surgical treatment for gastroparesis. *Am J Surg.* 2001;182:676–681.

Forster J, Sarosiek I, Lin Z, et al. Further experience with gastric stimulation to treat drug refractory gastroparesis. *Am J Surg.* 2003; 186:690–695.

Hejazi RA, McCallum RW. Treatment of refractory gastroparesis: Gastric and jejunal tubes, botox, gastric electrical stimulation, and surgery. *Gastrointest Endosc Clin N Am.* 2009;19:73–82.

Jones MP, Maganti K. A systematic review of surgical therapy for gastroparesis. *Am J Gastroenterol.* 2003;98:2122–2129.

Lin Z, Forster J, Sarosiek I, et al. Treatment of gastroparesis with electrical stimulation. *Dig Dis Sci.* 2003;48:837–848.

Lin Z, Forster J, Sarosiek I, et al. Treatment of diabetic gastroparesis by high-frequency gastric electrical stimulation. *Diabetes Care.* 2004;27:1071–1076.

Masaoka T, Tack J. Gastroparesis, Current Concepts and Management. *Gut Liver.* 2009;3:166–173.

McCallum RW, Lin Z, Forster J, et al. Gastric electrical stimulation improves outcomes of patients with gastroparesis for up to 10 years. *Clin Gastroenterol Hepatol.* 2011;9:314–319.

Parkman HP, Hasler WL, Fisher RS. American Gastroenterological Association: American Gastroenterological Association technical review on the diagnosis and treatment of gastroparesis. *Gastroenterology.* 2004;124:1592–1622.

Tougas G, Eaker EY, Abell TL, et al. Assessment of gastric emptying using a low fat meal: Establishment of international control values. *Am J Gastroenterol.* 2000;95:1456–1462.

Index

Note: Page number followed by f and t indicates figure and table respectively.